Surgeon General's Warning

The publisher gratefully acknowledges the generous support of Jamie Rosenthal Wolf, David Wolf, Rick Rosenthal, and Nancy Stephens as members of the Publisher's Circle of the University of California Press Foundation.

The publisher also gratefully acknowledges the generous support of the General Endowment Fund of the University of California Press Foundation.

Surgeon General's Warning

*How Politics Crippled
the Nation's Doctor*

Mike Stobbe

UNIVERSITY OF CALIFORNIA PRESS

University of California Press, one of the most
distinguished university presses in the United States,
enriches lives around the world by advancing scholarship
in the humanities, social sciences, and natural sciences. Its
activities are supported by the UC Press Foundation and
by philanthropic contributions from individuals and
institutions. For more information, visit www.ucpress.edu.

University of California Press
Oakland, California

Library of Congress Cataloging-in-Publication Data

Stobbe, Mike, 1966– author.
   Surgeon General's warning: how politics crippled the
nation's doctor / Mike Stobbe.
       p. ; cm.
   How politics crippled the nation's doctor.
   Includes bibliographical references and index.
   ISBN 978-0-520-27229-3 (cloth : alk. paper)
   ISBN 978-0-520-95839-5 (e-book)
   I. Title.   II. Title: How politics crippled the nation's
doctor. [DNLM: 1. United States. Public Health
Service. Office of the Surgeon General.   2. Physicians—
United States.   3. Public Health Administration—United
States.   4. Administrative Personnel—United States.
5. Politics—United States.   6. Science—United States.
7. United States Government Agencies—United States.
WA 540 AA1
   R152
   610.69'50973—dc23
                                          2014002379

Manufactured in the United States of America
23 22 21 20 19 18 17 16 15 14
10 9 8 7 6 5 4 3 2 1

In keeping with a commitment to support
environmentally responsible and sustainable printing
practices, UC Press has printed this book on Natures
Natural, a fiber that contains 30% post-consumer waste
and meets the minimum requirements of ANSI/NISO
Z39.48-1992 (R 1997) (*Permanence of Paper*).

To Hoss

Contents

PART FOUR. PLUMMET, 2002–PRESENT

Acknowledgments

This book took more than seven years to complete and involved interviews with more than one hundred people and research trips to a variety of university libraries, presidential libraries, and federal archives. That means a lot of people generously shared their time, memories, and expertise to help me complete this volume. I wish I had room to thank them all. But at least some have to be recognized here.

This book started as a doctoral dissertation, and my dissertation committee was pivotal in the early development of this project. The group included the journalist Karl Stark and University of North Carolina faculty members Jon Oberlander, Tom Ricketts, and Bryan Weiner. Most important was my committee chair, the canny Ned Brooks. Sue Hobbs was another key supporter at UNC.

Thanks also to my bosses and colleagues at the Associated Press who supported me in pursuing the doctorate and this project. Special mention goes to Kit Frieden, the AP's former national health and science editor; to Barry Bedlan, my initial supervisor in AP's Atlanta bureau; and to AP photographer John Bazemore.

My first real interview for this project, appropriately, was with former surgeon general C. Everett Koop in July 2006 at his home in Hanover, New Hampshire. (Perhaps also appropriately, my last book-related research trip was to his funeral service in Woodstock, Vermont, in March 2013.) Koop was hugely insightful, and his nod of support opened doors to other important interviews. My gratitude goes to him and to his longtime assistant, Susan Wills.

While working on this book I lived in Atlanta, and my unfunded research required repeated trips to Washington, D.C. So I'm grateful to Jeff Mains, an old high school friend who helped me save a lot of money by letting me crash at his company's condo in D.C.

My appreciation also goes to Alexandra Lord and John Parascandola, former historians of the U.S. Public Health Service, and the staff of that now defunct office. Jerry Farrell, of the Commissioned Officers Associations of the U.S. Public Health Service, answered questions no one else could. Fitzhugh Mullan, who had written the go-to reference on the PHS, was an important early source.

At UC Press, a big thanks to acquisitions editor Hannah Love for enthusiastically bringing me on board, to Naomi Schneider and Christopher Lura for getting me through the process, and to Steven Baker for his thorough and thoughtful copy editing. I'm also very grateful to Brooks, Parascandola, Paul Erwin, Glen Nowak, Jill Center, Dan Haney, Maryn McKenna, and James Morone for their important feedback on drafts of the initial proposal or subsequent manuscript.

I am indebted to my parents, Ed and Pat Stobbe. They taught me the work ethic necessary to pull off something like this, and kindly sent a check to help with my research expenses. A conversation with my mom led me to ponder the vacuum caused by absence of a strong surgeon general and the pop-culture healers who had rushed in to fill it.

Kudos to Rick Broadhead. I can't imagine a better agent. Honestly, I'm not sure this book would have come into being without his sage advice and tireless advocacy.

Lastly, love to my sons, Isaac and Luc, and to my wife, the superb journalist (and discerning editor) Heather Vogell. She helped me in a thousand ways, from the opening pitch to late-inning edits. This book is dedicated to her.

CHAPTER I

The Monarch of Public Health

Regina Benjamin took her place in front of dark velvet curtains, set her smile, and waited.

The scene was a bit like "Pictures with Santa" at a busy shopping mall on the Saturday before Christmas. More than 150 people patiently stood in line to have their photo taken with Benjamin, some with emotions akin to the awe of a child about to meet St. Nicholas. They craned their necks to see her up ahead; some were even a little giggly. Benjamin's helpers, wearing uniforms like hers, managed the crowd.

But the similarities stopped there. This was weeks after the holiday (January 11, 2010, to be exact). These were adults standing in line. The venue was the foyer of a federal building in downtown Washington, D.C. And this wasn't Kris Kringle they were waiting to see; it was the new U.S. surgeon general.

Minutes earlier, in a packed, 625-seat auditorium, Benjamin had been formally sworn in as the nation's eighteenth surgeon general. It had been an unusually florid affair, even by Washington's standards. Rows of federal health officials dressed in the formal, militaristic uniforms of the Commissioned Corps of the U.S. Public Health Service. Some formed a saluting gantlet that Benjamin passed through at the end. A passerby might have mistaken the event for some kind of war-hero homage.

Benjamin had many supporters there that day, and they were thrilled.

"It's wonderful to know that someone whose values you respect is in such a position of leadership," said Brenda Smith, an American University law professor standing in line with a group of friends.

"This is a great day for our state. For the world," said Betty Ruth Speir, an elderly gynecologist who, like Benjamin, was from Alabama.[1]

Was it, though?

The surgeon general is indeed a public health celebrity, a post rooted in a rich history and automatically held in high esteem. Surgeon general reports remain hallmark documents in our society, cited in everything from student term papers to legislative policy debates. Surgeon general warnings are fixtures on magazine liquor ads and cigarette packaging. Polls assessing the surgeon general's credibility award the position higher marks than most other government health officials. Indeed, the surgeon general is commonly perceived (or, rather, misperceived) to be the government official responsible for the health and well-being of the general public.[2] The surgeon general stars in public service announcement commercials and speaks frequently at university commencements and national conferences. The uniform and title still conjure importance and wisdom, and—for some Americans—a belief that there is still such a thing as a government health official who will level with the public when other bureaucrats won't.

Some of that aura comes from dewy memories of the surgeon general's power, independence, and integrity as it was many decades ago (when the federal health bureaucracy was much smaller). "He did not have to kowtow to the administration," said Daniel Whiteside, a dentist who served for years in the Public Health Service. "He could say, 'I don't care what the administration's policy is on any health issue. I'm going to tell you what is in the best interest of the American public, so far as a health issue is concerned. I don't care who likes it. I don't care who doesn't like it. I'm here for four years and you can't touch me.' And we had Surgeon Generals who did that; I mean, who went up against the administration and said 'Kiss off.'"[3]

Whiteside was speaking mainly about the men who held the position in the early twentieth century—the long-ago kings of U.S. public health who served multiple terms while presidents came and went. But the perception that surgeons general are science-above-politics monarchs, acting as the uncensored health consciences of the nation, occasionally has resurfaced. Jesse Steinfeld, who held the job in the early 1970s, angered Nixon administration officials by attacking the cigarette and television industries. C. Everett Koop, in place through most of the

1980s, led a benevolent education campaign on the emerging AIDS epidemic when some Reagan White House officials disdainfully considered it a gay disease. Joycelyn Elders, surgeon general in the early 1990s, dismayed the Clinton administration with her frank remarks about whether to legalize marijuana or teach kids to masturbate.

But in truth, tolerance for outspoken surgeons general has always been limited. Elders was fired. Steinfeld was forced to resign early. Even the powerful surgeons general of old were careful not to cross certain political overlords. An example: Hugh Cumming, who held the job from 1920 to 1936, was considered one of the most powerful surgeons general of all time. In 1925, after a rash of industrial worker poisonings tied to leaded gasoline, Cumming was publicly pressured to look into it. But he declined to take any action until he first discussed it with Secretary of the Treasury Andrew Mellon—whose family had financial interests in the oil industry. (Mellon, to his credit, recused himself and told Cumming to use his own judgment.)[4]

Surgeon General's Warning is a brief history of the office that includes the proud moments and the despicable ones, the perception and realities, the heroes and the scoundrels. The book explains how the surgeon general became the most powerful and influential public health officer in the country and how those powers were later stripped away. It discusses the unique bully pulpit role the post retained, and the prowess of some surgeons general in that pulpit and the meekness of others. It examines how the office reached its current nadir. And it concludes that it no longer makes sense to have a surgeon general.

"WHAT IS IT?"

In January 2009, just weeks before President Barack Obama's inauguration, the media buzzed with reports that the president-elect was considering CNN medical journalist Sanjay Gupta for surgeon general. The telegenic Gupta, a young Atlanta-based neurosurgeon, had once been voted one of *People* magazine's "Sexiest People" and was a television superstar. He promised to be the kind of head-turning persona not seen since the days of Koop and Elders. *The Daily Show,* the popular late-night comedy/news program, took note with an exchange between host Jon Stewart and Indian American correspondent Aasif Mandvi.

In the segment, Mandvi crowed about the prospect of Gupta taking the job, and how it would mean Indian Americans would have as prominent a place in the new Cabinet as Chinese Americans and other ethnic groups.

Stewart interrupted, "Aasif, surgeon general is technically not a Cabinet position."

"It's not?" Mandvi said, surprised.

"No."

"Oh. What is it?"

"It's the head of the Public Health Service. It's a lot of informal duties and—"

"So it's *beneath* the Cabinet," Mandvi said, a look of disgust erupting on his face.

"Well those are your words, Aasif. It's a very high level . . ."

Mandvi, however, acted devastated. Such a position was not worthy of an accomplished physician representing a talented and proud people, he lamented. Looking at the camera, addressing Gupta, he cried; "*Surgeon General?* You should be ashamed of yourself!"[5]

The bit was dead-on. Yes, the office is esteemed. And yes, many people don't really know what the surgeon general does.

During the flurry of attention over Gupta, the Harris Poll surveyed 2,848 U.S. adults about the surgeon general and 14 federal agencies. Participants were asked if they understood each entity's role. The surgeon general ranked near the bottom of the list—only the workings of the National Institutes of Health and Securities and Exchange Commission were bigger mysteries. Yet in the same survey, the surgeon general came out near the top of the list when participants were asked which entities were doing a good job.[6]

So what *does* the surgeon general do?

At one time, he oversaw nearly all of the federal government's civilian health agencies. It was a surgeon general in the 1870s who resurrected the first federal hospital system. His successors instituted quarantines to fight deadly yellow fever and cholera epidemics and calmed the nation during the deadly Spanish flu epidemic of 1918–1919. They handled the medical care of hundreds of thousands of veterans at the end of World War I, and spearheaded the desegregation of U.S. hospitals in the 1960s. They also issued warnings to the public about health dangers ranging from unpasteurized milk to laundry detergent. Perhaps most famously, Surgeon General Luther Terry in 1964 released the report that finally settled the question of whether smoking causes lung cancer. Arguably, no government official has had a greater personal influence on the public's health than the U.S. surgeon general.[7]

Such activities caused politicians and journalists to gradually start referring to the surgeon general as "the nation's doctor." The position retains a tremendous cachet today. If imitation is the sincerest form of flattery, note that since 2003, three states—Michigan, Arkansas and Florida—have created surgeon general positions to revitalize public health efforts.[8] The job descriptions differed somewhat, but each state surgeon general official has been expected to give accurate and objective reports and benefited from a title that confers a kind of instant credibility. "The name 'surgeon general' conveys a certain respect," said Arkansas surgeon general Joe Thompson.[9]

Although the U.S. surgeon general's stature endures, the office's powers are long gone. Federal reorganizations in the 1960s stripped away most of the job's responsibilities and gave them to people appointed by whoever was in the White House at the time. "It was really the politicization of the Public Health Service," said the late David Sencer, who was director of the federal Center for Disease Control when the most substantial reorganizations took place.[10] The surgeon general became a bench-riding bureaucrat and glorified health educator. As early as 1973, the political scientist Eric Redman likened the position to a once-powerful European king who had been reduced to a figurehead, "a pathetic shadow of authority who traveled around the country lecturing high school students on the hazards of smoking."[11]

Today, those speeches are the surgeon general's main job, at least as far as the public is concerned. Not all the men and women who have held the job enjoyed public speaking, but most have seen it as an important duty. Key to that duty, several have said, is being a guardian of scientific truth and steering clear of ideology and propaganda. "The surgeon general's responsibility is to communicate directly with the American people based on the best available science," said David Satcher, who held the job in the late 1990s and early 2000s.[12]

(Interestingly, there is no requirement that a surgeon general be a medical doctor of any kind, much less a surgeon. Federal law dictates that the main requirement for anyone aspiring to the job is that they have specialized training or experience in public health. And even that requirement has been repeatedly ignored—three of the eighteen surgeons general did not come from public health backgrounds, including Dr. Benjamin.[13])

The surgeon general also has some supervisory duties over the Commissioned Corps, a subgroup of uniformed health professionals within the 65,000-person U.S. Department of Health and Human Services. The quasi-military corps is a remarkable collection of doctors, nurses, and other health professionals trained to be deployed to disease outbreaks, disaster sites, and other emergencies. The Corps is most apparently modeled after the navy, and the surgeon general is treated as a three-star admiral and the organization's ceremonial leader. But most of the actual decisions about deployment are made by others, including the surgeon general's boss, the HHS assistant secretary of health (or ASH, in the parlance of the federal health bureaucracy). The ASH holds the rank of *four*-star admiral, but doesn't bother to wear the uniform.

In other words, the surgeon general is more a symbol than a job. To some, it's also an irritation.

Some politicos and commentators have accused surgeons general of being "nanny" figures whose reports and lectures about appropriate health behaviors amount to a taxpayer-funded annoyance. "I've been flipping through my copy of the Constitution, and I can't find the part where the federal government is charged with making our kids eat better," wrote the libertarian writer Michael D. Tanner in 2007.[14] Critics find it vexing that the position has built-in gravitas and a travel budget, and there have been a number of legislative attempts to eliminate the surgeon general or the Commissioned Corps, or both. Some presidents opted to just leave the job unfilled, sometimes for stretches as long as four years. "The last thing we wanted was a surgeon general to deal with; we had enough problems," groused Charles Edwards, a top Nixon health official, explaining why the job was left vacant after Steinfeld was tricked into resigning.[15]

Indeed, no presidential administration has been at ease with a free-wheeling, press-garnering surgeon general—not even Josiah Bartlet's. Recall that Bartlet was the idealized chief executive on the once popular television drama *The West Wing*. In an episode that aired in February 2001, President Bartlet called for the resignation of a surgeon general whom he admired but who caused a political headache by discussing the legalization of marijuana. (A storyline inspired by Bill Clinton's termination of Joycelyn Elders less than seven years earlier.)[16]

"If a surgeon general is doing the job correctly, they will eventually fall out of favor with the administration that appointed them, because they develop an allegiance to the science first," said David Rutstein, a former deputy surgeon general who resigned his job in frustration in 2010.[17]

CRUSADERS NO MORE

The genesis of this book was a class discussion among public health doctoral students at the University of North Carolina in the fall of 2005.

The topic was something like "What is the story of public health these days, and who are its protagonists?" One student said the president was sometimes a leader on public health matters. Another said the Institute of Medicine had an influential voice. Someone opined that trial lawyers had done a great deal to shape public health discourse. A fourth ventured that the rock singer Bono could qualify as a hero, for his work drawing attention to AIDS in the developing world.

I was one of those students, and as I sat listening, a thought began to nag me: why aren't they talking about the surgeon general? As someone who grew up in the 1980s, I had clear memories of Surgeon General C. Everett Koop, with a prophet's beard and an admiral's uniform, shaking his finger at tobacco companies and leading a compassionate public education campaign on AIDS at a time when fear and stigma about the disease was at its worst. Koop was perhaps the closest thing to a hero in that field I'd ever seen, but he and his successors apparently were nowhere on my classmates' radar. What happened to the surgeon general?

This book will offer an answer.

Surgeon General's Warning shows that the Office of the Surgeon General was always a bit of an anomaly within the federal government, and that odd status provided a unique potential for influencing the public health. Specifically, it afforded surgeons general the ability to speak more candidly and powerfully about the nation's problems than other health officials. But that potential was realized only occasionally. When it occurred, it was the result of a confluence of factors, including the determination and savvy of the surgeon general, the support of his or her political bosses, and a dearth of competing voices.

But the equation that could produce a Koop or Elders or Thomas Parran seems to have irrevocably changed. And that is to the public's detriment.

Surgeons general have always had to take orders from their political bosses. What's changed is that other federal health officials—like the HHS secretary and the CDC director—have developed an enduring taste for the bully pulpit, and have come to see surgeons general as unworthy competitors for it. They have a point: some surgeons general have been quota-filling, just-happy-to-be-here appointees with little expertise in influenza or some of the myriad other topics they were expected to speak about to a worried public. That was as much a failing of the surgeon general selection process as of the people who held the office.

In the past decade, in both Republican and Democratic administrations, surgeons general have become essentially invisible. Benjamin's predecessor, Richard Carmona, was repeatedly muzzled by the George W. Bush administration, and important reports he worked on were never allowed to see the light of day. Benjamin had an even lower profile, partly because of how she was controlled by her bosses and partly because of her own diffidence. "The general public, if you said Dr. Regina Benjamin, they wouldn't even know who you're talking about," said Laurence Grummer-Strawn, a federal expert on breast-feeding who has worked with Benjamin's office. "The surgeon general could have much more influence on the health of the nation if people were paying attention to her."[18]

There's no longer a realistic expectation that lawmakers or executive branch officials will restore the Office of the Surgeon General to its past status. In an era of perennial government budget shortfalls, when local public health departments have eliminated tens of thousands of jobs—including care-providing nurses and outbreak-controlling epidemiologists—an invisible surgeon general is an indefensible waste of money.[19]

But it is also the purpose of this book to mourn what has happened. The weakening of the office has led to a vacuum in health policy leadership. The federal bureaucrats who have taken the surgeon general's place in the spotlight have tended to walk a politically correct line and to steer clear of controversies that might trigger "Nanny state" complaints that the government is meddling in the lives of individuals. They almost refuse to openly acknowledge a central tenet of public health—that the state's responsibility is to look after the health of everyone, which sometimes means guiding or restricting people's choices. Their aversion to risk and confrontation has allowed a parade of misinformed talkers to fill the airwaves and Internet with wrongheaded theories that, left unchallenged, harm public health. Rantings about vaccines as a cause of autism have contributed to a resurgence of measles and other infectious diseases in areas where vaccination rates have been low.[20] Manufacturers of sugary and fatty foods and beverages have persisted in marketing campaigns that propel the nation's obesity problem. And gun makers and their enthusiastic customers have so far cowed every substantial attempt to limit the purchase of firearms and ammunition, as U.S. gun-related deaths continue to surpass 30,000 each year.

A Koop or Elders would have said something about such shenanigans, and their strong words would undoubtedly have emboldened some lawmakers and policymakers to take action. But the last couple of surgeons general were wimps. In recent years the bold, speak-truth-to-power public health figures in government have resided at the local level. Take former New York City mayor Michael Bloomberg and his city health commissioners, for example, who pushed for complete smoking bans, limitations on serving sizes of sugary sodas, and a variety of other measures irritating to libertarians and certain corporate interests.[21]

It was William Stewart, the ill-fated surgeon general of the late 1960s, who perhaps best described the historical standard for true public health leaders. "From the 1880s onward," he once said, "the public health movement always included rebels: men and women ready to strike out with new approaches at the roots of evil; crusaders who never lost faith that the movement possessed the breadth of vision, as well as the spirit and competence to meet the health needs of a growing and changing society."[22] Surgeons general have played that crusader role better and more often than any other national public health figure. Absent such a crusader, the public's health is prey to the misinformation and self-interest of tobacco companies, snake-oil salesmen, and other malefactors. There are other heroes at work, to be sure, some with substantial resources and policymaking powers. But the traditional leader is no longer up on the parapet, and the fight has suffered as a result.

I was struck by how much the role of surgeon general has deteriorated during a 2008 interview with Anthony Fauci, a potently articulate federal scientist with a job most people have never heard of—director of the National Institute of Allergy and Infectious Diseases. For decades, Fauci has been a de facto surgeon general, educating the public and speaking to the press about a range of health issues. Several people I interviewed said that if anyone had the smarts, passion, and oratorical skills to be a great surgeon general, it's Tony Fauci.

But when asked if he would ever want the job of surgeon general, he did not pause in answering no. He sees himself as a scientist who has maintained a high degree of prominence by being apolitical. Surgeons general talk about being apolitical, too, he said, but that's now more an aspiration than a reality. Surgeons general are too subject to the push and pull of the people in the White House and in the nearby Humphrey Building, where the HHS secretary and other top politically appointed health officials work.

"I love my job, and I'm more visible, and better known," he said. "Why would I want to be surgeon general?"[23]

RISE, FALL, AND STRUGGLE

This book traces the story of the surgeon general through the stories of the eighteen individuals who have held the post.

The Office of the U.S. Surgeon General was created simply as a house-cleaning administrator for a beleaguered string of marine hospitals. But the first surgeon general, John Woodworth, was an ambitious Civil War veteran with bigger plans. Intent on becoming the sole leader of a nascent federal bureaucracy with authority over sanitation and epidemic control, he died while vying for power against a gang of the great public health leaders of his era. The second man to hold the office, John Hamilton, was a nasty political fighter who picked up the sword and defeated Woodworth's competitors. He and his successor, Walter Wyman, cemented the surgeon general's position as the federal doctor in charge of the nation's health.

The surgeon general and his staff came to be heroes. Dressed in military uniforms, the doctors and sanitarians of the U.S. Public Health Service battled yellow fever, cholera, and other nineteenth-century scourges, some of them losing their lives to disease in the line of duty. In the early decades of the twentieth century, books and articles were written about their wisdom and valor. Burnishing that reputation was the fourth surgeon general, a mustache-twirling amateur boxer named Rupert Blue, who entered the office revered for his role in beating back plague in San Francisco. Blue was an instinctively quiet man who nevertheless built up the surgeon general's bully pulpit, leading health education campaigns and speaking out on the need for national health insurance. His eventual replacement, Hugh Cumming, reigned for an astonishing sixteen years through careful alliances and personal friendships with presidents and other power brokers.

Cumming was succeeded by Thomas Parran, who for many years afterward was regarded as the greatest surgeon general of all time. Parran worked the bully pulpit like no one before him, reaching celebrity status in the 1930s and 1940s as he forcefully worked to change social mores and stop the spread of sexually transmitted diseases. He wrote a best-selling book, graced the cover of *Time* magazine, and starred in radio broadcasts—all in his attempts to address a public health problem that even ham-fisted reporters had deemed too coarse a topic for polite company.

But the end of Parran's tenure also saw the first signs of an eclipse of the Office of the Surgeon General. He was attacked in a congressional hearing for supporting President Truman's health reform—an assault that had the long-term effect of discouraging Public Health Service leaders from taking on certain controversial topics. Despite his many accomplishments and near-celebrity status, Parran was ushered out of office following a petty disagreement with a hot-tempered political boss.

So began a decline that continues to this day.

The seventh and eighth surgeons general—Leonard Scheele and Leroy Burney—started to lose power in the 1950s, following the creation of a cabinet-level federal health department during the Eisenhower administration. They also blundered in dealing with cigarette smoking, problematic vaccines, and rival bureaucrats.

The early 1960s saw the office's pinnacle moment, when Surgeon General Luther Terry released a report that would cause a turnabout in the American public's regard for the dangers of smoking. But even as Terry changed the lives of generations of Americans, his power too was slipping away. The erosion of the once vaunted surgeon general's powers became complete during the term of Terry's successor, William Stewart. Those powers would never come back.

In the 1970s, two very different personalities—the feisty Jesse Steinfeld and the more accommodating Julius Richmond—served as surgeon general. Both endured political bosses who tried to push them upstage or offstage, but succeeded in making important contributions to public health. Steinfeld ignited a movement to ban smoking in public places, and Richmond set new societal goals for healthy living.

The surgeon general experienced a resurgence with Richmond's successor—C. Everett Koop, easily the most famous surgeon general of the past half-century. An outsized personality who managed to surprise nearly everyone in Washington, D.C., Koop elevated a moribund position into superstar status. He was the Reagan era's sage and unwavering voice of public health, educating and influencing the public on matters ranging from AIDS to zoonoses, and so good at it that he could not be hushed by the assorted political, business, and religious interests that disagreed with him. If Parran's reign was the golden age, Koop's represented the silver—a glorious era that suffered in comparison only because Koop was never given the administrative powers that were the standard in Parran's time.

However, Koop succeeded through a rare alignment of events and personalities that unfortunately would not be seen again.

His replacement—Antonia Novello, the first woman appointed to the position—was a just-happy-to-be-here team player who was a disappointment as surgeon general and a figure of ignominy years later. Then came Joycelyn Elders, perhaps the most inspiring public speaker to hold the office, but tone deaf to the political fallout from her confrontational candor about controversial topics like the teaching of masturbation or the legalization of marijuana. Elders's meteoric tenure ended after barely a year—the shortest ever for a surgeon general—after President Bill Clinton deemed her too much of a political liability. Her firing (by a liberal chief executive, no less) seemed to permanently brand the position as expendable, and cast a pall over it that cowed some of Elders's successors.

Elders was followed by David Satcher, the last important surgeon general. Borrowing a trick from Julius Richmond, the low-key Satcher secured a second appointment within HHS, which afforded him resources that bolstered his work as surgeon general. With subtle determination, he produced groundbreaking and agenda-setting reports on obesity, sexual health, mental health, suicide, and a range of other topics. He restored dignity, visibility, and influence to the office. People who were turned off either by Novello or by Elders were again listening to the surgeon general.

It's been downhill ever since. Richard Carmona was a brash former war hero who as surgeon general followed orders to dissolve into the woodwork. Even more discouraging is the story of the most recent officeholder, Regina Benjamin. In an earlier life, Benjamin was likened to a living saint, overcoming fire and hurricanes to serve poor patients in an Alabama fishing village. But she was ill-equipped for life in Washington, and has become the most underachieving surgeon general to date. The blame for her failings rests as much with the system that selected and suppressed her as with Regina Benjamin herself. A few legislators have ventured proposals to fix that system—good proposals that could work. However, there has been no political will to enact them. Federal power brokers occupied with constituent demands, political fights, and personal peccadillos tend to have little time or interest in the surgeon general's problems.

This book analyzes and celebrates the importance of Benjamin and her predecessors in the nation's public health history. But it comes with a warning of its own: Unless something changes, we can expect—and, frankly, should expect—the surgeon general's demise.

PART ONE

Rise, 1871–1948

CHAPTER 2

Coming to Power

John Woodworth was disgusted.

A year earlier, the thirty-three-year-old Woodworth had won a plum assignment—a newly created job to rebuild the Marine Hospital Service, the U.S. government's hospital system for seamen. Created in 1798, it was a pioneering federal venture into providing health care, embodied in grand structures across the young nation.

But now it was 1872, and as the young doctor from Chicago surveyed his new domain, he saw calamity nearly everywhere. Of thirty-one government-built marine hospitals, only ten were still used, some just barely. The hospitals in Detroit, Cleveland, Louisville, and Portland needed extensive repairs. The one in Key West had been badly battered by hurricanes. The overcrowded St. Louis hospital needed to be extensively disinfected or burned down.[1] The Pittsburgh facility seemed as if it was located in Hades, sandwiched between a blast furnace and a railway-iron rolling mill. "No matter which way the wind blows, the hospital is continually filled with soot and smoke," Woodworth wrote, in an early report on the situation. "That the marine hospital service had suffered from the lack of proper medical supervision is a fact too apparent to be controverted."[2]

The energetic, bushy-mustached Woodworth seemed the right man to turn the system around. He already had a reputation for able medical management, some of it coming from his Civil War service as the chief medical officer for General William Tecumseh Sherman. Woodworth had received commendations for running the Union Army ambulance train during Sherman's famous "March to the Sea," which put more than one hundred wounded soldiers in wagons bound for Savannah hospitals. Every one of the soldiers survived the trip, a miraculous achievement in an era before disinfection of wounds was common medical practice.[3]

Woodworth proved to be something of a miracle worker at the Marine Hospital Service as well. He brought the service out of debt, improved and redesigned the marine hospitals, and created an elite corps of physicians to staff them. Beyond that, he took steps to turn the service into the nation's preeminent public health agency, responsible for disease investigations, quarantines, and a range of other duties.

He and the two men who succeeded him—John Hamilton and Walter Wyman—were empire builders who built the core of what became the U.S. Department of Health and Human Services. They brought power and prestige to the job Woodworth established, a position initially known as supervising surgeon of the Marine Hospital Service but eventually renamed the U.S. surgeon general. To many, the job would become known simply as the nation's doctor.

ORIGINS

Woodworth and his successors were civilian officials focused mainly on merchant seamen, but "surgeon general" is a title from the military world. It refers to a chief medical officer, "general" being the rank part of the title. The French infantry is believed to have had such a position in the 1500s. Oliver Cromwell's New Model Army appropriated the title decades later, during the English Civil War. There were also appointments such as "physician general" and "apothecary general," but surgeons historically led in the treatment of battlefield injuries and were considered the most essential medical personnel.[4] Americans borrowed the term from the English, and "surgeon general" became the title for the chief doctor of the U.S. Army around 1813. The U.S. Navy's top doctor has had that title since the early 1800s as well. Today, the senior-most medical officers in the army, navy, and air force all have the title surgeon general. (But it's the official within the federal public health department who is known as the U.S. surgeon general.)

The Marine Hospital Service had its roots in the defeat of the Spanish Armada in 1588, one of the most famous events in English history. English sailors stunned an invading Spanish naval force considered the world's mightiest. A grateful England rewarded its sailors by establishing a hospital for them in Greenwich, giving birth to a hospital system for sick and injured sailors in the Royal Navy and merchant marine. The idea that seamen deserved special treatment became entrenched in England.[5] When the American colonies were founded, colonists chose to continue the custom of providing care for their seamen, and marine hospitals were opened under charter from King George.[6] The U.S. government created the Marine Hospital Service in 1798, placing it directly under the secretary of the treasury.

Why the Treasury Department? It had an organized presence in seaports, collecting customs and looking out for smugglers. So it was a sensible home for a health service focused on seamen.

The first marine hospital was in Norfolk, Virginia, and others were quickly established in Boston, Newport, and Charleston. As the nation grew, additional facilities were built or established on rivers and lakes in the nation's interior. An "orgy" of marine hospital construction began in the late 1830s.[7] Politicians in western states and territories were especially interested. An 1855 report by a Treasury Department inspector noted the prevalent absurdity: "In some towns, there appears to be a desire, on the part of some of the inhabitants, to have marine hospitals erected, not because they are actually wanted for the relief of sick sailors or sick boatmen, but simply that additional sums of public money may be there expended. If this feeling be not checked, we shall have sinecure surgeons, sinecure stewards, sinecure matrons, sinecure nurses, without number. We have too many such already."[8]

Hospitals were built in obscure places where few seamen could use them, such as Paducah, Kentucky; Burlington, Iowa; and Galena, Illinois. Marine hospitals of the era were exquisite brick buildings, often three stories high with cypress porches, mahogany doors, and a small cupola at the top. Expensive structures built as political pork, some were later sold off at greatly reduced prices. Others had darker fates. One hospital was built in the 1850s in Napoleon, Arkansas, a flood-prone town on the bank of the Mississippi River. By 1868, the marine hospital had caved into the river, and a flood in 1874 finished off the town itself.[9]

Other problems plagued the hospital system. The buildings were mainly under local control, in keeping with the prevalent political belief that public health and health services were a natural responsibility of state and local officials. The Marine Hospital Service was financed through a tax on the master or owner of every American ship arriving from a foreign port, but the federal government had little oversight of how the money was spent. Local collectors of customs gathered and spent the tax money, and local politicians influenced the hospitals' staffing, using it as a patronage system. (The president was authorized to appoint the directors of the marine hospitals, but Congress did not set aside funding for hospital directors' salaries. The hospitals' medical officers had no control over finances or the hospital property.)

The result? Graft and disorganization reigned, deficits were common, and seamen suffered. The hospitals sensibly located near bustling ports were so busy that only a small percentage of applying sailors could be admitted. As a rule, chronic and incurable cases were turned away, as were any patients who needed care for more than four months.[10]

As early as the 1830s, federal officials were fielding complaints about how the system was managed. In 1849, the government assigned George Loring and Thomas Edwards to inspect the hospitals and recommend improvements. The Harvard-trained Loring was a surgeon at the marine hospital in Chelsea, Massachusetts. Edwards, also a doctor, was an Ohio congressman who had lost a reelection bid in 1848. The two decided a new tonnage tax was needed to ensure adequate funding, and recommended a chief surgeon be put in charge of the service.[11] Their proposals were shelved, however. The service continued to limp along as mismanagement and other problems took their toll, including the Civil War, during which both the Union and Confederate Armies occupied and destroyed marine hospitals.

When President Ulysses S. Grant took office in 1869, his administration vowed to clean up the marine hospital wreckage. Grant's treasury secretary, George Boutwell, a committed reformer from Massachusetts, had led the impeachment of President Andrew Johnson and the drive for a constitutional amendment to give African Americans the right to vote. Boutwell assigned a new team to assess the marine hospital problem. One member was W.D. Stewart, a member of Boutwell's staff. Another was John Shaw Billings, a brilliant young military physician who would become a savior of the Marine Hospital Service and then, later, its bitterest enemy.

THE BILLINGS REPORT

Billings, in his early thirties when Boutwell placed him on the marine hospital study team, was already something of a medical hero. Raised on an Indiana farm, he was an intense young man with clear blue eyes and a Napoleonic nose who had taught himself Latin and Greek. He joined the Union Army in the early days of the Civil War and distinguished himself in field hospitals at Chancellorsville and Gettysburg, where he cared for wounded soldiers under artillery fire. He became a sought-after military medical expert, and in 1864 was transferred to a desk job in the Office of the Army Surgeon General in Washington.[12]

In his new assignment, he developed two kinds of expertise that would earn him lasting fame. First, he became a medical librarian, indexing and cataloging the army surgeon general's modest collection of medical books and pamphlets and then systematically building it into one of the leading medical libraries in the world. (It was the foundation of what is now the National Library of Medicine in Bethesda, Maryland.) Second, Billings became a leading authority on the construction of hospitals, and years later would design the renowned Johns Hopkins Hospital and Medical School at Baltimore, which opened in 1889.

Billings and Stewart began their tour of the marine hospitals in 1869. The exact details of what they saw may be lost to history; historians have not yet located their reports to Boutwell.[13] But the two recommended, as had Loring and Edwards, that a strong surgeon be placed in charge of the hospital service. On June 29, 1870, President Grant signed a bill enabling the treasury secretary to make that change and to increase the tax that supported the hospital fund.[14]

Some historians believe Billings wanted to be the first to head the reformed Marine Hospital Service, in a position titled at the time "supervising surgeon." Boutwell wanted to give him the job—Billings had toured the facilities and had a firsthand understanding of what needed to be done. But it's not clear the treasury secretary actually offered Billings the job.[15] Legally, he couldn't: Billings was an army officer and the Senate Commerce Committee had pointedly put a provision in the law that the supervising surgeon had to be a civilian.[16] (The historian Bess Furman, who wrote one of the best-known histories of the Marine Hospital Service, suggested that Billings could be something of a pill and some senators had grown weary of him during his frequent congressional testimonies. Billings had no intention of leaving his army job, and they were not interested in giving him a second salary.)[17]

The Treasury Secretary continued to push for Billings for nearly a year after the Marine Hospital Service legislation passed, but finally abandoned that fight and appointed someone else: a physician from Chicago named John Woodworth.

JOHN WOODWORTH
The Reformer

Billings and Woodworth had much in common. They were about the same age. Both were ambitious and keenly interested in the latest European medical advances. Both had been esteemed surgeons in the Union Army during the Civil War (though Billings was the bigger star). They also were acquainted: Billings knew Woodworth well and probably was the one who recommended Woodworth for the marine hospital system position.[18]

John Maynard Woodworth was born August 15, 1837, in Big Flats, a small river town in western New York. His family moved a short time later to Illinois, where he spent the rest of his childhood. Woodworth went to grade school in Warrenville, a small town near Chicago, and attended the University of Chicago to become a pharmacist. He grew dissatisfied with that field and started pursuing other interests. After helping organize the Chicago Academy of Science, he was appointed curator of its museum in 1858, around the time he turned twenty-one. The next year, the University of Chicago hired him to establish a museum of natural history, and he spent the winters of 1859, 1860, and 1861 at the Smithsonian Institute in Washington, D.C., studying with the great naturalist Spencer Fullerton Baird.[19]

But Woodworth's interests changed again. He earned a medical degree in 1862, and immediately after graduation joined the army during the early days of the Civil War.[20] He started as an assistant surgeon at a Union training camp in Chicago. Promotions came quickly: surgeon, then medical inspector of the Fifteenth Army Corps, then medical director of the Army of the Tennessee.[21] He rose to chief medical officer for General Sherman, meaning Woodworth was responsible for the care of the soldiers in one of the Union's most important forces. This last appointment permanently placed the young physician in an important orbit. Ulysses Grant, general-in-chief of the Union Army (and future president), considered Sherman a trusted friend. Sherman and his brothers went on to prominent government positions after the war, and Woodworth's Civil War service gave him good standing with those powerful men.

The highlight of Woodworth's service under Sherman came during the infamous "March to the Sea," a devastating military campaign through the heart of Dixie that was one of the Civil War's turning points. Sherman was a hard man who believed in crushing the Confederacy so completely that the idea of armed rebellion would sicken Southerners for generations to come. Sherman's troops laid siege to Atlanta for four days and captured the city in September 1864, then began a march southeast to Savannah. The general purged his troops of every sick and ailing man, and told the healthy 60,000 remaining that they were cut off from Union supplies. They would have to forage for themselves along the route, meaning they were free to take or destroy what they found. This scorched-earth policy terrified Southerners and broke them of their belief that the Confederate Army could protect the home front.

Woodworth's job was to manage the six hundred ambulances set aside for casualties and illnesses. Luck was with him: most of Sherman's soldiers ate very well during the campaign—better than they had during the rest of the war, in fact—and were in good spirits because of it. They saw just two battles of significance, and suffered only about one hundred casualties. But to Woodworth's credit, all of the hundred made it to Savannah hospitals alive. (He attributed his success to strict hygiene practices.) He received commendations and mustered out of the army in 1865, when the war ended, with the rank of lieutenant colonel.[22]

Woodworth visited Berlin and Vienna, cities at the forefront of medicine at the time, and studied German and Austrian hospitals. He returned to Chicago in 1866. For the next five years, he was attending surgeon at a Chicago soldier's home, an inspector for the Chicago Board of Health, and a professor of anatomy at Chicago Medical College. Photographs of him from the time show a trim man with a receding hairline and a large bushy mustache—almost comical by today's standards—that flared out to bracket his chin and all but cover his lips. His other most striking feature was his dark eyes, sharply fixed in each portrait.

History texts do not say how Woodworth became aware of the opening for a supervising surgeon of the Marine Hospital Service. Appointed to the post in April 1871, he tackled the job with intensity.

His first task was overhauling the organization. Following Billings's advice, he sold off facilities in small inland ports and focused on hospitals in the large port cities of New York, Philadelphia, Baltimore, New Orleans, and San Francisco. He worked on replacing the sooty Pittsburgh hospital. And he took steps to improve the thirteen-year-old hospital in Chelsea, plagued by poor ventilation and a chronically high rate of erysipelas (a fiery skin infection caused by bacteria that were no doubt abundant in the filthy facility).[23]

Woodworth also championed a new, "pavilion" style of hospital construction. Instead of tall brick and stone structures, he called for single-story, well-ventilated wards made of wood that fanned out from a central office (California redwood, in the case of a hospital planned for San Francisco). He believed it was impossible to keep any facility hygienic for long in that era, and argued that the pavilion hospitals could—and should—be destroyed and replaced every ten or fifteen years. His idea of disposable hospitals was never adopted, however. He was overruled by officials in the government who believed the old design had significant merits, once sewage and disinfection were better addressed.[24]

Woodworth also had to fix the Service's finances. The tax increase passed in 1870 was not enough, and Woodworth sought not only more money but also a larger clientele. He requested that eligibility for marine hospital care be extended to sailors on revenue cutters—known today as the U.S. Coast Guard. He also invited in those who worked on Army Corps of Engineers vessels and even yachts. He asked that the Treasury Department be granted greater flexibility in setting the charge for care of foreign sailors.[25]

He also moved to reform his workforce. He knew he needed to recruit capable physicians and hospital administrators, but saw an opportunity to build prestige for the service by setting a standard higher than mere competence. Woodworth envisioned a quasi-militaristic, nationally mobile corps of doctors who could be moved from location to location to meet the most pressing medical needs and to break the entrenched patronage system that had long afflicted the service. He empowered his doctors through regulations that gave them say over whether seamen seeking care should be admitted to marine hospitals, a medical decision that—astonishingly—had previously been made by port collectors of customs.[26]

Woodworth's new regulations, approved by the Treasury Department, decreed that physician appointments were to be made to the general service rather than to any specific hospital, and doctors would be selected only after passing an examination by a board of surgeons. The physicians who passed these rigorous exams—who would come to be known as the Commissioned Corps—advanced through regular grades comparable to military officer ranks.

This was all fairly novel. Medicine at the time was still emerging from its Dark Ages. Homeopathy was a dominant form of medicine, and antiseptic surgery and the germ theory of disease were only beginning to catch on.[27] The medical education system was a scattershot collection of quality institutions and quack factories, with no national competency standards to speak of. Many doctors received their degrees after two years or less, and formal analytical reasoning had not yet become a widely taught foundation of medical science. The Flexner Report of 1910 would shine a harsh light on these inadequacies and lead to overdue reforms in medical education, but when Woodworth took over the Marine Hospital Service, the Flexner report was thirty-nine years in the future.

Given that context, Woodworth's staffing reforms were remarkable. What's more, they came when the Grant administration was plagued by graft, and they presaged by a decade the federal government's first laws to institute a merit system for federal employees and end the political spoils system that had fostered mediocrity and corruption in many corners of the government.[28]

To go with these professionalization measures, Woodworth introduced the trappings of a military system. He designed a seal to be emblazoned on Marine Hospital Service flags and publications. The seal, still used today, is a ship's anchor crossed with the caduceus of Mercury (two snakes wrapped around a staff—a symbol of both commerce and medicine). He hyphenated "Marine-Hospital Service" to make it distinctive. He put together a reference book for his doctors, *Nomenclature of Diseases* published in 1874, that was one of the first volumes published in this country that comprehensively listed the names and spellings of known illnesses.[29] And he required his troops to dress in small-lapel military uniforms with flat-topped caps, modeled on the navy style.[30]

Congress recognized Woodworth's progress and in 1875 doubled his annual salary from $2,000 to $4,000 and changed his title to "supervising surgeon general." The legislators also decided that the president would name Woodworth's successors, with the advice and consent of the Senate.[31] That appointment process is still in place today.

In his annual report for the fiscal year 1876–1877, Woodworth announced that the Marine Hospital Service was solvent, with a surplus of more than $4,000 following expenditures of about $369,000. Revenues were up, and so was business: in 1877–1878, a total of 18,223 sick and disabled seamen were cared for—breaking the previous record by more than 1,400.[32]

Success in hand, Woodworth moved to expand his mission. The Service's reorganization coincided with a push for stepped-up governmental measures to fight infectious diseases. Deadly outbreaks of yellow fever in the South and cholera in the North had sparked the sanitary reform movement. The Louisiana State Board of Health—the first state health department—organized in 1853, following a terrible yellow fever epidemic that killed 9,000 in New Orleans. National and international public health conventions began springing up in the 1850s, too, attended by leading physicians who debated regulatory proposals for quarantines and other sanitary measures. The Civil War halted all that, but the movement reignited in the late 1860s.[33]

In September 1872, little more than a year after Woodworth took office, Stephen Smith of the New York City Board of Health and a few other movement leaders met in Long Branch, New Jersey, to create a national organization focused on such matters. Woodworth was among the dignitaries invited, and joined the group.[34] He thus became a founder of the American Public Health Association (APHA), the flagship professional organization for sanitarians and other public health workers.

The APHA advocated for a strong federal agency to administer quarantines and other disease-control measures. Woodworth loved the idea, and believed the Marine Hospital Service should be that agency. But John Shaw Billings, Woodworth's former benefactor, wanted another agency to handle it.

So began a bitter rift.

Battling Billings

In Woodworth's first years on the job, he and Billings were friendly and respectful to each other. In his first annual report on the Marine Hospital Service, Woodworth acknowledged Billings's "valuable" preparatory work on the reorganization. Woodworth quoted and praised Billings at an APHA annual meeting in November 1874.[35]

But Woodworth had already begun to establish his own voice. Also in 1874, Congress and the Grant administration assigned Woodworth and army medical officer Ely McClellan to investigate a cholera outbreak in the Mississippi Valley. The resulting 1,025-page report concluded that U.S. ports hadn't received enough warning about cholera spreading from Europe. (It's noteworthy that most of the work was done by McClellan, but only Woodworth's name was on the cover and title page. That kind of billing foreshadowed the surgeon general reports issued a century later, which also were published under the surgeon general's name but were actually written by others.) The American

Medical Association called it one of the most valuable contributions to the literature of the disease.[36]

Despite the AMA's praise, the report shows how little doctors understood about infectious diseases. At the time, many doctors still held to the "miasma theory," that illnesses like cholera and plague were caused by filth and inhaled stench. That theory had begun to crumble after the British physician John Snow deduced that an 1854 outbreak of cholera in London could be traced to tainted drinking water. But at the time of Woodworth's report, the germ theory had not yet completely taken hold. It was not until 1884—ten years after the Woodworth-McClellan report— that the German physician Robert Koch altered conventional scientific thinking with his identification of the bacteria that causes cholera.[37]

Woodworth realized cholera flourished in dirty environments and could be spread through the stools of an infected person, but believed the main mode of transmission was through dried particles carried on clothes and luggage and spread through the air. He concluded that the best way to stop cholera was to spot it overseas and impose inspections and quarantines before it could spread to U.S. ports and then inland.[38] He also argued that since the Marine Hospital Service already handled the care of merchant sailors, it made sense that the Service's doctors should be put in charge of inspecting and quarantining incoming vessels and their passengers.

By volunteering the Marine Hospital Service, Woodworth ended up picking two fights.

One was with Billings and other APHA leaders, who believed in greater federal public health powers but felt Woodworth's agency was the wrong place to put those powers. They thought a new government agency should be created for that purpose. The other fight was with congressmen and state officials who thought no federal agency of any kind should be handling such matters.

The idea that the federal government should be in charge of quarantines was still revolutionary, since public health powers in the United States—by law and tradition—had been the responsibility of state and local authorities. Politicians worried about an infringement on states' rights had defeated the Evans-Ramsey bill of 1865–1866, which would have given the secretaries of the treasury, war, and navy power over national quarantines at all ports.

Fortunately for Woodworth, that kind of opposition had begun to wane, especially after devastating outbreaks that had repeatedly proved that states were not up to the task of preventing deadly illnesses from entering and radiating across the country. Congress began seriously discussing creation of a federal disease prevention agency in 1871 after the South was hit by epidemics of yellow fever—a ghastly illness that came on like flu but could lead to liver failure, jaundice, black vomit, bleeding from the gums and nose, and a quick death. Talk of a national health agency gained new momentum after another epidemic in 1873. By that time, even rebellious southern states began to stand in favor, with the Louisiana Board of Health asking the state's congressional delegation to lobby for federal officials to take over quarantines.[39]

Woodworth kept pushing for the responsibility. In 1876, he read a paper at the International Medical Congress in Philadelphia, arguing that he should be the one to write rules concerning the quarantine of vessels from other ports, and that the Service should collect reports from U.S. consular officers on outbreaks and sanitary conditions overseas. He recommended inspecting U.S.-bound ships in foreign ports— the first federal official to make such a suggestion publicly. He also proposed that his troops be charged with investigating the causes of U.S. outbreaks of cholera and yellow fever.[40]

He found he had a lot of supporters in the South, where yellow fever was a leading menace and quarantines were considered the best way to stop that scourge.[41] The zealous Woodworth worked closely with southern congressmen, including Julian Hartridge of Georgia, who on March 9, 1878, introduced a bill containing the proposals Woodworth had made in his 1876 speech in Philadelphia. The bill initially granted the Service the authority to set and enforce quarantines, but later was reworked to say that Woodworth's staff should act as an auxiliary to the states and no federal regulation should supersede state quarantine policy. The bill passed both the House and the Senate in April, aided in part by ominous reports that a new yellow fever epidemic was burning through Havana and the West Indies and might arrive soon.[42]

The National Quarantine Act of 1878, as the law was called, was actually not much of a victory for Woodworth. The Service was officially made the leading federal agency in quarantine efforts, but Congress did not give the Service additional funding or any substantive new power. (Indeed, in his State of the Union address of December 1878, President Rutherford B. Hayes acknowledged that the law "was passed too late in the last session of Congress to provide the means for carrying it into practical operation.") Local governments still had primacy, meaning the same crazy-quilt system was in place that had proved a sieve against yellow fever infections.

Just a few months after the legislation passed, yellow fever hit the South again. This epidemic killed a staggering 20,000 people over five months. Memphis was hit particularly hard, after city officials, business leaders, and dozens of doctors rejected a proposed quarantine because of concerns about its impact on commerce. Woodworth could do little, given his limited authority and resources. In September 1878, he organized a commission to go to the South, investigate the origins of the epidemic, and advise how to prevent another in the future. But he was able to do so only after securing a $250 pledge from the New York philanthropist Elizabeth Thompson to pay for the group's expenses.

As Woodworth floundered, his opponents organized. They saw in the 1878 yellow fever calamity an opportunity to revive their plans for a new, stronger federal agency—a National Board of Health—to lead quarantine efforts and disease investigation. They pushed their plan at the APHA meeting in Richmond that November. Woodworth fought back, and some historians believe he tried to sabotage the meeting by ignoring a preset agenda and distributing a program that promised a full hearing to every yellow fever theorist, thereby fostering chaos and perhaps enabling him to emerge with a strengthened claim to being the nation's leading public health authority. However, the APHA's executive committee denounced his action and restored order.[43]

While these squabbles raged in the public health community, the panicked public demanded the government do something—anything—to tame yellow fever. In December 1878, at the urging of President Hayes, the House and Senate agreed to allocate $50,000 to an expert panel overseen by Woodworth to report on the epidemic. The panel began meeting in late December and hurried a report to Congress on January 30, 1879, but it was an incomplete document, with the authors begging for more time and unable to say whether the epidemic was imported or endemic.

Meanwhile, U.S. Senator L.Q.C. Lamar of Mississippi had introduced a bill that would essentially turn the Marine Hospital Service into a federal bureau of public health, with greater power over quarantines. He had Woodworth's enthusiastic support, but Billings and his allies fought the bill bitterly. They loathed the idea of so much power in Woodworth's eager hands. Said one physicians' periodical, "We feel required to state that the great mass of the thinking portion of the profession would at once recognize the unfitness of Dr. Woodworth for such a position." Arguments about Woodworth's suitability aside, the specter of one federal official having so much power over public health frightened enough senators that Lamar's bill was rejected.[44]

APHA leaders were working with others in Congress to establish a National Board of Health. The National Board was to have the same scope of powers Woodworth had proposed for his agency, but in this version a director general and a seven-member panel of leading sanitarians would be in control. Many members of Congress fought this proposal, as well. Congress was under public pressure to respond to the yellow fever epidemic, but faith in states' rights was far too ingrained for such bold leaps.

Woodworth and Billings both battled on, furiously lobbying for their respective proposals and picking at each other's. On March 3, in the final hours of the last day of the legislative session, Billings and his allies won. Congress passed a watered-down version of an APHA-supported bill creating the National Board of Health. The final legislation did not provide for a director general to be chief administrator of the agency, nor did it give the National Board the authority to supersede states and localities in setting quarantines. Even a clause for a $500,000 appropriation to fund the new agency was deleted. The new agency's purpose was mainly to gather information about epidemics and advise others on health matters.[45]

But Woodworth was crushed. The National Board took over all the quarantine and disease investigations roles he had gained a year earlier. The Service's health-care duties to seamen would continue, but he had lost his bid at establishing the Marine Hospital Service as the nation's first federal public health agency.

Two days after the bill's passage, Woodworth broke out with erysipelas, the terrible bacterial skin infection that had plagued marine hospitals when he first became surgeon general. A few days later he was diagnosed with pneumonia. He deteriorated rapidly and died at 4 A.M. on Friday, March 14, just eleven days after the National Board legislation passed. Woodworth was forty-one and left a wife and no children.[46]

One medical journal attributed his death to overwork. But John B. Hamilton, the Marine Hospital Service physician who would succeed Woodworth as surgeon general, blamed Billings and his clique of APHA associates. Speaking years later at a hearing on Capitol Hill, Hamilton said Woodworth "was hounded to his grave by some of the same 'sanitarians' who became the temporary beneficiaries of that cessation of opposition."[47]

Hamilton took up his predecessor's fight, vowing to torpedo the National Board of Health and bring to the Service the powers Woodworth had dreamt of.

JOHN HAMILTON
The Avenger

Woodworth's funeral was held Sunday, March 16, at the home of the successful businessman Andrew Langdon. Every parlor was packed. President Hayes was there, as was Treasury Secretary John Sherman and his brother General William Tecumseh Sherman. The president's wife contributed an elaborate floral cross that was placed on top of the surgeon general's black walnut casket. Articles about the funeral in the *Washington Post* and the *National Republican* named about two dozen of the dignitaries present, but did not note whether Billings attended.[48]

The president needed to replace Woodworth, and within a few weeks chose John Hamilton, a thirty-one-year-old physician who had joined the Marine Hospital Service only three years earlier and had hardly any experience in Washington. Billings and his associates were initially relieved; they saw Hamilton as a political neophyte who would tend to marine hospital duties while leaving larger public health matters to the new National Board.

They completely misjudged him. Hamilton quickly developed into a shrewd political tactician, outfoxing the APHA's brightest minds and ensuring the demise of the National Board of Health by 1884. Hamilton was no saint—in some fights, he opposed National Board efforts that were the wisest path to saving lives. His goal, pure and simple, was to grow the Marine Hospital Service into the federal government's public health agency. Billings quickly grew wary of him. "He is an ass to meddle but he may do a good deal of mischief and forewarned is forearmed," Billings wrote in a letter to an acquaintance a year after Hamilton took office.[49]

John Brown Hamilton was born December 1, 1847, in Otter Creek, Illinois. He was a descendant of Miles Standish and other passengers on the *Mayflower,* his great-great-grandfathers were soldiers in the American Revolution, and his father was the Reverend Benjamin Brown Hamilton—known as "the fighting chaplain" of the 61st Illinois Volunteers during the Civil War. Hamilton attended a school operated by his family and by his teen years was infatuated with medicine. At age fifteen he worked part-time in a sawmill during the day and at night pored over books like Carpenter's *Physiology* and Gross's *Pathological Anatomy*. At age sixteen, he became an apprentice to an uncle who was a physician.[50]

Around the time of his seventeenth birthday, Hamilton enlisted in the Union Army to fight in the Civil War. He served about two months, part of the time guarding railroad bridges in Missouri, before his father persuaded army officials to honorably discharge him because of his young age. Hamilton returned to his medical studies and attended Rush Medical College in Chicago, where he earned his medical degree in 1869. He then married and settled into private practice in a village near St. Louis.[51]

It wasn't enough; he was restless and ambitious. In 1874, Hamilton rejoined the army, as an assistant surgeon, serving two years. He briefly returned to private practice, but then learned of the competitive examination to join the Marine Hospital Service. Intrigued, he signed up and scored the highest grade among the fifteen doctors who took the test that year. He was assigned to the marine hospital in Chelsea, Massachusetts, where he soon made his mark.

The Chelsea hospital, serving the port of Boston, was the oldest marine hospital and had the finest reputation. It also had some of the most serious problems. Its poorly constructed sewage system emptied into a nearby salt marsh, causing a stench that angered nearby residents. The hospital also had an extremely high rate of erysipelas and postoperative infections. When Hamilton took over, he relocated all patients to the third floor and ordered an extensive renovation to update the sewage system and ventilation. Chelsea became a model facility, and a delighted Woodworth rewarded Hamilton with a transfer to headquarters in Washington, D.C.[52]

Hamilton was in the capital during the Woodworth's final legislative battles. On his deathbed, the dying surgeon general implored Vice President William Wheeler to make sure Hamilton was named his successor. Treasury Secretary Sherman hesitated over the boyish-looking Hamilton, reportedly saying, "His credentials seem to be the best, but his youth and even more his youthful appearance seem to make his appointment open to just criticism." But the nomination went forward, and Hamilton became surgeon general on April 3, 1879.[53]

As Hamilton began his new job, Billings was trying to build up the new National Board of Health, lobbying Congress to expand the nascent agency's resources and better define its responsibilities. Two bills passed in early June helped. Congress appropriated $500,000 for the Board and gave it the authority to rent office space, hire clerical help, and use government printing services. It also transferred from the Marine Hospital Service to the National Board the oversight of information-gathering about disease conditions in foreign and domestic ports. Nevertheless, Congress still considered the National Board an experiment, and set a four-year sunset on the agency's enabling legislation (which could be modified at a later time, if Congress was satisfied with the agency's progress). Congress also stressed that the Board must cooperate with state and local authorities in setting quarantines.[54]

The National Board had seven members appointed by the president, as well as representatives from the army, navy, Marine Hospital Service, and Department of Justice. The president was James Lawrence Cabell of the University of Virginia, one of the most distinguished physicians of his day.[55] But Billings was the real boss. Cabell made only occasional trips to Washington and was often absent for crucial decisions. Billings, the Board's vice president and guiding hand, led most of the organization's initiatives.

The new agency immediately focused on yellow fever. The disease's cause was still a mystery, but Billings and his associates were wise (wiser than Woodworth and Hamilton) about pursuing the right theories of infectious disease transmission and control. The National Board sent a commission to Havana to work with a Cuban scientist named Carlos Finlay who was exploring the idea—later proven correct—that mosquitoes spread the disease. Billings also pursued the observation that yellow fever seemed to arrive on ships in the hottest months of the year and end with the frost. He worked with a British veterinarian, John Gamgee, who had proposed building a refrigeration ship to fight yellow fever. The idea: cargo and luggage from incoming vessels could be placed in the refrigeration vessel's chilling compartments to kill whatever might be breeding infection. Billings convinced Congress to appropriate $200,000 to make it happen.[56]

The matter was immediately plunged into controversy. Gamgee was a professional associate and friend of Billings (they had co-authored a book on cattle diseases), and other companies protested what appeared to be a sweetheart deal between the two men. The United States Ice and Refrigerating Company claimed Gamgee's proposal violated two of its patents. Gamgee, meanwhile, said it was his private design and must not be opened to the review of outside companies that also wanted to bid on the contract. The Senate quickly passed a resolution directing Treasury Secretary Sherman to look into the matter. Sherman handed the matter over to his new surgeon general.[57]

This was balm for a seething man. In his first few months on the job, Hamilton had been forced to watch as the Service's limited quarantine powers and epidemic-response functions were stripped away. He also had to turn over to the National Board the weekly bulletin of disease conditions that the Service had been publishing since 1878.[58] In late May, when Billings had summoned the surgeon general to discuss transferring responsibilities, he had refused to go. Ah, but this refrigeration ship controversy gave Hamilton new leverage. He was ready to speak to the Board now.

He appeared before the Board on June 23. (Billings was absent that day due to illness.) The surgeon general was gruff, saying the new agency's quarantine regulations were too vague and that he and Secretary Sherman had just proposed a more sensible proposal to the president's cabinet. The next day, Sherman ruled—per Hamilton's advice—that the plans and specifications for the refrigeration ship would be publicly advertised and opened for bid. That decision begat a mess of proposals and counterproposals, and the ship was never built.

Hamilton was just getting started. He spent the next four years doggedly undermining Billings's agency. More cunning than Woodworth, he worked behind the scenes, buttonholing legislators and administration officials as he pushed for legislation and policies that would favor the Service and weaken the Board. He was good at this sort of lobbying, winning the backing of several key members of the House Appropriations Committee and enjoying the firm support of his superiors at the Treasury Department.

The National Board, meanwhile, had other problems on its hands. Congress had not given the new agency power to enforce its quarantine rules on states that resisted (only the president could do that), and Billings and his colleagues found a significant lack of state cooperation. One obstacle was Joseph Jones of the Louisiana Board of Health, a former Confederate Army officer and fervent believer in states' rights. Louisiana was a particularly unfortunate place for the Board to encounter such resistance; the state was a constant launching pad for yellow fever epidemics that ravaged the South. But Jones insisted that his staff had everything under control, and resisted requests by the national agency to station federal quarantine officers in Louisiana or to even allow them to see death reports.[59]

Public relations blunders compounded the problem. The National Board's members, and some of the men who worked for them, came off as elitists who believed they knew better than the rest of the country how to practice public health. One of the Board's inspectors, A. N. Bell, disparaged southerners in an 1879 interview with the *New York Herald*. "They assume, whenever I have been in the South, that they cannot have yellow fever unless it is brought to them from somewhere else. In the seaport towns they insist that the disease never reaches them except by ship, yet some of these very towns have filth in their midst to infect every ship's crew in the world."[60]

Meanwhile, Hamilton pressed his attacks, and the haughty reputation of the National Board—coupled with the agency's growing requests for money—made more congressmen sympathetic to the surgeon general's arguments. In 1882, the House of Representatives put the Marine Hospital Service in charge of a $100,000 appropriation for preventing the entry and spread of infectious disease. Hamilton spent the money almost immediately, to combat a yellow fever outbreak in Brownsville, Texas. He used armed guards to set up a cordon sanitaire of quarantine stations on the Mexican border where travelers were detained for ten days and watched to see if they had the illness. (This was an era when public health officials carried badges and regularly exercised police powers, something Hamilton did his best to promote.)[61] Probably only a fraction of the $100,000 was necessary to handle the situation, but Hamilton liberally shared the money with officials in affected regions to buy their support.[62] He used the same strategy during a yellow fever outbreak in Pensacola in 1883.

The Brownsville and Pensacola outbreaks seemed to be quickly controlled, and Hamilton celebrated. George Waring, secretary of the National Board, issued a press release in 1884 to ridicule the surgeon general's chest thumping. He said that Hamilton had misrepresented what happened in those cities and the Service actually had taken the wrong approach. Waring ultimately proved correct. Science would later show that controlling the conditions that allow the proliferation of disease-spreading mosquitoes—the Board's approach—was more important than using guards to fence off travelers from an outbreak area.[63]

But it didn't matter. By the time Waring issued his release, Hamilton had already won. The National Board's enabling legislation sunsetted on June 2, 1883. The Marine Hospital Service took over national quarantine and public health matters. The Board lingered for a little while in weakened form; retaining a few supporters on Capitol Hill, it won a small grant to continue some disease investigations for a few years. But the agency was dead by 1886.

Power and Pride

In 1888, Billings tried again, testifying to the House Commerce Committee that a new agency could do the kinds of scientific disease investigations that were lacking. But Hamilton torpedoed Billings's bid by quickly rebutting that the Marine Hospital Service had already set up the permanent Hygienic Laboratory, which was doing exactly the kind of work Billings proposed. One year earlier, the Staten Island Marine Hospital had turned over a room to a young physician named Joseph Kinyoun who had studied with leading scientists in Germany and France, copied their techniques and equipment, and begun to study infectious microbes and experiment with gases that might be effective disinfectants.[64] The lab was moved to Washington, D.C., in 1891, to a building near the Capitol. By then Kinyoun was turning into something of a star within the agency, preparing diphtheria antitoxin, testing wells during a typhoid fever outbreak, and teaching his techniques to representatives from state and local health agencies across the country. The lab would keep growing, eventually becoming the National Institutes of Health.

Hamilton looked to grow the Service in other ways. In 1884, he prodded Congress to approve a new tonnage tax on vessels arriving to the United States from foreign ports—as Loring and Edwards had recommended thirty-five years earlier—as a new funding source for the Service. By 1890, the tax was bringing in nearly $600,000 a year, more than covering Service expenditures. Hamilton also took steps to build prestige for his medical officers. In January 1889, he won passage of a congressional act that formally authorized the Commissioned Corps as a uniformed, physicians-only component of the Service.[65]

By 1890, Hamilton's agency had achieved record growth, with eighteen marine hospitals serving more than 50,000 patients. The Service also operated seven quarantine stations, and Congress that year directed Hamilton to draw up any necessary regulations to stop the spread of a disease from one state to another, and to employ whatever manpower was needed to enforce them.[66] Hamilton regarded the Service as much more than a system of hospitals for seamen, and asked legislators to change his organization's name to the U.S. Public Health Service. Congress declined.

In late May 1891, Hamilton abruptly resigned to accept a position at Rush Medical College in Chicago. The newspapers called it a surprise, but noted he had been unhappy with his $4,000 annual salary and wanted it increased to equal what the surgeons general of the army and navy were paid. His successor was named immediately—Walter Wyman, the doctor who had run the Staten Island Marine Hospital (home of Kinyoun's lab) before becoming Hamilton's chief assistant in Washington.[67]

Hamilton may never have intended to give up the surgeon general post permanently. The journalist and historian Bess Furman wrote that

Hamilton struck a deal with Wyman that, after a year, Hamilton would come back to Washington and reassume the top job. But when the year passed, Wyman reneged (or so the story goes).[68]

When he first resigned as surgeon general, Hamilton worked out an agreement that he would run the marine hospital in Chicago and supervise the Service exhibit planned for the upcoming World's Fair. But he quit the service altogether in 1896, when Wyman tried to transfer him to San Francisco. In his final years, he was the administrator of a state insane asylum in Elgin, near Chicago.

During a trip to New York in December 1898, Hamilton came down with what was initially labeled a severe cold. Upon his return, he was diagnosed with something more dire—an abdominal infection called peritonitis. A prominent surgeon tried to save him, but the operation failed and Hamilton died in the Elgin asylum that Christmas Eve.[69] He was fifty-one. Hamilton's body was buried at the National Cemetery at Arlington, with military honors. The newspapers carried little detail of what was said at the interment, but others have since memorialized him as the greatest enemy the American Public Health Association ever had, and the schemer who destroyed the National Board of Health.[70]

WALTER WYMAN

A Rule for Everything

Walter Wyman was a walruslike man and longtime bachelor who regarded the Service as his family. He could be a gruff and difficult patriarch, however, prone to making abrupt and seemingly callous assignment transfers. (As one Service veteran commented, "He found out where you didn't want to go—and then he sent you there."[71]) And the rules! Wyman set rules about even the tiniest details of Service life, authoring a ninety-four-page manual that specified exactly how to wear a sword belt and what wording to use when addressing a memo.[72]

He did not become such a stickler through army training—unlike his two predecessors, Wyman never served in the military. He was born in St. Louis on August 17, 1848, the son of a teacher. He earned a bachelor's degree from Amherst College in 1870 and his medical degree from St. Louis Medical College. He joined the Marine Hospital Service in 1876—the same year Hamilton did—and rapidly cycled through a series of administrative positions at Service facilities in St. Louis, Cincinnati, Baltimore, and New York.

He had a fateful experience one night in May 1881, while working at a Cincinnati Catholic hospital in which the Service operated a ward. Wyman admitted a roustabout who had been pulled out of the Ohio River. The man was violent, foul-mouthed, and irrational, and arrangements were made for the straightjacketed man to be treated at a federal hospital for the insane in Washington, D.C. Wyman wanted to see the Service headquarters, so he decided to personally escort the patient, in a railroad baggage car. After Wyman delivered the patient, he went to see Surgeon General Hamilton. As it happened, Hamilton was looking for a Service physician to send on a two-and-a-half-month assignment to Spain and the Azores. "Send me!" Wyman said. Hamilton agreed, and from then on would frequently tap Wyman for unusual opportunities and ultimately choose him as his successor.[73]

The Wyman administration began with a wave of energetic transformation. The Service relocated its headquarters from Washington's F Street to a mansion just off the grounds of the Capitol. The Service also bulked up its quarantine operations, in the wake of a March 1891 law that mandated immigrant health inspections and specified that Service doctors were to do the task. Service inspectors were detailed to Boston, Philadelphia, Baltimore, and to an immigration portal in New York's harbor—opened in 1892—called Ellis Island.

Wyman ordered his men to watch for signs of problems like defective eyesight, trachoma, rheumatism, odd behavior, and "loathsome diseases" like syphilis, gonorrhea, and leprosy. Service inspectors had the power to send an immigrant back to his or her origin country, on the grounds that such people were likely to become a public charge.[74]

The call for inspection and quarantine of immigrants became more acute in February 1892, when an epidemic of delirium-inducing typhus fever emerged in New York among recently arrived Russian Jewish immigrants. Six months later, cholera erupted in the same population. Yellow fever may have been the terror of the South, but cholera was more feared in New York. The painful and ghastly bacterial illness spread through feces and literally drained its victims to death as they gushed diarrhea speckled with gray (which was mucous, but for years was assumed to be bits of shredded intestines).

Wyman advised President Benjamin Harrison to encourage every state to quarantine all immigration ships for twenty days. (This was a backdoor ban on immigration—having a ship in quarantine for twenty days was too much of a financial burden for shipping companies.) Harrison approved. New York officials had initially taken the lead in the cholera outbreak, but by late September, Wyman was deemed the ultimate health authority. At about that time, the cholera outbreak was subsiding, with the death toll in New York and at its quarantine stations holding to fewer than fifty-five. Wyman was hailed for the success, though perhaps at least as much credit should have been given to such factors as a safe New York City water supply and quick isolation and sanitation measures imposed by the city leaders.[75]

The New York harbor success story fed interest in a tougher national quarantine law. Lawmakers also were concerned about the upcoming 1893 Chicago World's Fair, for an epidemic could kill the event. In February 1893, President Harrison signed a law directing the surgeon general to evaluate and strengthen U.S. quarantine laws and ordering that no arriving ship could unload its cargo or disembark its passengers until a federal quarantine officer gave his approval.

Meanwhile, Wyman tried to strengthen relations with state health officials. He offered Kinyoun as a trainer and resource to state health departments, and scheduled a continuing slate of conferences with state officials. He was largely successful, and was elected president of the American Public Health Association in 1902, partially erasing the bitterness that had existed between the APHA and the Service during Hamilton's reign.[76]

Wyman also emerged as a Progressive who strongly believed in a proactive role for government in improving the public welfare, and sought a change from the traditional practice of society looking to charities to deal with calamities and societal woes. "Charity, as it is ordinarily understood, is insufficient. . . . The best physical charity is the establishment and enforcement of proper sanitary laws," Wyman wrote in 1907, in an article for Samuel Gompers's *American Federationist,* the official magazine of the American Federation of Labor.[77] He was in sync with the White House: the Progressive Teddy Roosevelt became president in 1901. He endorsed Wyman's legislative goals and, in 1902, a sympathetic Congress finally agreed to rename Wyman's agency the U.S. Public Health and Marine Hospital Service. The same congressional act shorted Wyman's formal title from supervising surgeon general to surgeon general. Wyman also won a pay bump, to $5,000 annually.[78]

Plague and Death

Wyman and his doctors handled U.S. outbreaks of cholera in 1892, yellow fever in 1893 and 1897–1898, smallpox in 1897, and typhoid fever in 1898. But more than that, as the new century dawned, Service investigators became noted not only for limiting epidemics but also for solving the medical mysteries behind them.

Wyman's staff included a Who's Who of public health legends, including Kinyoun, the laboratorian who planted the seeds for the National Institutes of Health; Milton Rosenau, Kinyoun's successor and a primary force behind the campaign for milk pasteurization; Henry Rose Carter, who played a key role in establishing that mosquitoes spread yellow fever; and Joseph Goldberger, who would deduce that the cause of the pellagra disease that annually killed hundreds in the South was not an infectious disease—as many doctors assumed—but rather the region's poverty-driven diet.

In assembling such an elite cadre, Wyman helped set the stage for a golden age of American public health. Sadly, he marred his legacy through his shameful handling of a plague outbreak in San Francisco.

No disease was as internationally terrifying as plague. In the 1300s, it wiped out a third of Europe's population in five years and earned the fearsome nickname "the Black Death" for the way it darkened its victims' skin. The very possibility of plague in a community could spur extreme and dramatic isolation measures.

Wyman came to deal with plague through an unfortunate string of occurrences in and near the booming metropolis of San Francisco. To help protect that city from invading pestilence, the Service operated a quarantine and inspection station on Angel Island in San Francisco Bay. In January 1900, Angel Island quarantine officers examined the steamship *Australia* as it arrived from Honolulu, a locale hit by plague the month before. The Angel Island officers failed to notice—or take action against—plague-infected rats on board the *Australia,* and the ship was allowed to proceed. It docked at a spot where the sewers of San Francisco's Chinatown district emptied, offering the rats a quick-and-dirty highway into the city. In early March a forty-one-year-old lumber salesman named Wong Chut King died and was diagnosed with plague—the first case of plague ever on U.S. soil.[79]

Wyman sent Joseph Kinyoun to San Francisco in 1899. It was one of Wyman's famous abrupt transfers, and it surprised and angered Kinyoun, a star with the Service who had a wife and four young children and no desire to move so far. But his talents proved valuable in San Francisco. As far back as 1895 he had predicted plague would likely enter the United States, and had started a plague research program in 1896.[80] He expertly identified plague in the salesman's tissue samples, and notified Wyman.

Then things got nasty. In March 1900, the city health department quarantined Chinatown after Kinyoun's diagnosis, but lifted the restriction after three days when no new cases appeared. Denialist newspapers and local businessmen criticized Kinyoun for raising the commerce-killing specter of plague. The Chinese community, meanwhile, was wary of the thousands of doses of the primitive Haffkine serum vaccine Wyman had shipped to San Francisco for plague control. The situation became volatile as Chinese people hid suspected cases of plague and began to leave the city. Wyman spoke with President William McKinley, who authorized the surgeon general to order the vaccinations and stop the Chinese from leaving without a health certificate from Kinyoun predicated on their immunization. Chinese residents chafed and federal vaccinators found almost no takers.[81] Kinyoun—who reported directly to Wyman—wanted to go further, and discussed with Wyman the idea of putting Chinese into plague detention camps.[82] Kinyoun also warned health officials in other states to be careful about passengers or freight from California.

The California State Board of Health stepped in and, in late May, forced city officials to quarantine Chinatown's twelve city blocks a second time. That sparked riots and anger in the Chinese community and prompted a lawsuit by a Chinese grocer named Jew Ho. His case went to the federal court of appeals, which sided with the plaintiff, calling the quarantine an unwarranted act of racial discrimination. Meanwhile, President McKinley—a Republican—nullified the travel ban after hearing bitter protests from California Republicans about its impact on commerce. The following January, California legislators (who had openly discussed the idea of lynching Kinyoun) passed a resolution asking McKinley to remove Kinyoun.[83]

Wyman, having firmly backed Kinyoun during the turbulent spring of 1900, now abandoned him as the politics of the situation became more severe. The surgeon general cut a deal with a group that included California's Governor Henry Gage. They promised to help clean up Chinatown if Wyman would get rid of Kinyoun—and suppress an independent investigative panel's report confirming at least six people in San Francisco had died from the plague. Wyman agreed, transferred Kinyoun to Detroit, and issued the gag order.[84] (The report got out anyway.) It was a disgraceful moment in the history of the Office of the Surgeon General. In caving to wrongheaded politicians, Wyman essentially violated a federal law that required him to report on health conditions at U.S. ports. It was one of the first times a surgeon general allowed politicians to hold his tongue. Sadly, it would not be the last.[85]

Wyman shrugged off news coverage of his compact with Governor Gage, and agreed to a request for more help by sending a young service officer named Rupert Blue. Blue held the plague in check for years before eradicating it with a rat extermination program in 1905. He returned to San Francisco when plague erupted again in 1907, and again stamped it out.

Wyman, meanwhile, grew old.

The 1908 election brought into office William Howard Taft, a massively obese man who proved a more lethargic president than Teddy Roosevelt. The tempo change at the White House coincided with Wyman's physical decline—he turned sixty that year, and was fat, diabetic, and prone to dozing at his desk. As a younger man he had worked hard to expand his agency's powers and responsibilities, but in his final years he flat-out rejected a proposal to create within the Service a Children's Bureau responsible for the welfare of mothers and infants, which he deemed a sentimental endeavor that would complicate his life.[86]

In late 1911, Wyman fell apart. He had boils and Bright's disease (a kidney condition), and then fell into a diabetic coma. He died just after midnight on November 21, 1911, at Providence Hospital in Washington. He was sixty-three.[87]

Wyman and his two predecessors had managed to build a ragged collection of decrepit marine hospitals and turn it into a small but widely respected federal agency that led the nation's efforts to prevent and control disease. The surgeon general had become a health leader in American society, and was about to become even more prominent.

CHAPTER 3

War and Prominence

When Walter Wyman died, the Office of the Surgeon General was forty years old, and an informal tradition regarding succession was already in place. Each surgeon general had chosen his replacement. Woodworth, on his deathbed, advocated for Hamilton. Hamilton engineered the selection of Wyman. But Wyman—that old controlling bachelor—made no arrangement for an heir.

President Taft was left to choose between two men. One was Rupert Blue, the forty-six-year-old hero of the San Francisco plague outbreaks. The other was Joseph H. White, an older veteran of the Service (he was fifty-three at the time) who had distinguished himself on a variety of assignments, including the nation's last yellow fever outbreak in 1905. The selection process dragged out for more than a month, and Taft enjoyed building a little suspense—he jokingly invited reporters to pick their favorite color, Blue or White.[1] The contest split opinion within the Service, with many officers considering White the more sensible choice. Among them was the brilliant epidemiologist Joseph Goldberger, who felt White had a moral courage that Blue lacked but believed Blue had the advantage of being more politically adept and—like Taft—a Republican.[2]

On the advice of Treasury Secretary Franklin MacVeagh, Taft in early January 1912 announced Blue won the job. The president also decided to limit the surgeon general to four-year appointments, instead of the unlimited terms Blue's predecessors had enjoyed.[3] The surgeon general and his staff in the Service saw themselves as being on an independent mission, practicing science and protecting the public health. They grew increasingly prominent in that undertaking, as they helped lead the nation's response to a global pandemic and a world war, and that growing prestige drew attention—both wanted and unwanted—from power brokers. Elected officials would occasionally intrude in the world of the Service; indeed, the whims of one politician would cost Blue his job.

RUPERT BLUE

The Shy Younger Brother

Blue was like a character out of a Rudyard Kipling novel: an imposing, mustached amateur boxer who had traveled the world in service of his country, retaining his optimism through a series of sometimes lonely and discouraging assignments. A female reporter for the *San Francisco Bulletin*, profiling Blue in 1908, seemed to nearly swoon in midsentence: "A man of action rather than word—big, broad-shouldered, handsome, commanding in his plain brown officer's uniform. Yet modest and unassuming . . . a quaintly drawn Southern wit and kindly sympathy always lurking in his eyes and under the slim mustache, one to inspire confidence and to make one feel if worse should come to worse, we would have a man at the helm."[4]

Not everyone was as impressed. Certain doctors gradually came to see Blue as a scientific lightweight, a public relations man who might do fine speaking to laymen but lacked the intellectual power to make timely decisions under challenging circumstances. The historical writer John Barry offers a particularly harsh assessment in his book *The Great Influenza*: "Blue became surgeon general simply by carrying out assigned tasks well, proving himself an adept and diplomatic maneuverer, and seizing his main chance. That was all."[5]

Blue was born on May 30, 1867, in Richmond County, North Carolina, a rural area along the border with South Carolina about sixty miles east of Charlotte.[6] His parents soon moved to his mother's hometown, Marion, South Carolina, not far from Myrtle Beach.

Rupert was on the losing end of a sibling rivalry. His father had been a colonel with the Confederate Army, and Rupert's outgoing older brother, Victor, attended the Naval Academy at Annapolis and became a hero for his surveillance of enemy ships during the Spanish-American War. The introverted Rupert became interested in medicine as an apprentice at a pharmacy in a town near his home.[7]

The future surgeon general attended the University of Virginia for two years, and then went on to the University of Maryland for his medical degree, where he was considered a middling but hardworking student. He graduated from Maryland in 1892 and began a nine-month internship with the Marine Hospital Service, working at the hospital in Baltimore. Blue applied for a regular position with the Service as his internship was ending, and was one of four selected out of twenty-five applicants. He was commissioned as an entry-level assistant surgeon in March 1893, in the early days of the Wyman regime.

Blue spent the following nineteen years in typical Service fashion, serving in a series of assignments in various cities. An early stop was Galveston, Texas, where he became smitten with an extroverted, stylish young actress named Juliette Downs. They married in 1895, and she was with him during a series of West Coast assignments, including at the Angel Island quarantine station in San Francisco. It was a nomadic life she was ill-suited for, and their marriage ended in 1902, despite it being an era in which divorce was commonly considered a shocking disgrace.[8]

During those early years, Blue's peers judged his work to be solid but unspectacular. Nevertheless, his reputation soared after his marriage ended, thanks to his involvement in successful assignments fighting yellow fever in New Orleans in 1905, handling sanitation at the international exposition in Jamestown, Virginia, in 1907, and his star turn eliminating plague in San Francisco in 1902–1904 and 1907–1908. Aided by the recent discovery that rat fleas spread the disease, Blue's San Francisco campaign succeeded in disinfecting 11,000 houses, trapping and killing hundreds of thousands of rats, and replacing millions of square feet of boardwalks and home, shop, and stable floors with rat-proof concrete. He cajoled local politicians and citizens to enact the sanitary measures, and at one point threatened to prevent a much anticipated visit from the navy's "Great White Fleet" of sixteen gleaming battleships unless the city could be deemed plague free.

Blue was lucky in that he missed much of the early plague battles in San Francisco—by the time he was in charge, it was settled that plague existed and something had to be done. Still, leading a public health education campaign wasn't easy for him. He remained a shy boy at heart, and had to work at appearing comfortable in front of large audiences and speaking with enough skill and passion to stir people to adopt hygienic measures. (Even at his most rousing, Blue lacked the folksy talent possessed by Colby Rucker, his handsome and lively second-in-command in San Francisco, who became known as "Garbage Can

Rucker" for his funny, popular presentation to women's groups about the proper disposal of trash.)[9] But Blue was no slouch. Like Rucker, he gave half-a-dozen speeches daily and spent nearly as much time winning the cooperation of people as they did killing rats and other plague-spreading vermin. Together, the two gradually convinced more and more people to clean up their properties and support their extermination campaign.

Blue and Rucker went on to other assignments. When Wyman died, Rucker—stationed in Washington, D.C., at the time—immediately lobbied for Blue to be the next surgeon general. Blue was stationed in Hawaii commanding a campaign against the yellow fever mosquito, but with Rucker's help and the legend of the San Francisco success, he swept in from the islands as a popular choice. Blue was a graceful victor, always happy to see any current or former colleague who made it to Washington. He helped create an "era of good feeling" at the Service headquarters on Capitol Hill, as one historian described it, and won friends on Capitol Hill. One of Blue's doctors gushed to a journalist about the high morale in the Service and the "corps spirit," which he described as "the spirit that makes every man on the corps go where he is ordered on a minute's notice and put in 24 hours a day instead of the regulation seven whenever there is the slightest public reason for it."[10]

The new surgeon general was well regarded on Capitol Hill and heartily supported by President Taft. In August 1912, Taft signed legislation that changed the name of Blue's agency—the U.S. Public Health and Marine Hospital Service—to, simply, the U.S. Public Health Service. The law also expanded the agency's focus to all "diseases of man," not just certain infectious illnesses. Woodrow Wilson became president in the November 1912 election, and he too was a friend to Blue (at least at first). In June 1913, Wilson signed an appropriation act that attached money to the name-changing legislation of the previous year. The Service received an additional $200,000 for expanded field work against various diseases. It was big money at the time, equal to more than a tenth of the agency's annual budget, and close to the amount spent to maintain the Service's twenty-three marine hospitals.[11]

At this point, the Service had a total budget of about $1.7 million and a staff of more than 1,000, including pharmacists, engineers, nurses, hospital attendants, quarantine station staff, and about 140 commissioned medical officers. Besides the government-owned marine hospitals, Blue oversaw 50 quarantine stations and 125 medical relief stations. Additional operations included a leprosy research center in Hawaii and a tuberculosis sanatorium in New Mexico.[12]

Service members were also busy policing quacks trying to peddle "cures" for tuberculosis and other diseases, investigating pollution in watershed areas, and checking industry compliance with worker safety laws. They were fighting outbreaks of typhoid fever in Iowa and Virginia, smallpox in Kentucky, dengue fever in Florida, polio in western New York, and the threat of plague coming in from Cuba and Puerto Rico. They were studying and battling trachoma, malaria, hookworm, and a variety of other maladies. And they began to focus on an emerging, mysterious scourge called pellagra.

Pellagra began like sunburn, with the skin turning crimson before peeling to reveal a shiny lower layer. It was especially common around the hands; crusty "pellagra gloves" were a telltale sign. Victims experienced malaise early on, then diarrhea, dementia, and sometimes death. No cases of pellagra had been reported in the United States before 1907, perhaps because the condition was not well recognized. But just eight years later there were an estimated 25,000 to 100,000 cases and the situation seemed to be getting worse.[13]

Blue assigned Joseph Goldberger to help determine the illness's prevalence and discover its cause. In December 1915, Goldberger made the surprising announcement that it wasn't an infectious disease causing the illnesses, but rather a nutritional deficiency.

With this finding, the disease investigation began to dovetail with a social movement. Goldberger worked with Edgar Sydenstricker, a pioneering public health statistician who happened to be the brother of the novelist Pearl S. Buck (the S in her name stood for Sydenstricker). The tall, handsome, and low-key Sydenstricker had been a newspaper editor in Lynchburg, Virginia, before switching to a career in public health, and had a Progressive idealism that served him well in both journalism and his new field. While in the Public Health Service, Sydenstricker reported that southerners had the worst diet in the nation. He attributed the problem to a rapid shift from farming to industrial life, and an industrial depression that began in 1907: the economic conditions left many southerners too poor to buy the beef, chicken, eggs, and milk that they'd had in the past. (Years later, the Service prescribed a balanced diet and supplemental brewer's yeast as preventive measures, and in the 1940s the advent of niacin-enriched flour helped bring an end to pellagra.)[14]

The pellagra research coincided with the Progressive era's focus on the social conditions associated with disease, and two Public Health

Service researchers became prominent in the movement to address poverty and provide health insurance. One was Sydenstricker. The other was Benjamin S. Warren, a Service medical officer who had studied dietary problems among girls in a Washington, D.C., reform school. Drawing from pellagra research and other studies, Sydenstricker and Warren authored a pamphlet arguing for a national system of compulsory health insurance. It basically agreed with a proposal by reformers to create state-based health insurance for lower-income industrial workers; England had recently adopted such a system. A joint meeting of U.S. Public Health Service officials and state and territorial health officers endorsed the principles in May 1916.[15]

Rupert Blue did too.

Blue was a big deal. He was elected president of the American Medical Association in 1915—the only surgeon general to win that position. The worlds of public health and organized medicine more closely overlapped at the time. It was an era when epidemic diseases were still common and private physicians and public health officials were closely allied in dealing with them. What's more, society still expected doctors—who were paid on a fee-for-service basis in those days—to be self-sacrificing heroes who (like public health workers) readily made house calls and cared for poor patients without payment or complaint.[16] The situation would soon change as the AMA became more powerful, more conservative, and more fiercely protective of its members' economic interests. But in 1915, organized medicine still welcomed someone like Blue and his talk of a growing government role in such areas as drug regulation, medical education, and health insurance. In fact, the AMA that year named Blue as the doctor who did the most good for humanity.[17]

At a Detroit meeting of the AMA in June 1916, Blue made a presidential address lamenting the toll of death and illness on workers who did not earn enough to follow a healthy diet or lifestyle. He described compulsory health insurance as impending—and welcome. "There are unmistakable signs that health insurance will constitute the next great step in social legislation," he said, to thunderous applause.[18] The movement toward European-like health reform seemed to be gaining velocity. The AMA's leadership supported it. The American Public Health Association was on board. Reformers were active at the state level, where traditional government health responsibilities resided.

However, fissures were already erupting in the movement's support. Organized labor was far from united on health reform; the labor leader

Samuel Gompers opposed it, believing resources should rather be focused on raising wages. Many private physicians disagreed with the AMA leadership's endorsement of compulsory health insurance, arguing that the proposals could hurt them financially if insurance company payments to doctors were set too low. There was even a rift within the Public Health Service, with some officers less interested in social insurance than in having government doctors and medical facilities care for the poor. Indeed, by 1919, Sydenstricker and Warren—who had written the 1916 pamphlet endorsing compulsory health insurance—were fretting that sickness insurance legislation would absorb public health funds and endanger state health departments. As support fragmented, opposition united. Conservative legislators, businessmen, insurance companies, and many physicians rallied together to fight an effort they termed "Bolshevism."[19]

Blue remained a believer. But his energies were diverted to two events that would undo his promising administration. The first was World War I; the second, the terrible Spanish flu pandemic of 1918 and 1919.

War and Pandemic

World War I began in 1914, but the United States stayed out of the European conflict for years. Blue focused his staff on fighting diseases at home, and used his bully pulpit to push the public toward better health. He helped make "Safety First" a national slogan in 1916, and joined with other federal agencies in creating a traveling locomotive exhibit with nine cars that showcased the government's efforts to improve health and welfare. The Public Health Service car focused on sanitation, displaying models of sanitary toilets and using motion pictures, lantern slides, and other media to teach people how to exterminate rats, mosquitoes, and other dangerous pests. An average of 6,500 people a day streamed through the Service car that summer.[20]

Meanwhile, the United States was tilting toward war. U.S. public opinion strongly turned against Germany in 1915, when a U-boat off the coast of Ireland sank the British ocean liner *Lusitania*. The *Lusitania* had been bound from New York to England, and about 120 of the 1,198 who died were Americans. Political and economic concerns also pushed President Wilson to consider allying with England and France in the war. The last straw came in early 1917. Germany had restricted its submarine warfare after the *Lusitania* incident, but returned to sinking any ship involved in trade with Britain, and in March it sank three

American ships. On April 2, 1917, President Wilson asked Congress for a declaration of war against Germany, and the next day ordered that the Public Health Service become a part of U.S. military forces. On April 4, Congress declared war.

Blue had prepared for war by assembling a plan to oversee sanitation around army and navy training camps and at weapons and war matériel factories. He also proposed to use Service hospitals to provide medical care to soldiers and sailors. But control of the situation quickly began to slip from his hands. Wilson's April 3 order—which may have been unconstitutional—initiated the transfer of more than a dozen key Public Health Service medical officers to the army and navy, and seventeen to war-zone duty with the Coast Guard. Among them was Colby Rucker, Blue's right-hand man.[21]

The war caused Blue other headaches, too. The surgeon general had to contend with an effort by some of his own men to dissolve the Service and merge the staff into the army or navy until the war was over. It was spurred by Service medical officers who had requested assignment with the army, navy, or Coast Guard and been denied. U.S. secretary of war Newton Baker wanted to take Blue's staff and raised the issue with President Wilson, saying Blue was not necessarily opposed to it. Wilson told Baker to get the opinion of Secretary of the Treasury William McAdoo, who oversaw Blue and the Service. McAdoo would have none of it.

McAdoo was a wiry and courageous administrator with a lot of personal and political capital. Much of it accrued in 1914, when he married one of Wilson's daughters and also managed to prevent a financial calamity; he closed the New York Stock Exchange for four months to avert a huge sell-off of American securities by war-panicked European investors. Presented with Baker's gambit, McAdoo told the war secretary he had no interest in giving up the Service, that such a transfer would be illegal, and that the Service should be allowed to increase its sanitation work around military training camps and its public health services for the civilian population.[22]

McAdoo did not discuss Blue's feelings about the matter in the letter. He didn't even mention the surgeon general. This was a battle over the fate of the Public Health Service, but it was fought at the cabinet level, and the surgeon general took care not to antagonize either combatant. It's not surprising that Blue stepped back: he was at heart a shy man who was always much better at genial politics than power struggles. Indeed, despite his love of boxing, Blue was the least pugilistic of the surgeons general up to that point, a man far less willing to throw a political punch than Woodworth, Hamilton, or even Wyman.

The episode demonstrated that even back then, when the surgeon general's powers were ascendant, the position was vulnerable to higher-level machinations. Surgeons general needed cabinet-level officials to protect and enable them. That was certainly true in Blue's case. President Wilson sided with his son-in-law, and in July 1918 issued an executive order making it clear that the Public Health Service was responsible for all civil health activities incident to the war.

Congress, meanwhile, had begun appropriating much more to the Service. It provided $3 million to the Service in 1917, then ballooned the amount to $50 million in 1918. Blue's overall staffing grew from 3,000 to 23,000.[23] But Congress also gave the agency more responsibilities, and none was as daunting as the care of sick and wounded veterans.

In October 1917, Congress passed a law establishing a War Risk Insurance Bureau within the Treasury Department to coordinate the care of disabled soldiers and sailors injured overseas. There were no veterans' hospitals in the United States at the time; they had to be established in a hurry. The War Risk Insurance Bureau contracted with the Public Health Service to use its two dozen marine hospitals to provide the care. In March 1919, shortly after the war ended, Congress put the Service in charge of care for all returning veterans, not just the disabled, and gave it a limited appropriation of $9.5 million to pull off the feat.[24]

Despite the rising budget and a dramatic expansion of the Service's ranks of nurses, dentists, pharmacists, and other health care professionals, Blue was still engaged in an underfunded scramble to find places for more than 200,000 wounded and disabled soldiers and sailors. The Service snatched up military barracks, old military hospitals, and a hodgepodge of other buildings. By 1921, it was operating sixty-two veterans care facilities, with only about a third of them marine hospitals.[25]

Just as the Service was grappling with veterans' care, another problem hit—the deadliest infectious disease epidemic in modern times. The Spanish flu, as it was called, in 1918 and 1919 sickened an estimated 5 million Americans and killed roughly 500,000. Doctors had never seen anything like it.

The worldwide epidemic hit the United States in three waves over the span of only a year.[26] The first wave began in March 1918 and spread unevenly across the country, causing many illnesses but not unusual numbers of deaths. A second, far deadlier wave hit the country in the fall of that year, and then a third in early 1919. In the two latter waves, simple flu infections quickly worsened into fatal pneumonia. But from the beginning to the end of the pandemic, healthy young adults were primary victims. The first and second waves hit while the United States was still at war. The Service was overburdened with war injuries, and Blue and his troops were slow to understand how large and severe the threat was. During the first wave, the Service did little to investigate reports in the late spring of flu death spikes in young people in Kentucky and a few other locations.[27]

If Blue was slow to react, he was hardly alone. More than twenty-five years had elapsed since the last flu pandemic (which was slower moving and far less lethal), and many doctors then saw flu as most people see it today—a recurring problem that may be dangerous to the elderly but for most others is more like an unwanted visitor that causes a few weeks of misery before going away. As the first edges of the deadly second wave began to appear in August, New York City health commissioner Royal Copeland told the press, "There is nothing alarming in the increase."[28] On September 13, Blue warned the public about a wave of a sudden-onset type of flu, along with advice to take aspirin and get bed rest, but he did not detail the illness's severity. The press took its cues from public health leaders like Blue and Copeland. On September 22, the *New York Times* ran a "calm down, everyone" article that said the disease can be "overcome without much difficulty" if properly treated with rest, fresh air, abundant food, and Dover's powder for pain relief.[29]

By the last week of September, it became clear that the second wave was shaping up to be far worse than the first and that this was a different type of flu—one that seemed particularly dangerous to young, healthy adults. On September 26, Massachusetts became the first state to ask the Public Health Service for doctors and nurses to help treat the mounting flu cases, and Blue and other health officials begged Congress for funding. On October 1, Congress voted to spend $1 million for flu response. A new scramble began, as the Service worked with the Red Cross to find and pay doctors and nurses to go to flu-ravaged cities at a time when many medical personnel were tied up in the war effort. Blue put sixty-four of his commissioned officers on flu duty, and his staff helped recruit in excess of a thousand more—not nearly enough, unfortunately, given the widespread suffering in so many cities.[30]

In early October, reports of thousands of flu deaths in a single week came in from Chicago, Philadelphia, and other large cities, and Blue took steps to better manage the crisis. He called on state and local health departments to telegraph the Public Health Service with case counts and deaths, so it could better track how bad the pandemic was getting. He also appointed officials in each state to distribute emergency funding and to direct doctors and nurses to the most needed areas, and established networks of emergency hospitals and soup kitchens.

Just as important, he was a steady and regular source of counsel and information for the nation. Through press interviews, posters, and pamphlets distributed nationally by the Red Cross, Post Office Department, and Federal Railroad Administration, Blue communicated some of the same messages that health officials would use nearly a century later during the swine flu pandemic of 2009: thoroughly wash your hands with soap and water, avoid crowded places, cover your coughs and sneezes, and stay home if you're sick. Six million copies of one informational pamphlet were printed and sent out under Blue's name. "If influenza could have been smothered by paper, many lives would have been saved," observed the historian Alfred Crosby in his 1989 book *America's Forgotten Pandemic*. Blue calmly preached good health practices to the public, but also urged local health authorities to shut down public gathering places. In an era before antiviral medications or effective flu vaccines, it was the best advice that could be offered. Some historians believe Blue's unruffled demeanor in the bully pulpit during the pandemic burnished the Service's reputation with the public.[31]

The last three months of 1918 would see more than 4 million flu illnesses and nearly 400,000 deaths; this wave accounted for roughly four-fifths of the pandemic's entire toll on the United States. But during the worst of the pandemic came a giant shot of psychological relief, when war ended in November 1918. The news prompted parades and widespread celebrations, despite the flu worries. Only a short time later, the second wave was over.

Ultimately, more than half a million Americans died from influenza on Blue's watch, but there was no public blame or ire against the surgeon general's handling of things. Americans, perhaps preoccupied by the Great War, were oddly accepting of the tragedy wrought by the killer virus. In November 1918, a *New York Times* editor wrote that "perhaps the most notable peculiarity of the influenza pandemic is the fact that it has been attended by no traces of panic or even of excitement."[32]

Blue's Final Days

In the nearly fifty years that the Office of the Surgeon General had existed, longevity was a given. Two of Blue's predecessors had died in office, and one left after a dozen years only because of an intemperate resignation. No one had pushed them out. When Blue took office, President Taft limited surgeons general to four-year terms, meaning they had to be reappointed to stay in office.

Blue, in good standing in 1916, had been reappointed to a second term with little fuss. But by the time he came up for a third term, things had changed. For two years he had been battered by simultaneously dealing with a world war and a historic pandemic. The overburdened Service's failings had become evident, and while there was little grumbling about the Service's handling of the flu, veterans' groups and others increasingly complained about the Service's hasty patchwork of medical care facilities for the war's wounded.

Still, Blue retained his characteristic optimism, and in March 1919 wrote an eleven-page memorandum outlining his ambitions for his next term. He envisioned the Service growing into a Cabinet-level national health agency, with Blue at its helm. He was already involved in discussions to create an international public health organization after the war, and saw himself as the U.S. representative to whatever group that would be formed. He also proposed more widespread milk pasteurization, limits on water pollution, establishment of clinics for sick children, and a renewed discussion about national health insurance.[33]

But political forces were aligning against him. Treasury Secretary McAdoo—Blue's protector—resigned three days after the war ended, saying he was fatigued. To replace McAdoo, President Wilson named U.S. Representative Carter Glass of Virginia, a son of the Confederacy who had supported a poll tax and other measures to disenfranchise black voters. Blue meant nothing to Glass, who wanted a new surgeon general, preferably a Virginian.

High on the new treasury secretary's list was Hugh Cumming, a twenty-five-year Service veteran who was part of the gang who had pushed to dissolve the Service into the military during the war. In 1919, while Blue was in Washington planning his third term, Cumming was in Europe making political connections. He toured historic medical centers in France with William Henry Welch and spent time with his old friend Cary T. Grayson, who was the personal physician to President Wilson (yet another Virginian).[34]

Wilson grew ill in September and a suffered a stroke in October, and for many months his wife and Grayson closely attended him, hid his condition from the public, and helped make executive decisions. In late 1919, Glass said he wanted Cumming to be appointed the next surgeon general, and there was no objection from the invalid president or Grayson.

Blue was bitter, but like Hamilton decided to remain in the Service, demoted. He was put in charge of Service operations in Europe, and in 1924 was put in charge of a campaign against plague in Los Angeles. He retired from active duty in 1932. In early April 1948 he grew seriously ill and was admitted to a hospital in Charleston, South Carolina. He died ten days later, at age eighty. Blue was buried in a graveyard in Marion, the town where he was raised, under a granite headstone decorated with the Public Health Service emblem.[35]

HUGH SMITH CUMMING
Proper Breeding

Hugh Cumming certainly looked the part of the nation's doctor. While Rupert Blue resembled a brawny heavyweight boxer, Cumming was like the captain of an Ivy League rowing team—tall and lean, with a sloping nose and spectacles. He had a distinguished air and courtly manner and was frequently described as a well-respected master of diplomacy.

In 1928, a *Time* magazine reporter wrote: "Most Congressman know Dr. Cumming personally. Few men are better known in Washington. When a telephone rings and his soft voice asks something for his Public Health Service, he gets that something very quickly."[36] Bess Furman, veteran Washington correspondent for the *New York Times,* wrote in her memoir that she found him "a courteous and charming Virginia gentleman whom I liked tremendously."[37] On March 10, 1920, when he took the oath of office as surgeon general, Cumming was fifty and had spent half his life in the Public Health Service. He was a year younger than Blue, the man he replaced, but had much better and more current political connections, owing in part to his Virginia roots.

He was born August 17, 1869, in Hampton, Virginia, a historic town on the Chesapeake Bay founded just a few years after the first permanent English settlement at Jamestown. Cumming's father was a previously married Scotsman named Samuel Cumming who at one point operated a saw mill and coal business. Cumming would have a lifelong interest in his father's lineage, fascinated by family fables of ancestral estates.

His mother Diana, a Virginian, was the daughter of a Confederate artillery captain and the widow of a soldier before she married Samuel

Cumming. She also was an invalid as long as her son could remember, usually served meals in her room. Hugh was devoted to her and grew interested in medicine when he accompanied his mother to Johns Hopkins Hospital in Baltimore and met the doctors there. Some maternal nudging helped. Cumming's mother, "one of the most intelligent women I have ever known, had always wanted me to be a doctor," he wrote in his unpublished memoir.[38]

He was placed on an education track that enabled him to pursue that dream. His parents sent him to finish grammar school in Baltimore, where he stayed with a relative who was a school principal. Cumming later went to Baltimore City College for two years, then attended the University of Virginia for his medical training.

The University of Virginia had a huge influence on Cumming. Founded by Thomas Jefferson in the city of Charlottesville, the university had long held a prominent place among the nation's most respected public institutions of higher education (one of the "public ivies," as it has been called). It had one of the country's oldest medical schools, with a historic roster of noted medical faculty that included James Lawrence Cabell, the early president of the National Board of Health. Cumming, throughout his career, was helped immeasurably by his Virginia training and connections.

But the university also bestowed on him something more unfortunate—a core belief in eugenics. Eugenics was a pseudo-science that borrowed from the agricultural model of breeding animals, encouraging reproduction of the strongest of the species and preventing reproduction of the weakest. It was popular in medical, scientific, and political circles in the early twentieth century—Teddy Roosevelt and Woodrow Wilson thought there was something to it, as did Rupert Blue. The eugenics culture resulted in increased immigration restrictions, laws prohibiting interracial marriage, and statutes allowing sterilization of people deemed feebleminded.[39]

Virginia was a center for the American eugenics movement from the late nineteenth to the mid-twentieth century, and U.Va. faculty provided the movement's intellectual heft. Cabell played a key role. He had owned slaves and believed in the principles of eugenics. He was a mentor to Paul Brandon Barringer, a leading eugenicist and popular professor. The eugenics perspective was built into the University of Virginia's medical school curriculum from 1900 to 1950, and was seen as scientific and consistent with the tenets of public health. Individual rights were seen as secondary to the good of society, and separating blacks and the feebleminded from healthy whites was equated to quarantining the sick from the healthy. Cumming graduated before eugenics was formally taught at the university, but not before Barringer and others had begun to share their views with students. Cumming acknowledged he was heavily influenced by Barringer, and once called him "one of the most brilliant intellects I know."[40]

Cumming was not the only one in the Service to absorb these views. Virginians made up 16 percent of the commissioned corps by 1923, and many were University of Virginia alums. Among them were leaders of the Service's venereal disease programs, and some historians see their embrace of eugenics as an explanation for the Tuskegee Syphilis Experiment, one of the most reprehensible scientific studies in U.S. history (more on that later).

Young Dr. Cumming joined the Marine Hospital Service in 1894, commissioned as an assistant surgeon when Walter Wyman was boss. He started at the marine hospital on Staten Island, working for Preston Bailhache, an old lion of the Service who had been Woodworth's spy on the old National Board of Health. While there, Cumming played tennis with Bailhache every afternoon.[41]

During an assignment to Norfolk in 1896, Cumming married Lucy Booth of Carter's Grove, Virginia, a community in the same corner of the state as Hampton. He'd met her shortly before Christmas, 1893. Her wedding picture shows a wasp-waisted, dark-haired, confident-looking woman posed on a thronelike chair. She was his equal in social acumen and would become a great asset to him in Washington circles later on.[42]

Cumming was transferred repeatedly, just like virtually everyone else in Wyman's Service. He was assigned to quarantine stations at Blackbeard Island, Georgia, and then Angel Island at San Francisco in the early 1900s. He went on to spend four years at a Service posting in Yokohama, Japan. In 1912, he was put in charge of a study of water pollution in the Potomac River. During all these assignments, he was exposed to a variety of illnesses, including diphtheria and yellow fever. But Cumming rarely got sick and gradually formed the opinion that he was largely immune to infectious diseases.[43]

During World War I, Cumming was among the Service officers assigned to branches of the military. He became a sanitation advisor to the navy, an assignment that sent him to Europe, where he was responsible for preventing the spread of typhus and other diseases to America through returning troops. He was in Versailles the day the peace treaty was signed, and stayed in Europe after the war, representing the Service in work with the League of Nations and other international organizations on postwar public health missions. As he worked on the continent, he took time to sail the Mediterranean and meet some of the most prominent people in Europe, including the pope.[44]

He had built powerful connections, but was still surprised to learn that Blue was not being reappointed and he was getting the nod instead. Cumming was in Rome when he learned from his wife that a London newspaper had reported he had been nominated surgeon general. "The hell I have!" Cumming replied.[45]

Scandals and Straightjackets

Hugh Cumming came into office with a full plate. Pellagra cases were mounting. Plague resurfaced in June 1920, with cases seen at U.S. ports on the Gulf of Mexico. Yellow fever seemed poised to invade from Mexico and Guatemala. And, of course, there were the ongoing complaints about the care of war veterans.

The Service's veterans hospitals included some hastily opened facilities in terrible old buildings that Cumming himself referred to as "flimsy and inflammable." The Service was operating about 20,000 beds by the end of 1920 (up from 2,000 in October 1919), but more than half were in structures deemed unsafe. Congress's failure to provide necessary funding was the real issue, but the Service caught most of the heat. One hospital, in an old army structure in Chicago, was such a maligned problem that Blue came to believe it cost him the job as surgeon general.[46]

In March 1921, Woodrow Wilson was succeeded by a Republican, Warren G. Harding. There was talk that Harding would replace Cumming (a Democrat) with a Republican physician, but such a move never materialized. It may have helped that Harding's sister—Mrs. Heber Votaw—was part of Cumming's staff, working on a study about absenteeism of young women in the public services.[47]

Cumming developed a good relationship with Harding and his treasury secretary, Andrew Mellon, but the patchwork care of veterans was clearly a problem. The new president decided to turn the issue over to Charles R. Forbes, a redheaded go-getter whom Harding had met during a vacation to Honolulu. Supremely unqualified, Forbes was a vice president of a Seattle engineering firm who had awarded himself the title of colonel. But in April 1921, Harding appointed him head of the War Risk Insurance Bureau. Forbes quickly began working with unhappy veterans' organizations to press for independence from Treasury Department oversight. The next year, Forbes took over from the Service the operation of the fifty-seven veterans' hospitals and their 17,000 beds. The Service was left with twenty-four marine hospitals with 3,000 beds.[48]

Forbes turned out to be a crook. He embezzled $250 million from the government through corrupt construction deals and through selling supplies from a warehouse jointly operated by the Public Health Service and the War Risk Insurance Bureau. Cumming learned from one of his men that Forbes was selling off large amounts of supplies from the warehouse, and drove down to the warehouse with White House physician Charles Sawyer to investigate. Finding supplies loaded onto an unauthorized train, they gathered some samples and took them to the president. But Harding, wary of scandal, declined to prosecute the scoundrel and instead told Forbes to resign and leave the country. Forbes did. However, after Harding unexpectedly died in office in August 1923, other federal officials caught and prosecuted Forbes. He was sentenced to two years in prison and fined $100,000 on charges of conspiracy to defraud the government.[49]

Cumming was untouched by the scandal and enjoyed a soaring reputation during what was a golden era for public health. Service officers were often portrayed as heroes in magazines and popular books. The writer Paul de Kruif generated a series of hot-selling volumes that chronicled the work of medical investigators, including *Men Against Death*, which featured chapters on the disease-sleuthing efforts of Hygienic Laboratory scientists and federal and state epidemiologists.[50] And for weeks in 1925, newspapers were filled with breathless accounts of a Service-initiated effort to use husky sled dogs to get life-saving medicine to diphtheria-ravaged Nome, Alaska—an effort led by a dog named Balto, and retold since in several books and a 1995 Universal Pictures cartoon movie.

To be sure, the surgeon general had his struggles. He worried about Harding's successor, Calvin Coolidge, who nixed budget requests and caused Cumming to worry about his prospects for reappointment. Cumming also fought off a bill to create a federal Department of Welfare that Cumming believed would have absorbed and obliterated the Public Health Service.[51]

But he managed to thrive, as the distinguished leader of the heroic Service, with a trusting Congress that gave him more and more responsibilities. Cumming expanded the Commissioned Corps to admit dentists, pharmacists, and sanitary engineers. He also established a Rocky Mounted Spotted Fever Laboratory in Montana, a Special Cancer Investigations Laboratory at Harvard University in Boston, and a National Leprosarium in Louisiana. He completed the turnover of state quarantine stations to the federal system. His doctors helped in the abolition of the common drinking cup at public water fountains. And he was quick to grasp the contagion-spreading potential of airplane travel, proposing health inspections of flight crews and passengers.[52]

Cumming also was the first surgeon general to warn about the dangers of cigarette smoking. Smoking rates had begun to skyrocket during World War I, when cigarettes were passed out as part of soldiers' rations and men began to prefer them over previously more socially acceptable forms of tobacco consumption, like pipe and cigar smoking. In 1929, Cumming sounded an alarm, proclaiming that smoking could lower the "physical tone" of the nation. "This is one of the most evil influences in American life today," Cumming said.[53] It was a remarkably bold statement for the nation's doctor to make, considering that the hallmark studies demonstrating a causal link between cigarette smoking and lung cancer would not be conducted for two more decades. But it was social propriety, not science, driving the surgeon general's concern. Smoking was becoming a fad among young women in the late 1920s, as Prohibition Era flappers wore higher skirts and enjoyed more social freedom. The surgeon general was a smoker himself. "The habit harms a woman more than it does a man," Cumming said, without a scrap of evidence to substantiate that claim.[54]

However, Cumming's words helped set an important precedent. The surgeon general was cited by several legislators making small, early attempts to restrict the sale and advertising of tobacco. It foreshadowed many hundreds of federal and state legislative hearings on tobacco dangers in the late-twentieth and early-twenty-first centuries, in which do-gooder legislators used the statements and reports of surgeons general to bolster tobacco-control proposals.

Given Cumming's prestige and willingness to take on new public health issues, it made perfect sense that he would take charge of another new health controversy that emerged in the 1920s—the debate over leaded gasoline.

Some background: A recurring problem with automobiles in the early twentieth century was a "knock" or sharp pinging sound from the engines, due to premature combustion of the mixture of gasoline and air in the tank. Chemists and engineers worked for years on the knock to make gasoline combustion more efficient, trying additives that ranged from alcohol to iodine to melted butter. In 1921, a young engineer with the General Motors Corporation discovered that tetraethyl lead—a colorless, sweet-smelling liquid—silenced the knock. It also seemed well suited to the kind of more powerful, long-distance machines that auto-makers were trying to produce. In 1923, GM and the chemical firm E. I. du Pont de Nemours & Company teamed up to manufacture the new gasoline. The next year, Standard Oil began producing it.

But tetraethyl lead was not benign. It was an extremely poisonous organic compound easily absorbed through the skin and harmful to the nervous system. The War Department had considered it for chemical warfare, but dropped the idea when mustard gas proved more efficient in combat conditions. Some public health leaders had misgivings about the idea of adding it to automobile exhaust gases, and Cumming wrote company leader Pierre du Pont in December 1922 raising concerns. The executive assured Cumming there would be little risk to the public health.[55] Aware that questions would persist, General Motors embarked on an unusual arrangement in which it funded the U.S. Bureau of Mines—the federal agency with the most experience with lead—to look at the issue. In the fall of 1924, the agency concluded there was no danger of lead poisoning from even prolonged exposure to exhaust from auto engines burning leaded gasoline.[56]

Meanwhile, events were unfolding that cast doubt on such a conclusion. In October 1924, in the days leading up to Halloween, five employees at Standard Oil's Bayway plant in New Jersey grew violently insane and quickly died. Their stories were like something out of a macabre novel: The first victim was a worker named Ernest Oelgert, who on a Thursday told his co-workers that someone was following him, then the next day screamed that three were coming at him. Oelgert ran from the factory and was caught and taken to a hospital, where he died in convulsions that Saturday. Four others died at the same plant within the next week, one of them taken off the job in a straightjacket. Autopsies found lead poisoning in their lungs and brains, and officials tied it to leaded gasoline. The press was all over the story. Reporters called the product "loony gas"—workers at a DuPont chemical plant in Deepwater, New Jersey, referred to their workplace as the "House of Butterflies" because of hallucinations about insects experienced by lead-poisoned workers there. Newspapers also reported that deaths associated with tetraethyl lead had occurred at a GM plant in Ohio and a DuPont facility in Delaware.[57]

The deaths led manufacturers to suspend sales of leaded gasoline, and Cumming was publicly pressured to set up a scientific committee to look into the matter. His immediate supervisor—an assistant treasury secretary named Moss—approved the investigation. But Cumming was acutely sensitive to both the politics and economics of the situation. He declined to convene anything until he first discussed it with Treasury Secretary Andrew Mellon. The auto and petrochemical industries had already become anchors of the U.S. economy, and Cumming knew that Mellon's family had significant financial interests in the oil industry especially. (Mellon, to his credit, recused himself and told Cumming to use his own judgment.)[58]

Cumming held a conference on tetraethyl lead in May 1925. It was a landmark event, the first time the Public Health Service really took on a national-level environmental danger. Manufacturers at the conference said the product was essential to the growth of their industry and the nation, and that they had already found a way to make the product safely. Cumming appointed a committee of seven scientists to investigate the arguments for and against leaded gasoline and gave them seven months. The panel studied 252 gasoline station attendants and chauffeurs in Ohio. The scientists found that lead absorption was common, and believed that it could induce lead poisoning or other problems. However, they did not find clear evidence of acute lead poisoning in the Ohio test subjects. (The panel called for more research that was never done.) The New York Times summarized the conclusions with the headline "Report: No Danger in Ethyl Gasoline."[59]

In 1926, Cumming issued new rules for the manufacturing and handling of leaded gasoline, but he argued against any bans on its general use, saying there was no good evidence for such measures. For the next several decades, the Public Health Service and the rest of the federal government left it at that.

The logic of Cumming's decision may seem defensible, based on the information in front of him. At that time, researchers hadn't developed the kind of epidemiological studies needed to show the harms leaded gasoline could cause the general public. Indeed, some of the most influential studies definitively showing lead's impact on children's intellectual development would not occur for another fifty years. Nevertheless, there was enough known about tetraethyl lead to cause some medical and chemistry experts to shudder. Among them was Yandell Henderson, a Yale physiologist, who predicted that hundreds of thousands of pounds of lead would be deposited on the streets of U.S. cities each year and would slowly and insidiously poison the public.[60] He and others said that as a matter of scientific common sense, leaded gasoline posed a danger and must not be permitted. But Cumming saw such a step as advocacy-like overstep by a government official, and rationalized his stance with the (flawed and limited) studies at hand.

Leaded gas would remain in common use in the United States until the 1970s, when federal officials—increasingly worried about the cumulative impact of lead from auto exhaust—launched a phaseout of leaded gas that was not declared completed until 1996. The phaseout contributed to a 30 percent drop in the level of lead in Americans' blood over five years.[61] To be sure, the phaseout of lead-based paint and other measures also had a huge impact, but some researchers argue that the phaseout of leaded gasoline was a key factor for that improvement and for the modest rise in the average IQ scores for school-age children that followed.[62] "Obviously, years later, we can say the decisions he [Cumming] made in the 1920s ended up costing the United States," said Tom Hatfield, a California State University, Northridge, researcher who has looked into the harms of leaded gasoline.[63]

The Tuskegee Experiment

An even more lamentable legacy of Cumming's decision making is the Tuskegee Syphilis Experiment.

Syphilis is a sexually transmitted infection caused by a corkscrewlike bacteria. It can, over many years, destroy the brain and other internal organs and kill the patient. The disease and its genital sores have always come with social baggage, but in Cumming's era it was especially associated with immigrants, philanderers, and others seen as immoral, mentally deficient, and low-class. African Americans were prominent in that grouping: many doctors in the South thought of blacks as a "notoriously syphilis-soaked race" and susceptible to other venereal diseases.[64] These perceptions fit snugly with the eugenicists' ethos. True, there were "innocent" victims of syphilis, such as soldiers from upstanding families who were infected by prostitutes during war. But prominent eugenicists felt the majority of people who got the infection—like promiscuous blacks—were committing a form of racial suicide that was perhaps a necessary step forward for the rest of the species.[65]

Cumming was not willing to go that far. In his memoirs, he maintained that he "had always been deeply interested in improving the health of the Negroes."[66] But from early in his administration, his actions suggested that in his view, disease-stricken blacks were as much a curiosity as a cause for empathy. In 1923, when a black leper was on trial for murder in Louisiana, Cumming volunteered to provide a glass cage for the suspect to sit in during the trial.[67] And of course there was the Tuskegee Study.

In 1929, the Julius Rosenwald Fund funded the Service to study the prevalence of syphilis among rural blacks in the South and look into potential mass treatments. The study focused on six counties and found particularly high rates in Macon County, Alabama, home of the town of Tuskegee. A shocking 40 percent of the Macon County men who took part in the study had syphilis. The study concluded that, given the proper funding and resources, it was possible to administer mass treatments to the syphilitic men in Alabama. A drug called arsphenamine (also known as Salvarsan), which became available in 1910, was shown by European researchers to be successful against the disease. Mercury and arsenic compounds, less effective and more toxic, were also available. The report was authored by Taliaferro Clark of the Service's Venereal Disease Division—another U.Va. man and disciple of Professor Barringer.

But the U.S. economy collapsed in 1929, government funding became tight, and the Service made no attempt to begin the kind of mass treatments called for by the Rosenwald Fund. Still, Clark was fascinated by the hotbed of syphilis he'd found in Macon County. He saw it as an opportunity to study how latent disease progressed in untreated individuals, information some scientists believed could provide a useful comparison to study populations that were treated. Clark sought cooperation from Alabama health officials and from leaders at the Tuskegee Institute, which operated a Macon County hospital that cared for blacks. The institute was a private, historically black college founded by former slaves and initially led by Booker T. Washington, and its leaders were keenly aware of the devastating impact syphilis had on their community. Washington himself was rumored to have had it.[68]

The surgeon general not only approved the project but helped Clark win cooperation from the locals. Cumming wrote the Tuskegee Institute's principal, Robert Russa Moton, on September 20, 1932. He solicited Moton's support and framed the study as one that would focus on treatment. In the letter, Cumming noted the Rosenwald Fund study not only found an astonishingly high rate of syphilis in Macon County but also revealed that 99 percent of the syphilitic study participants there had not previously been treated. "This combination, together with the expected cooperation of your hospital, offers an unparalleled opportunity for carrying on this scientific research which probably cannot be duplicated anywhere else in the world."[69] The letter, coming from the nation's top health official and hinting at increased federal health resources and future treatments, was persuasive.

The study began that year and would run for forty years. Consistent with Clark's design, the four hundred syphilitic sharecroppers enlisted in the study were denied effective treatment—deprived of the Salvarsan available before the study started and, later, the penicillin that became available in the 1940s.

In 1933, the Service misled the men who participated by offering a "last chance" at a "special free treatment" if they came in for a hospital examination, but instead gave them painful and dangerous diagnostic lumbar punctures ("spinal taps"). At other points in the study, the cost-conscious Service shipped medicines to Tuskegee, but most of it was pink aspirins along with some small, inadequate amounts of mercury and arsenic compounds. Men in the study received some medicine, but not in any systematic manner. Those who were treated got whatever was available. What's more, the Service never sent public health doctors to Macon County, except for occasional visits to do blood draws and physical examinations.

Cumming not only blessed the Tuskegee Syphilis Experiment but actively supported it, right to the end of his administration, with no apparent qualms. In 1935, he successfully lobbied for Milbank Memorial Fund money to enable the Service to offer $50 to the family of each study participant that consented to an autopsy—a powerful enticement to poor people hard-pressed to provide a loved one with a decent funeral. Around the same time, the surgeon general authored a study that used Tuskegee data to discuss serological tests for syphilis.[70]

The Tuskegee Experiment, once fully revealed to the public in 1972, engendered a deep mistrust of government physicians by the black community that continues to this day.

Cumming's Departure

The surgeon general's power was greatest during the Coolidge and Hoover presidencies in the late 1920s and early 1930s. He was well known to the public for his annual reports to Congress on the health of the nation, and newspaper and magazine articles featured Cumming's guidance on public health matters. And he and his wife had close relationships with an array of leading politicians. Cumming's daughter Diana in 1929 married Manville Kendrick, the son of a former U.S. senator from Wyoming. (First Lady Grace Anna Goodhue Coolidge attended even though the wedding fell on her birthday.) Cumming's wife was a good friend of Lou Henry Hoover, wife of the commerce secretary who became president in 1929. Lucy and Mrs. Hoover had a dramatic bonding moment on a cold March evening in 1928 when their chauffeur-driven auto skidded on an icy Virginia road and came to a stop on the edge of a bridge, perilously hanging thirty feet over the Shenandoah River.[71] "Surgeon General Cumming knows virtually every one in Washington and has friends throughout the United States and abroad. When a problem arises that requires for its solution the cooperation of someone outside of the service, he can often count that person as a personal friend," a *New York Times* reporter wrote in 1928.[72]

But Cumming gradually found himself on the outs, thanks to his conservative stance on the question of health reform and to a 1932 election that brought a more liberal set of power brokers to Washington.

The surgeon general viewed himself as a close ally of organized medicine and frequently worked with AMA leaders. In a March 1927 speech to doctors that was published in the *Journal of the American Medical Association* (*JAMA*), he groused about organizations pushing for "the socialization of medicine" and called on private physicians to help head off such efforts by solving problems like insufficient numbers of doctors and facilities for middle-class patients. Cumming also joined with the AMA in fighting congressional appropriations to the Children's Bureau, which provided grants to states for maternal and child care. Cumming's position was that any funds be the responsibility of public health professionals, not social workers. The AMA's position was that the medical care grants posed a threat to the future livelihood of physicians. Together, in 1929 they ensured the expiration of the Sheppard-Towner Act, the 1921 legislation that had provided for the Children's Bureau's grant program.[73]

Cumming even campaigned—twice—to become president of the AMA, losing the second time, in 1934, by only fourteen votes. Some believed Cumming's AMA ambitions prompted some bad administrative decisions, including the 1930 transfer of Service officer Leslie Lumsden from a national rural sanitation improvement project. The brilliant, tough-minded Lumsden wanted a stronger federal role in public health, a goal the AMA opposed. Lumsden told friends he believed he was reassigned because of Cumming's AMA aspirations.[74]

But circumstances at work began to change for Cumming in 1932, when Franklin Delano Roosevelt was elected president. FDR appointed Josephine Roche as assistant secretary of the treasury in charge of public health in October 1934. That made her Cumming's boss, and she did not share his worldview.

The modest-mannered Roche had a fiery belief in liberal causes. She had been a crusader for the United Mine Workers earlier in her career, and was a strong believer in the idea of compulsory health insurance and in government moving further into the world of clinical medicine. Roche was involved in the debates about whether to include national health insurance as part of the Social Security Act of 1935. Roosevelt left it out, concerned that its inclusion would provoke AMA opposition, but Roche subsequently went to work on Social Security Act amendments that took the form of the Wagner-Murray-Dingell bill for compulsory health insurance.[75] She was well aware of Cumming's opposition to national health coverage and considered him a hindering presence in an important job.

As soon as Roche was appointed, rumors began swirling that she would push Cumming out and that the president would replace him with Thomas Parran. While governor of New York, Roosevelt had made Parran the state's health officer, and the two had a good relationship. The rumors were consistently denied, but wore on Cumming. In 1935, he also began to deteriorate physically, suffering a painful bout of sciatica, cystitis, and a debilitating cold. After he spent two weeks in a hospital, his doctors told him to restrict his frequent traveling and even to find a gentler place to winter than Washington, D.C. Cumming, now sixty-six years old and close to the end of his fourth term, decided to call it quits.[76]

Roosevelt praised Cumming to the newspapers: "I am happy to recall that your labors in protecting humanity against disease and in advancing health standards everywhere have brought you deserved recognition and honor not only in your own country but throughout the world," Roosevelt said in a statement to Cumming that was released to the press.[77] Cumming was allowed to remain director of the Pan American Sanitary Bureau, an organization of about twenty Western Hemisphere nations. He'd led the organization for years, bringing nations together to fight and prevent disease. That work made him something of a global public health celebrity, and he cherished it. But Cumming was quietly bitter about his successor, and in a 1939 letter to his son called Parran "a menace" and warned that "the main danger now is Parran himself and his half-baked socialistic schemes."[78]

Cumming had a stroke in November 1947 and spent the last year of his life in poor health. He died at his home in Washington, D.C., on December 20, 1948, of a heart attack. He was seventy-nine.[79]

The tall, mannered Cumming was a poster-boy surgeon general who was at the Public Health Service's helm at a time when the agency enjoyed some of its greatest prestige and talent. He was a capable and well-connected administrator who helped the agency grow and gain international acclaim. But he also set an unfortunate precedent. Public health is by its origin and proper nature a field for progressives—people intent on making government-led changes to reduce health risks and improve the general welfare. Cumming—professing to be a disinterested scientist—was at heart a conservative shaped by a daughter of the Confederacy (his mother) and by a proponent of eugenics (University of Virginia professor Paul Barringer). Unfailingly pleasant to those in power, Cumming had a cold heart in matters concerning black people and others he considered undeserving. Other surgeons general would later use his "scientist first" rationale to shirk an advocacy role, to the detriment of the job and the nation.

CHAPTER 4

The Best Seller

Thomas Parran grew up shy, with a tendency to stutter that he had to suppress, and as an adult was an unimposing five feet, eight inches and 150 pounds. But he was a giant in the surgeon general's bully pulpit, and raised the job to a level of national and international influence never seen before.

Parran bullied prudish journalists to carry frank discussions about venereal disease, and spoke forcefully about mental illness in an age when psychiatric disorders were still kept in the closet. He used newspapers, magazines, radio, and even motion pictures to push messages about a range of topics, some of them quite sensitive. His handsome, mustached visage was on the cover of *Time* magazine and he penned a best-selling book within two years of taking office. He also established a reputation as a bogeyman to organized medicine.[1] Except for C. Everett Koop in the 1980s, no other surgeon general had as large a persona in popular culture or was so willing to take on controversial topics.

Admirers singled out his campaign against venereal disease, confessing in letters that they were thrilled by his courageous pulpiteering. "I have wanted to tell you in person what I think of you and your magnificently courageous frontal attack on syphilis," wrote Roy Flannagan, Virginia's assistant state health commissioner, in one of many fan letters to Parran from within the public health community. "I extravagantly admire your boldness in facing the scandalously neglected public health problem of syphilis and forcing it into the open."[2] From another letter: "I have been impressed by other radio speeches, but this is the first time I feel impelled to play the role of radio 'fan.' I don't see how your educational work could be done any better," wrote Joseph V. DePorte, director of vital statistics at the New York State Department of Health.[3] From one more: "I have long been deeply impressed by your splendid leadership in the campaign to combat venereal diseases. I think it is one of the most humanitarian campaigns I have ever known and I would like for you to feel that in my limited way you will have all of the support and encouragement I can give you," wrote U.S. Representative Louis Ludlow of Indiana, an important member of the House Appropriations Committee.[4]

Ludlow's words would later carry unintended irony, however. Parran's "humanitarian campaign" was really a crusade and, like other crusades, had a terrible ends-justify-the-means underside to it. Parran condoned the arrest of women deemed promiscuous spreaders of venereal disease. And he sanctioned some of the most notoriously unethical federal medical experiments in the nation's history, including not only the expansion of the Tuskegee Experiment but the initiation of an even more repugnant set of studies in Guatemala.

THE RABBIT'S FOOT

Parran's convictions came, in part, from a family history of medical duty and government service. He was named for a great-great-grandfather who was a surgeon in the Revolutionary War. Two of his uncles were physicians. His father was a gentleman farmer and politician, who served briefly in the U.S. House of Representatives and for longer terms in the Maryland legislature. But everyone in the family assumed young Thomas would grow up to be a doctor, per the family tradition.[5]

Thomas J. Parran Jr. was born September 28, 1892, and grew up in rural Maryland near the town of St. Leonard's, on an isolated farm his family had owned since 1655. He was essentially schooled by an aunt, but was taught well. He won a scholarship to attend the St. John's College, a military school in Annapolis that included drilling and uniforms as well as rigorous teaching of the liberal arts. After four years there, he went to Georgetown University, where he earned his medical degree in 1915.[6]

During medical school, Parran spent two summers working at a local public health laboratory operated by the District of Columbia. There, he worked under Joseph Kinyoun, the legendary—and now elderly—founder of the Hygienic Laboratory (renamed the National Institute of

Health in 1930). Kinyoun took a shine to young Parran and presented him with a lucky rabbit's foot wrapped in tissue paper just before Parran took the Public Health Service entrance examination. Decades earlier, Kinyoun had carried the good luck charm when he took the examination, and had passed with flying colors. Parran used the rabbit's foot to similar success, scoring the highest in his group. "But Dr. Kinyoun wouldn't give me the rabbit's foot. I had to give it back to him," Parran later recalled.[7]

Parran really wanted to be a lab researcher, like his mentor. But Kinyoun suggested work under Leslie Lumsden, an old friend of Kinyoun's who at the time was leading the Service's campaign in the South to improve sanitary conditions. In March 1917, Parran reported to his first assignment in Okmulgee, Oklahoma. Then came stops in Chattanooga, Tennessee, and Muscle Shoals, Alabama. He worked not only on sewage improvement and sanitation but also outbreaks of malaria, smallpox, venereal disease, and influenza. He was chief medical officer for the Service operation at Muscle Shoals during the worst of the Spanish flu outbreak, and helped manage the care of thousands, including hundreds who died. His time as a "privy builder"—as the job was known within the Service—gave him a good feel for the value of county health departments. It also practiced him in speaking to the public at churches and other places about the importance of sanitation. "It was in effect an educational job," he later recalled.[8]

Next came a series of assignments in Washington, D.C. In September 1926, he was appointed chief of the Service's Division of Venereal Diseases, a job he would hold for four years. The division was established in 1918, when Surgeon General Rupert Blue was calling venereal disease "a national menace" and Congress worried about a tide of sexually transmitted infections as a result of wartime craziness. Funds were appropriated for Public Health Service public education campaigns, for work by state health departments, and for detention homes for women deemed to be spreading the diseases to doughboys and other men.[9]

But congressional interest in funding venereal disease programs waned after the war ended. Hugh Cumming did little to help, opposing campaigns on using condoms to stop the spread of such infections, believing the people who most needed to use prophylaxis—including black people—were too irresponsible to use it. The division's annual spending plummeted from $4 million in 1920 to less than $60,000 in 1926—the year Parran took over. "It was dying on its feet from lack of appropriations," Parran later recalled.[10]

(The new job was not his only challenge. Shortly after his appointment to the division, Parran's wife, Angela, died; they had married in 1918. Her passing left him grief-stricken and faced with the challenge of raising four young sons.[11])

In the new job, Parran pushed for funding research on syphilis treatments. He focused on working with—and strengthening—local health departments. And he formed strong opinions about how venereal disease should be attacked, views influenced by a trip to Scandinavia in 1926, where sexually transmitted diseases were openly discussed in the same way as other illnesses. "My approach to the problem was a pragmatic one," he later said, "being less concerned about [trying to change] the moral behavior of individuals than about finding cases and contacts and bringing cases under treatment."[12]

Parran left the division by the time the Tuskegee Study had started, but he was involved in some of the activities that led up to the project. Parran's staff surveyed Mississippi plantation workers to understand the prevalence of syphilis in parts of the South and worked on a project there to treat poor black laborers with neoarsphenamine and mercury. After Parran left the division in 1930, he was succeeded by Taliaferro Clark, the man who would ignite the forty-year experiment in Tuskegee.[13]

A RADIO SMACKDOWN

The year 1930 contained several turning points for Parran. In his personal life, he married a woman he had worked with, a writer named Buda Carroll Keller. At about the same time, he accepted an offer—from New York's jovial governor, Franklin Delano Roosevelt—to run the state's Department of Health.[14]

Roosevelt did not know Parran personally; he selected Parran on several recommendations. An important voice was Edgar Sydenstricker, the pioneering statistician and health reform advocate, who had left the Service and taken a job at the Milbank Memorial Fund. Sydenstricker had raved about Parran to the Milbank Fund's director, John Kingsbury, a good friend of Roosevelt's. Parran hesitated, telling Roosevelt he did not want to leave the Service. He agreed to take the New York job only if he could do it through a leave of absence from the federal agency. The arrangement was worked out, and Parran started in New York in April 1930.[15]

He jumped into the pressing task of reorganizing the state's public health services, but never lost his passion for fighting venereal disease.

He gained notoriety for a radio address he was scheduled to give in November 1934 at the Columbia Broadcasting System studios. Shortly before he was to go on the air, a young CBS employee who had seen an advance copy of the remarks told Parran he could not utter the words "syphilis" or "gonorrhea." Parran grew angry and refused to go on; listeners heard piano music instead. The next day, Parran sent a telegram to CBS deploring the censorship and resigning from a CBS health education committee. He also sent a copy of the telegram to press associations, other radio networks, and the New York newspapers. The media relished the controversy, and the public heard much more about venereal diseases than if CBS had allowed Parran to make his original address.[16]

Media prudishness reared its head again two years later, at Parran's first conference as surgeon general. When Parran cited syphilis and tuberculosis as two major preventable illnesses, an Associated Press reporter commented that the wire service wouldn't use the word "syphilis." Parran harrumphed, "The Associated Press will use it from now on or it probably will have to omit all pronouncements of the Surgeon General of the Public Health Service."[17] (Indeed, it was only during Parran's time that "syphilis" came to be commonly used in newspapers and that medical leaders came to discuss the disease in public without a blush and apology for seeming crude.[18])

Roosevelt—elected president in 1932—liked Parran, and had him in mind for the surgeon general job. (Parran initially demurred, saying he respected Cumming and felt the surgeon general should be allowed to finish his term.) In 1934, FDR appointed Parran to the Committee on Economic Security, which helped put together the Social Security Act of 1935. Parran was influential in garnering $2 million for disease research and sanitation, $8 million for grants to states for maternal and child welfare, and another $8 million in additional assistance for the Public Health Service to dole out to state and local health departments. (About $1 million from that last pot of money was devoted to syphilis control.) Those funds would invigorate public health programs across the country as the nation attempted to pull out of the Great Depression.[19]

When Cumming stepped down, Parran was named the new surgeon general. He was sworn in on April 6, 1936, and was in place to administer the public health grant programs he'd helped create earlier.

As surgeon general, Parran immediately focused his bully pulpit on venereal disease. By the summer of 1936, he had written an article that laid out the venereal disease situation in the United States. Published both in *Survey Graphic* and the widely read *Reader's Digest,* Parran's piece argued in plain terms that problems like syphilis had to be talked about openly, and described how the nation could control and cure the problem. He made a similar case in an August 1937 article he coauthored with Paul de Kruif in *Ladies Home Journal.* Parran was on a roll, and in 1937 published a book—*Shadow on the Land*—that became a surprise best seller.[20]

Parran never forgot what he had seen in Scandinavia and argued for de-moralizing and destigmatizing venereal diseases. He often seemed to be trying to depersonalize it, as well. The statistics and illustrations that went with his popular writings featured faceless, abstract human figures and emphasized, for example, that syphilis was striking one in ten U.S. adults. The implied message now was "We're the same, more or less, and are all vulnerable to a twist of unfortunate biological circumstances that could make us that diseased tenth person." Even the great discoverer Christopher Columbus was not immune, Parran said.[21]

But Parran—a Roman Catholic—occasionally sermonized a bit too, and urged his audiences not to become too abstract in how they thought of venereal diseases. In *Shadow on the Land,* Parran argued that in the case of syphilis,

> we are so apt to think we know nobody who, conceivably, might be suffering from it. It is so easy to slip into the fallacy that this is a plague of the lower classes, the submerged tenth. . . . Before we can generalize about syphilis or understand it in the mass, we must see it in the flesh and pity it in the misery of its victims. There are situations in which any emotion, even pity, muddies our intellectual clarity. But I think it is characteristic of the really great men and women whom I have known in the fight for human welfare, that they could think more clearly because they could feel first.[22]

Parran advocated that testing become routine at hospitals, in prisons, and as part of the application process for public service and private-sector jobs. He pushed for more treatment funds. And he wanted more syphilis education for private physicians and the general public.

In 1938, Congress—pushed by the popular surgeon general—passed the National Venereal Disease Control Act, which provided $3 million in matching grants to states for the first year and increased that funding over the following two years. Parran's campaign was spotlighted by *Time* in October 1936 when the magazine put the surgeon general on the cover. A few months later, *Time* named Parran a finalist for Man of the Year.[23]

Movies and radio broadcasts continued to bar venereal disease terminology, but print reporters were coming around. Before 1929, no large

U.S. newspapers printed the word "syphilis." But "the ice of journalistic reticence"—as *Time* phrased it—was completely melting in 1936, when 125 U.S. newspapers were mentioning "venereal disease" and "syphilis" and some were even featuring the topic in Sunday-edition featured articles. The Pulitzer Prize Committee in 1937 bestowed an honorable mention on the *New York Daily News* for its campaign covering venereal disease and prophylaxis.[24]

Yes, prophylaxis. Under Cumming, the Public Health Service had left condoms out of its public campaigns against venereal diseases, focusing instead on abstinence as the way to stay safe and healthy. That remained the message, even as technological innovations in the 1920s made it easier for manufacturers to make condoms faster, cheaper, and in much larger quantities. Laws in the mid-1930s added regulations to make sure condoms were effective.

In 1937, the Service released new pamphlets on syphilis and gonorrhea that broke new ground by noting that "the use of the rubber (condom) during sexual intercourse . . . protects both the man and the woman." It was a paradigm shift. Abstinence was still the safest course, public health officials said. "But," as the historian Alexandra Lord notes, "the careful reader would now learn that he or she could have sex and still avoid venereal disease."[25] Parran thus blazed the condom-embracing trail followed in the late twentieth century by surgeons general like Joycelyn Elders and David Satcher.

The message seemed frank, sensible and humane. It also appeared to be successful, with syphilis rates falling even before the availability of penicillin. The army reported declining cases of venereal disease among recruits. The infant mortality rate from syphilis dropped dramatically in some places, thanks in part to state laws that tested pregnant women for the disease. Parran's push for testing helped make blood tests before marriage a standard experience for American couples.[26]

For decades after his tenure as surgeon general, Parran was remembered as a hero in the battle against venereal diseases. But in more recent years, revelations about other actions by Parran and his Service officers have muddied the picture.

The Tuskegee Syphilis Experiment started while Parran was New York's health commissioner, but he propelled it after he became surgeon general. Service officers still believed there was value in a study that showed how the untreated disease progresses. Penicillin, the syphilis-curing antibiotic, became available in the early 1940s, and public health officials urged it on most infected Americans—but denied it to the Tuskegee test subjects.

In 1941, when the army drafted some of the Tuskegee test subjects and took steps to get them treated for syphilis, the Public Health Service approached the draft board and succeeded in getting the men excluded from treatment.[27]

Parran believed in the study and asked the Milbank Fund to continue to provide funding for burials of the study participants. He wrote: "This study, with its careful and complete physical examinations and subsequent observation up to and including autopsy at death, forms a necessary control against which to project not only the results obtained with the rapid schedules of therapy for syphilis but also the costs involved in finding and placing under treatment the infected individuals."[28]

Another black mark: Parran established hospitals for the detention and treatment of prostitutes and other women deemed promiscuous. In 1941, Congress passed the Lanham Act to fund defense housing and community facilities in war areas. Some of that money went to build and operate venereal disease quarantine hospitals near army and navy training facilities, under the rationale that such facilities were necessary to keeping the military healthy and disease-free. More than twenty were built in 1943, and nearly fifty were open by 1947. Some of the largest could handle three hundred patients at a time. Officially, they were called rapid treatment centers (though some newspapers referred to them as women's prison hospitals). Initially they used toxic arsenical compounds, and gave the drugs to women through IV drip or multiple injections rather than through the occasional-injection regimen more common for patients in other settings.[29]

The idea for special measures against VD-infected women was not new. During World War I, thirty-two states had laws authorizing the arrest and examination of prostitutes and others for venereal diseases. The Lanham Act venereal disease hospitals were an extension of that policy: police and health officials arrested women for prostitution or "suspect behavior" and detained them in the hospitals, frequently against the women's will. One woman—a married waitress—was arrested when she stopped to get something to eat on her way home from work. She was pressured to commit herself to the local VD hospital but was released when she tested negative.[30]

Parran was on a crusade against venereal disease, clearly, and health officials marching under his orders were making judgments about women and their behaviors. Parran believed women were "prolific spreaders" who kept syphilis alive by transmitting it through a succession of localized epidemics. And despite the surgeon general's previously stated intention of taking a dispassionate, scientific approach to stamping out the problem and of not trying to judge or change the sex habits of the population, his campaign purposefully attempted to supplant ignorance of syphilis and other venereal diseases with fear of it. The historian Allan Brandt has argued that Parran's endorsement of "syphilophobia" encouraged stigma and denial, fostered by wartime posters and other campaign materials that depicted vamps and even the slightly-too-friendly girl-next-door as disease-carrying menaces. Parran, in a 1962 interview, acknowledged the tactic as hardball designed to break the chain of infection. "Oh, yes," he said. "We played upon the fear motif."[31]

Health officials today look back at the approach and shake their heads. "They, in fact, used fairly stigmatic images as a way of basically frightening people into concern about STDs. We've gotten smarter about it," said John Douglas of the U.S. Centers for Disease Control and Prevention. He later added that the HIV epidemic taught health officials that stigma can hinder prevention efforts by making people reluctant to be tested.[32]

Parran and his men, so intent on their war on syphilis, made other decisions that were—by today's standards—even more abhorrent.

From 1946 to 1948, the Public Health Service ran a series of experiments in Guatemala in which they deliberately tried to infect more than thirteen hundred people with sexually transmitted diseases. The human guinea pigs included soldiers, prostitutes, prisoners, and—most lamentably—mental patients. The purpose was to see if penicillin, then relatively new, could prevent infections.

The researchers included some of the same doctors who had run a similar experiment with prisoners in Terre Haute, Indiana, during World War II. But unlike the Terre Haute subjects, the Guatemalans were not told what was being done to them. In Guatemala, but not in Terre Haute, some children were infected as part of the study. And in Guatemala, many test subjects—perhaps several hundred—were not given treatment after the infection. Syphilis was injected into cerebrospinal fluid of seven epileptic women in the mental asylum through cisternal puncture beneath the base of their skulls, a risky procedure that caused each to suffer bacterial meningitis from contaminated needles. In an even more horrific experiment, Cutler ordered that gonorrhea pus be injected into the eyes, urethra, and rectum of one woman who was dying (probably, the records suggest, from a terminal illness unrelated to the experiments).

The experiments were run by John Cutler, a Service physician, and historical records indicate he was no renegade. Parran knew about the experiments and was excited about them, though he sensed that frank reports about the Guatemala experiments would not play well with the public. The medical historian Susan Reverby, who first brought the Guatemala experiments to light, adduces a letter from malaria specialist G. Robert Coatney, who visited the Guatemala researchers in 1947 and then briefed Parran on what he saw. According to Coatney, a "merry twinkle came into [Parran's] eye," and he said, "You know, we couldn't do such an experiment in this country."[33]

WORLD WAR II

The United States entered World War II in December 1941, following the Japanese attack on Pearl Harbor. The nation had been gearing up for possible entry into the war for years, as Nazi Germany invaded neighboring nations and threatened England and other U.S. allies.

In 1940, Secretary of War Harry Woodring formally asked for the Public Health Service to work with the army in overseeing food inspection, sewage disposal, and other sanitation work around training facilities. Woodring also asked the Service to organize efforts to prevent venereal disease in the military. Parran agreed, and made other preparations, like assembling a national roster of nurses who could be pressed into service and planning how to provide and safeguard malaria treatments and other drugs that might be needed by troops.[34]

Meanwhile, the Public Health Service gained responsibility for the medical care of another group of Americans—those in internment camps. In the spring of 1942, the army ordered 110,000 U.S. citizens of Japanese ancestry from their homes in California, Oregon, Washington, and Arizona and placed them in internment camps. The government was worried about distinguishing loyal from disloyal Japanese Americas citizens and herded them into camps under the guard of the Border Patrol. Initially, camps were hastily set up at fairgrounds, horse-racing tracks, and other large and available facilities. Thousands of people were packed into unsanitary conditions, some of them forced to bed down in whitewashed animal stalls that still reeked of manure.[35]

The army began to worry that the camps could become launching pads for disease outbreaks that could spread to the rest of the population. The Public Health Service seemed the logical agency to handle medical care and infection control at the camps; it already had been handling medical services for Axis seamen and enemy aliens, under a program operated by the Immigration and Naturalization Service. At the Japanese internment camps, Parran's doctors provided vaccinations, dealt with food poisoning from spoiled foods, and set up hospitals and infirmaries largely staffed by detainees (some of whom were health professionals).

Parran's doctors were able to rationalize their participation in the internment camps this way: About 285 Japanese Americans died at the camps from April 1 to September 1, 1942—a small number given circumstances that included chronic lack of equipment and supplies. Moreover, most of the fatalities were people who had been hospitalized and been in fragile health when the evacuations first began. Many healthier detainees, meanwhile, got better health services than they had ever seen. Pregnant Japanese American women received pre- and postnatal care that they otherwise couldn't have afforded. Some detainees received dental care for the first time in their lives. "No one died because they couldn't get access to medical care. If it was necessary, we found a way to do it," recalled Henry Taira, a Japanese American physician from Fresno who was involved in internment camp care.[36]

As the Public Health Service took on more and more tasks, Parran saw a need for reorganization and administrative streamlining. In 1943, he set all Service functions into four divisions—the Office of the Surgeon General, the National Institute of Health, the Bureau of State Services, and the Bureau of Medical Services. The marine hospitals, once the Service's core, were rapidly shrinking in importance and now were a subunit of the Hospital Division of the Bureau of Medical Services.

There had been an earlier reorganization of the federal government in 1939, with oversight of the Public Health Service switching from the Treasury Department to the Federal Security Administration, a forerunner of today's U.S. Department of Health and Human Services. The Public Health Service had enjoyed a nice home and a long leash within the Treasury Department—Parran once called the placement "quite an independent and comfortable position."[37] The change in oversight initially had little impact on Parran's power. Indeed, Congress passed a law in 1944 that streamlined and expanded the surgeon general's authority in several areas, including research and training grants.[38]

One of Parran's new programs would expand dramatically. It was a malaria-control program for military bases and the war industry in the South, led by public health visionary Joseph W. Mountin. Parran decided the program's headquarters should be in Atlanta and gave the program its first name, Malaria Control in War Areas. Parran also began to pile other responsibilities on the program such as controlling murine typhus at airfields. In 1946, with Parran's hearty support, the program was expanded and rechristened the Communicable Disease Center. And so was born what we know today at the U.S. Centers for Disease Control and Prevention, the federal government's primary disease investigation and prevention agency.[39]

Another Parran creation success story: he was a driving force in the creation of the World Health Organization (WHO), the Geneva-based entity that coordinates and directs international health measures for the United Nations. In 1943, the surgeon general began working with U.S. State Department staff who would help create the United Nations in 1945. Parran pushed for the creation of an international health organization adjunct to the UN, and chaired the 1946 conference where the WHO's draft constitution was adopted. The surgeon general also proposed that the WHO be decentralized, using, for example, the Pan American Sanitary Bureau—now known as the Pan American Health Organization—as the WHO regional office for the Americas. He was a founding father of the WHO, and later counted his involvement in it as one of his proudest accomplishments.[40]

While pursuing these efforts, Parran continued to work the bully pulpit, warning about the dangers of venereal disease as well as speaking on other health topics. A practiced veteran of public speeches, published discourse, and radio addresses, the surgeon general now started turning to motion pictures.

The Public Health Service was behind several movies released during the war. The first, *Know for Sure,* was produced for the Service by the Research Council of the Academy of Motion Picture Arts and Sciences. Several Hollywood actors donated their time, including Ward Bond. The short film began with an Italian immigrant shopkeeper, an accordion-playing stereotype named Tony Midroni, who is devastated when he learns he has infected his wife with syphilis and caused their baby to be stillborn. He goes to a public health clinic, and the doctor sees him and two other men (one of them Bond) who come in complaining of the same telltale sores. The film was meant for male factory workers in war industries, but other groups used it, including the military.[41]

Parran did not appear in that movie, but he was on screen twice in another film, a twenty-one-minute short completed in late 1943 entitled *To the People of the United States.* Essentially, it was a very long public service commercial, to be shown in movie theaters across the country. It encapsulated many of Parran's arguments. The film is worth discussing in detail, because it was a perfect representation of what Parran was trying to communicate.

The film begins with introductory comments from Army Surgeon General Norman Kirk, stiff, squinting and obviously reading cue cards. Parran appears next, suave in comparison, with an actor's manner and elocution. Then the film cuts to an airfield where a ground crew worker played by Robert Mitchum grouses that a B-17 was grounded from the big mission because the pilot got yanked from duty. It turns out the pilot has syphilis, and soon the diseased flyboy comes on screen as a colonel explains to him the illness can be cured with fifty-six painless shots.

The colonel has an accent and says he was born in Denmark. The character spends several minutes of the film discussing how open and progressive people in Scandinavia are about venereal disease compared to Americans—who by the way, he notes, have a much worse syphilis problem. Next comes a scene with the colonel and an American doctor. The U.S. physician concludes the exchange by addressing the camera and saying, "I don't know about you, but I hate the idea of the Swedes, Norwegians, and Danes thinking we're a bunch of superstitious idiots. Let's show them we're as adult and intelligent as they are!" Then the Danish colonel's voice returns to chide any audience member who might be squeamish about the terminology: "Syphilis. Say it. Syphilis. Learn about it. Have a blood test to make sure you haven't got it."

The film ends with Parran on screen one more time. Churches, schools, and social agencies need to be applauded for preventing promiscuity, he says. "Learn the facts. With knowledge and intelligent action, the people of America can eradicate the venereal diseases."[42]

This kind of film was bound to be controversial, and before its 1944 release it came under fire from the Legion of Decency, an organization established by the Catholic Church to judge films by moral standards. Although *To the People of the United States* was not a commercial film, the Legion felt it should comply with Hollywood's Motion Picture Code, which restricted films on venereal disease and sex hygiene. Legion officials also believed Parran's movie did not focus enough on promiscuity as a cause for the disease's spread. Catholic organizations also criticized as "indecent, repulsive and un-American" a Public Health Service brochure on venereal disease.[43]

Parran dispatched one of his officers, Leroy Burney, to meet with the Legion's monsignor director. Burney—who would become surgeon general himself in the late 1950s—served as a technical advisor on the film. The meeting did not go well. "I'd never talked with someone and it just bounced back, as if it makes no penetration," Burney later recalled. In an interview more than forty years later, Burney said the exchange went like this:

> He said, "This is health education, and health education on venereal diseases must be done by the home or the family."
> I said, "But home and family aren't doing it."
> He said, "That's just too bad. I'd rather see a mother get syphilis than to have education by this fashion."
> I said, "Yes, but look at the progress that the Scandinavian countries have made against venereal diseases by having very thorough and well-developed health education."
> His reply to that was, "Well, everybody knows that Scandinavians are the most immoral people in the world."[44]

Parran then turned to a Public Health Service advisory committee that included clergymen as well as health officials and teachers, but had no more luck. The committee counseled Parran not to release the film, fearing it would provoke enough opposition to torpedo the whole venereal disease education effort. Parran expected a fight, but must have been shaken to his Catholic core when even his advisors shook their heads at provoking the Legion. Parran took his committee's advice and decided to keep the film out of commercial theaters and distribute it only through health departments and like organizations.[45]

Parran's decision to restrict release of the film, though perhaps pragmatic, set a cowardly precedent. Decades later, some of Parran's successors—especially C. Everett Koop and Joycelyn Elders—would also find themselves in conflict with social conservatives over sexual health issues. They had to decide how far to push science-backed public health messages in the face of fierce moral opposition. A few surgeons general would charge hard, with one (Elders) pushing so hard it led to her dismissal. But many others would choose not to roil the water.

Much of Parran's campaign rolled out intact, and the effort did have its supporters—including the AMA. In the 1930s, AMA leaders worked with Parran on a venereal disease film for doctors, and went to the mayor of Chicago to successfully steamroll an attempt by the Chicago censorship board to stop the film from being shown to medical audiences.[46] However, their interests would soon collide on the subject of health reform.

HEALTH SECURITY UNDER ATTACK

Indirectly, national health insurance was the issue that elevated Parran to U.S. surgeon general. It was also the issue that helped force him out.

Parran's ascension to the national office was aided by Edgar Sydenstricker, the Service alumnus and health reform advocate who helped get Parran's name in front of Roosevelt in the first place. Sydenstricker at the time was working for the Milbank Memorial Fund, founded in 1921 to promote public health. Parran shared the Milbank leaders' conviction that government intervention was needed to help the people who could not afford health care. The surgeon general also felt both social insurance and public medicine were necessary parts of any changes.[47] "We have now reached a stage in the evolution of citizenship when all the people, rich and poor alike, are beginning to demand at least a minimum of health protection as a right. . . . To the informed mind, this opportunity for health is beginning to rank with the other basic qualities of American life—freedom of speech, of faith, of assembly, of franchise," Parran said in one speech in 1939.[48]

The surgeon general had been close to the reformers for a long time and had worked with them on the Committee on Economic Security. The group had drafted the Social Security Act of 1935, but the majority of the members were cautious about including national health insurance in the bill and plunging into a political battle with organized medicine. The AMA already viewed some members as enemies, particularly Sydenstricker. In 1935, Morris Fishbein—the AMA's loud-barking attack dog on the issue of health reform—wrote in the pages of the *Journal of the American Medical Association* that Sydenstricker was "completely antagonistic to the medical point of view." Sydenstricker turned to Parran and asked him to persuade President Roosevelt to pursue health insurance.[49]

Despite the career boosts he'd received from Sydenstricker and other reformers, Parran actually came down somewhere in the middle. He was certainly no Hugh Cumming, who eschewed national health insurance proposals and dreamed of being counted among the AMA's elite. But he questioned whether national health insurance was the best way to provide health security, and he preferred not to alienate private physicians; he was recruiting them to join his venereal disease campaign.

In 1938, Parran was appointed to the Interdepartmental Committee to Coordinate Health and Welfare Activities, a group charged with considering amendments to the Social Security Act. In July of that year, the group held a national health conference in Washington, D.C., that was a turning point in the push for medical reform. The organizers brought in the AMA and other traditional players in the debate, but also invited advocates representing the interests of mothers and children, the unemployed, labor, and others with a stake in the debate. The committee put out a program that became the basis for health reform initiatives for years afterward. It discussed expanding federal public health and maternal and child services, aiding hospitals through federal grants, promoting federally assisted disability insurance, and adding new funding—perhaps through general taxation or social insurance contributions—to provide medical care to all who needed it.[50]

In a radio address broadcast to the nation during the meeting, Parran noted what seemed a sea change, with so many people pressing for better access to health care. He told the conference attendees: "People in general are beginning to take it for granted that an equal opportunity for health is a basic American right. They are thinking just a little ahead of the lawmakers and even, I fear, ahead of the practitioners of public health and clinical medicine."[51] Often cast as a leader of reform, the surgeon general tried to portray himself more as an observer of change than as its instigator.

Others took the conference as a clear sign of widespread demand for government action. U.S. Senator Robert Wagner, a Democrat from New York, introduced a bill in early 1939 that encapsulated the committee's main recommendations. Parran spoke in favor of it, while taking care to address concerns of organized medicine. "This is not a measure to socialize medicine, but one that will free medical practice," he said.[52]

But the powerful AMA was having none of it. The organization's delegates felt ambushed at the 1938 conference, confronted by labor leaders and others impatient for change. AMA leaders dug in and lobbied hard against the proposal. Labor leaders undermined it a bit too, actually. Understandably, they believed public health agencies were under the sway of doctors' groups, and complained about provisions that would give the Public Health Service a major say over state medical programs. Roosevelt, preoccupied with the worsening situation in Europe, chose not to endorse the bill and take on the whole headache.

World War II put health reform on the back burner, just as World War I had roughly twenty-five years earlier. In 1943, Wagner teamed with two other legislators, Montana senator James Murray and Michigan representative John Dingell, to introduce a bill that dropped the state medicine component and focused on national health insurance.

Roosevelt was consumed with the war, and the most support he would offer was a "good luck with it" comment to Wagner.[53] The Wagner-Murray-Dingell bill died in Congress in 1944.

Privately, Parran was a bit relieved by the bill's demise. He gradually came to believe national health insurance was the wrong way to go—indeed, despite his comments to the press in support of the Wagner bill in the late 1930s, he had reservations. The surgeon general worried such an approach would put too much emphasis on taking care of people after they got sick and make short shrift of measures to prevent illness. He also worried it would leave him with huge responsibilities for running a national health system but with only limited authority over how services were delivered. Parran preferred the idea of using public health doctors to broaden preventive services as well as fill in gaps in the medical system.[54]

All along, the surgeon general remained a good soldier, staying true to the president's position on health reform. (That wasn't difficult, because Parran was nearly as ambivalent about it as Roosevelt was.) But Parran's job grew more complicated when Roosevelt died in April 1945 and Vice President Harry Truman took over the Oval Office. Whereas the aristocratic Roosevelt had been noncommittal on the question of national health insurance, the Missouri-bred Truman was an ardent believer, a prairie-populist who, as a county judge earlier in life, had frequently seen struggling families financially devastated by illness. Truman often said that those who opposed national health insurance "really want to go back to the horse and buggy days."[55] Calling for a national health program, Truman assigned the job of putting it together to Parran's boss—Watson Miller, head of the Federal Security Agency.

As Truman championed a revived Wagner-Murray-Dingell bill, Miller and Parran were called on to lead the push. Conflict with the AMA escalated, and Parran soon found himself under attack. The onslaught started with a fearmonger named Marjorie Shearon. A former employee of both the Public Health Service and the Social Security Board, in 1944 Shearon went to work for Republicans in Congress. She was passionately opposed to national health insurance and put out a pamphlet in which she said the Social Security Board was the "mecca for socialization efforts." She did not see Parran as part of the conspiracy to socialize American medicine, believing he was double-crossed by the people at Social Security. But her account cast him as an accomplice, and AMA attack dogs and Republican opponents of Wagner-Murray-Dingell seized on it.[56]

At an AMA House of Delegates meeting in December 1946, doctors from Colorado introduced a resolution to prohibit political activity by the surgeon general and the Public Health Service. The measure focused on a January 1946 letter from Parran to Service officers urging support for Truman's health program. It was propaganda, the Colorado delegates argued, "a perversion of function and dereliction of duty" by Parran. The House of Delegates debated the proposal, then passed a less incendiary resolution expressing disappointment in Parran's conduct.[57]

The resolution triggered a hearing by the House Subcommittee on Government Publicity and Propaganda in July 1947 that also sought to condemn Parran. Forest Harness, an Indiana Republican, led the inquiry. Harness complained that in late 1945, Parran had disseminated to public health doctors a special message from Truman on national health reform. The Indiana legislator also decried a series of Service-sponsored public health workshops in 1946 that he called a government-funded attempt to generate public sentiment for socialized medicine.[58] It was part of a political witch hunt that presaged the "Red Scare" tactics used by Senator Joseph McCarthy a few years later. Harness was never able to gather hard evidence to support some of his key claims against Parran. The surgeon general continued on in his job as Harness moved on to other targets.

"Parran was absolutely superb" in handling the bitter battle over health insurance, said Warren Palmer Dearing, a Service physician who served under Parran. "He didn't battle it, but he also didn't give any ground."[59] Parran no doubt was troubled by the attack. He had supported—but didn't truly believe in—Truman's quest for a form of health reform. But Truman had not risen to Parran's defense during the Harness mess, choosing instead to ignore the Republican attacks on his surgeon general.

The situation then went from bad to worse. In August 1947, Truman replaced Watson Miller, a capable administrator, with the more pugnacious Oscar Ewing as head of the FSA. Ewing had led a group at the 1944 Democratic convention that got Truman named vice president on the ticket with Roosevelt. He relished political fights and aggressively took the reins of the campaign for national health insurance.

PARRAN'S DEPARTURE

Oscar Ewing and Thomas Parran had little in common. Parran was a career health bureaucrat focused on scientific details, while Ewing played loose with the facts as he pursued political goals. In 1948, Ewing argued for national health insurance by estimating that 300,000 Americans were dying each year for lack of national health insurance. It was an unsubstantiated claim with no known connection to public health data. How Ewing came up with the number was a mystery.[60]

The static between the men was personal, as well. It started at their first meeting, when Parran stopped by to congratulate Ewing on the FSA appointment. The initial conversation was pleasant, with Ewing expressing his interest in health issues and mentioning that his wife had received terrific care for her high blood pressure from Walter Kempner at Duke University Hospital. In the days that followed, Ewing said he felt the National Institutes of Health—which Parran oversaw—should provide a research grant to Kempner. "It just so happened that because of this experience with Mrs. Ewing I knew more about Dr. Kempner's work than anyone in the Public Health Service, and I felt, therefore, justified in insisting they make Kempner a research grant," Ewing recalled in an interview years later.[61]

Parran said he'd look into it, and then reported that an NIH advisory committee had reviewed Kempner's application for funding and turned it down. Ewing wasn't interested in hearing about the scientific reasons for the denial. He believed the Duke doctor should get federal money and viewed Parran's inaction as disobedience. Ewing became less cooperative with Parran on other matters, such as refusing to fill appointments to NIH advisory committees that should have been pro forma. One day the two had a sharp exchange about it in Ewing's office; Ewing said he would not make the appointments until Parran found a way to fund Kempner. Parran stormed out. Within a week, the grant for Kempner was approved. But it was too late; Ewing had decided Parran was not a team player. "That whole experience annoyed me so much that when Dr. Parran's term as Surgeon General expired, . . . I did not recommend him for reappointment," Ewing recalled.[62]

That's not what Ewing said at the time, however. Ewing held a press conference in February 1948 to announce he would recommend not reappointing Parran when the surgeon general's third term expired in April, because it was important to periodically bring new blood into the position. "If you don't rotate it, you to a certain extent kill ambition" within the Public Health Service, Ewing told reporters.[63]

The press didn't buy Ewing's explanation, and mourned the decision. "Whatever the reason for Mr. Truman's failure to reappoint Dr. Parran, there will be nation-wide regret at his departure from an office which he administered with zeal and distinction," said an editorial in the *New York Times* the next day.[64] Service physicians had a similar opinion. "He was a brilliant, precise, tough-minded, imaginative, courageous guy . . . we worshipped him," Dearing said.[65]

Parran was only fifty-five when he was forced into retirement. He continued to work with the World Health Organization and helped establish the Graduate School of Public Health at the University of Pittsburgh, where he was dean for ten years.

He died of pneumonia on February 16, 1968, in Pittsburgh. He was seventy-five. "Few have done more to bring modern medicine to the nation's poor than this gentlemanly physician," *Time* magazine wrote, in tribute on Parran's passing.[66]

Since Parran's death, however, revelations about research conducted during his time in office have complicated his legacy. In early 2013, Parran became the focus of an agonizing debate within the American Sexually Transmitted Diseases Association (ASTDA), which for decades had named its most prestigious achievement award after him. The revelations about the Guatemala study, particularly, prompted the association's members to re-evaluate whether the Thomas Parran award should be renamed.

In postings on the ASTDA Web site, three of Parran's grandsons defended the former surgeon general, suggesting he won the war on syphilis and urging association members to interpret past events within the context of the ethical standards (and inherent racism) of the era in which they occurred. That argument was echoed by others. "I am confident that if Dr. Parran was around today, he would certainly not approve of or participating [*sic*] in any research work that would even remotely resemble what happened in Guatemala," typed one commentator, Chang Lee.[67]

But when the association conducted a straw poll of its members, only 20 percent voted to keep Parran's name on the award. The organization's leaders removed it, partly out of concern that future recipients might turn down the award because of the controversy surrounding the former surgeon general.[68] "It's always shattering to realize that our 'hero' was all too human," wrote Khalil Ghanem, a Johns Hopkins University physician who sided with the majority. "Was he a product of his time or should he have known better? There's no easy answer. For me, he's still a hero—albeit a flawed one. I can live with that. I don't think the ASTDA award has to."[69]

Parran can be judged harshly in other respects as well. A supremely skilled government administrator and public communicator, he nevertheless failed to achieve the kind of national health reforms he and Rupert Blue had spoken about from their bully pulpits. Their opportunities passed, lost in international war preparations and domestic political skirmishes. No surgeons general after them would come as close to being major voices for health reform.

Indeed, after Parran, surgeons general gradually lost power as a federal health bureaucracy grew up around them and politics played an increasingly larger role in public health decision making. The slide began in earnest with Parran's replacement, Leonard Scheele.

PART TWO

Decline, 1949–1980

CHAPTER 5

The Quicksand Bureaucracy

It was once said that Leonard Scheele was the last happy surgeon general.[1]

Scheele did have more reason to be chipper than any of his successors. He reigned when the office was still steeped in prestige and significant power, and he was not fazed by the lobbyists, congressmen, or executive branch political appointees who would have growing influence over the Public Health Service through the 1950s and beyond. They were only just beginning to push in when Scheele became surgeon general.

The tall and jowly Scheele served eight years as America's doctor, some of them tumultuous and involving the assimilation of the Public Health Service into a new federal entity, the Department of Health, Education, and Welfare.

The advent of HEW, as it was called, marked a significant change. For decades, surgeons general had stood tall in the government. They often brushed elbows with presidents: Hugh Cumming had close personal ties to Herbert Hoover, and Thomas Parran was known as a friend of FDR.[2] Such status—along with the tradition that surgeons general served multiple terms, through multiple presidencies—had caused Public Health Service physicians to believe their commander was beyond the reach of petty politics.

But those days were over. For surgeons general, life within HEW coincided with their increasing remove from the White House and the growing meddling in Service affairs by politicians and advocates. Scheele and his successor, Leroy Burney, strove to safeguard a science-based integrity for the office, even as they saw their power and influence begin to wane. Like some Dr. Livingstone–esque British jungle explorer caught in quicksand, each tried to maintain the semblance of dignified professionalism as he sank into the new bureaucratic quagmire.

LEONARD SCHEELE

Important Allies

Leonard Andrew Scheele was born July 25, 1907, in Fort Wayne, Indiana. He grew interested in medical school when he was in high school and was working in a pharmacy run by his father, Martin Scheele. Leonard traveled north for college to the University of Michigan, where he earned a bachelor's degree and met and married a future dentist named Frances K. McCormick. Scheele went on to get his medical degree from the Wayne State University School of Medicine in 1934.

Attending medical school in the midst of the Great Depression, he became interested in public health through the inspiration of a medical school professor who ran the Michigan state health department's laboratories. Scheele applied for—and got—an internship at the U.S. Marine Hospital in Chicago, and after graduation signed on with the Public Health Service full-time.[3]

Like others in the Service, he worked a variety of posts, including at quarantine stations in San Francisco and San Pedro, California, and at Pearl Harbor in Honolulu. In 1936, he was assigned to Washington, D.C., where he gained the attention of one of Parran's top lieutenants, Joseph Mountin. Mountin—a legendary figure in the Service who would later create the CDC—became a guiding hand in Scheele's career.

Traditionally, the bright young stars of the Public Health Service had worked on infectious diseases—the leading causes of death of the late nineteenth and early twentieth centuries. But Scheele joined the Service at a time when contagious killers had receded, life expectancy had improved, and diseases associated with older age were coming to the fore. In 1938, heart disease and cancer took their place as the nation's top two causes of death.[4] Recognizing the shift taking place, Mountin sent Scheele for two years of specialized training at the New York City cancer hospital known today as Memorial Sloan-Kettering. In 1939, Mountin put Scheele in charge of a new national cancer control program at the NIH's National Cancer Institute. In that post, Scheele spearheaded a unique national effort to systematically evaluate the causes, distribution, and control of cancer and to examine how well various cancer treatments worked.[5] The assignment put Scheele on a path to becoming a champion of NIH's cause.

World War II interrupted Scheele's work in cancer research, but gave his career a different kind of boost. The day after Pearl Harbor, he was assigned to the Office of Civilian Defense in Washington, D.C., to plan for casualties that might take place in the United States if there were a major invasion. In 1943, he was lent to the army and sent to the Mediterranean to oversee public health issues in North Africa, Sicily, and southern Italy. Then he served in Western Europe, including a stint as a junior officer on the staff of General Dwight D. Eisenhower. Scheele met Ike only a few times, including a small social gathering the night before the Germans surrendered.[6] But Scheele's wartime experience would serve him in good stead years later when Eisenhower would become president.

His war duty ended with a reposting to the National Cancer Institute as assistant director. Two years later, in 1947, Parran promoted him to director of the NCI and also gave him the title of assistant surgeon general. It was at the NCI that he got to know a couple who would become his great patrons—Albert and Mary Lasker.

The Laskers had extraordinary connections, tremendous charm, and the drive to engineer a boom in American medical research. Albert was a wealthy, Chicago-based advertising pioneer known for cigarette campaigns designed to get more women to smoke—his hit ads for Lucky Strike carried slogans like "Cigarettes Are Kind to Your Throat" and "Reach for a Lucky instead of a Sweet." But even as he shilled cigarettes, he also had a growing interest in medical philanthropy. That humanitarian bent magnified after he married his third wife in 1940. She was Mary Woodard Reinhardt Lasker, a persuasive, raven-haired divorcée with a keen interest in health issues who became focused on cancer when her longtime housekeeper fell ill with the disease.[7] The Laskers essentially took over the American Cancer Society, reorganizing it, redefining its mission, and dramatically boosting its financial strength and prominence.[8] They set up their own influential foundation too, and cultivated friendships with a variety of important congressmen like Senators Lister Hill of Alabama and Claude Pepper of Florida. As they pushed for more research funding, they targeted the NIH—and, particularly, Scheele's National Cancer Institute.

So Scheele was in the right place at the right time, and recognized that fact. Unlike Parran, who had only casual contact with the Laskers,

Scheele made a point of being accessible to them. He planned a clinical center for the NCI, to the couple's delight. And at their suggestion, he drew up proposed legislation for what would become the NIH's National Heart Institute. Mary Lasker—who knew President Truman and visited him in the White House—thought the cooperative Scheele would make an excellent surgeon general, and his name rose to the top of the list when Parran left.[9] When FSA administrator Oscar Ewing called Scheele in to give him the news, Ewing was clear that Scheele's selection had been arranged by powers higher than himself. "Say, they told me up at the White House that they want you to be Surgeon General. . . . I haven't got anything against you. I guess it's all right if they want you," Scheele later recalled Ewing saying.[10]

The Senate quickly confirmed Scheele's nomination, and the new surgeon general made the growth of the NIH and medical research an immediate priority. He helped to more than triple the NIH budget, growing it from $29 million in 1948 (when Scheele became surgeon general) to $98 million in 1955 (Scheele's last full year in office). What's more, in 1955 he named his protégé, James Shannon, to become director of the NIH. Shannon was a gifted and politically savvy administrator who would create headaches for subsequent surgeons general, but in the late 1940s and early 1950s the agency was still firmly under Scheele. Service veterans have said the NIH's boom was his main interest and proudest accomplishment.[11]

Scheele believed he succeeded by being apolitical. Since John Woodworth, surgeons general had been building and maintaining a professional public health corps and were supposed to act like eunuchs when it came to politics—disinterested in election excitement, simply there to do a job. It was to some extent a myth: surgeons general like John Hamilton and Hugh Cumming were quietly cunning Washington operators, and Thomas Parran openly campaigned for Democratic health reform. But the ideal still existed, and when Ewing wanted Scheele at his side for televised debates on national health insurance proposals, the new surgeon general invoked it. "I said, 'The minute I do that I'm finished as a professional officer for you, and you want the Surgeon General's job to stay a professional officer's job, so I think you've got to find somebody else," Scheele later recounted. "He [Ewing] was, as I say, pretty upset, but he came to accept this view as a very proper one, and we became fast friends."[12] Political realities may have helped bring about Ewing's acquiescence. After all, it was one thing to oust Parran, who was at the end of his term and no longer under Roosevelt's protection. But Scheele was new and well liked by the Laskers and other powerful insiders. Besides, Ewing did need a professional to attend to a crowd of public health problems, many of them having to do with air and water.

Smoke, Water, and Smoking

In late October 1948, six months after Scheele was appointed, the first major deadly air pollution incident in U.S. history occurred. It was in Donora, Pennsylvania, a small steel town about twenty miles south of Pittsburgh. The Pittsburgh area had long been known as something of an atmospheric hellhole (recall the smoky conditions reported at the Pittsburgh marine hospital in the 1870s, when Woodworth had just become the first surgeon general). For decades, smoke from steel mills had turned sunny afternoons into acrid dusk, but most people thought of air pollution as a nuisance—not a health threat.

Donora was a turning point. During a windless week leading up to Halloween, a temperature inversion trapped pollutants from the town's concentration of mills (a steel plant, wire plant, and zinc smelting plant, all operated by a subsidiary of the United States Steel Corporation). The resulting smog blanketed the town and hung in the air for days. The esteemed medical journalist Berton Roueché would later report that it was the second smoke-contaminated fog in history to reach toxic density, after a killer smog that struck an industrial valley in Belgium in 1930 and left sixty people dead.[13] The Donora smog was easily the worst ever seen in America. Nearly half the populace got sick within two days, reporting headaches, vomiting, coughing up blood, and irritation of the eyes, nose, and throat. Some suffered much worse. At least twenty people died, all age fifty-two or older.[14]

Donora drew national headlines and prompted a call for more aggressive regulation. The town's residents resisted the push for more government oversight, worrying that any new restrictions would hurt U.S. Steel, which ran the mills that were the economic lifeblood of the community.[15]

The Public Health Service started an investigation within a week of the first death, and soon twenty-five PHS workers were studying the site and looking for residual health effects in Donora residents. They announced their findings in October 1949, fingering air pollution as the cause while acknowledging they simply didn't know what the toxic effects were of mixing sulfur dioxide, fluoride, chloride, and other stack gases in Donora's air. "One of the most important results of the study is to show us what we do not know," Scheele said.[16] Ewing and Scheele jointly spoke to the media, with Scheele asking Congress for $250,000 toward additional research. A call for more research was perhaps a weak response to a tragedy that had killed so many people. But the Donora incident generated a push that years later led to the first formal federal air pollution program. Although states were expected to regulate air pollution, the Air Pollution Control Act—passed by Congress in 1955—gave the Public Health Service responsibility for studying air pollution and providing training and technical assistance.[17]

Meanwhile, Scheele was dealing with an even more controversial topic: water fluoridation.

For decades dentists had noticed stained or mottled teeth in people who lived in certain areas (the condition was known as "Colorado brown stain"). By the 1920s, some researchers had pinned the condition to naturally elevated levels of fluoride, a mineral in the drinking water. By the early 1940s, scientists concluded it wasn't necessarily bad—fluoride reduced the incidence of cavities in those same areas with naturally elevated levels of fluoride. In the right amounts, it could be a boon to a nation plagued by cavities and where pulling teeth was the common treatment.

In 1945, Grand Rapids, Michigan, became the first city to adjust fluoride levels in its water supply with the intent of promoting the community's dental health. In 1950, the American Dental Association endorsed fluoridation of community water supplies. And at an April 1951 hearing, Scheele told the U.S. Senate that fluoridation was an official policy of the Public Health Service.[18]

Scheele backed fluoridation after studies in Grand Rapids and five other communities showed reductions in childhood cavities. In so doing, he showed a little of the old Parran backbone—a willingness to throw the credibility of his office behind an important but controversial initiative. Opposition to fluoridation was common. Adversaries ranged from thoughtful people to paranoids who thought fluoridation was a Communist plot to soften the minds of Americans. But the surgeon general's endorsement was influential, and by 1954, about 15 million people in roughly eight hundred communities were receiving fluoridated water.[19] In the decades to come, fluoridation would be common and be labeled one of the ten great public health accomplishments of the century.[20]

Scheele's handling of cigarette smoking was not as laudable.

For decades, some scientific studies had been pointing to cigarette smoking as a possible cause of lung cancer, and Surgeon General Hugh

Cumming in 1929 had warned that tobacco was a threat to the "physical tone" of the nation. But the science was inconclusive. The medical literature contained speculative animal studies and retrospective human studies that frequently could not clearly differentiate the impact of cigarette smoking from that of car exhaust, mill dust, or other potential causes.[21]

The 1950s saw a wave of better-designed efforts that turned heads in the scientific community. It began with a study by Ernst Wynder, a German-born researcher fresh out of medical school, and Evarts Graham, a heavy-smoking thoracic surgeon. During a summer internship, Wynder had become fascinated with the idea that smoking caused lung cancer after watching the autopsy of a two-pack-a-day smoker. He and Graham assembled a study of 684 cases that in design sophistication, population size, and conclusiveness, set a new standard for human tobacco studies. It was published in the esteemed *Journal of the American Medical Association* in May 1950. Using a large control group of cancer-free patients for comparison, Wynder and Graham found 96.5 percent of lung cancer patients were smokers, while only 73 percent of patients who did not have lung cancer were smokers.[22] Four months later, the *British Medical Journal* published a paper by the researchers Richard Doll and A. Bradford Hill. They looked at lung cancer patients at twenty London hospitals and, based on their findings, estimated that people who smoked twenty-five cigarettes a day or more had a risk of developing lung cancer fifty times greater than that of nonsmokers.

Such research burst on the public's radar in December 1952, when *Reader's Digest* published an article on the topic by Roy Norr, the gadfly editor of a little-known newsletter on smoking and health. *Reader's Digest* was the nation's primary consumer magazine at a time when magazines and newspapers were far and away the most influential media. Indeed, *Reader's Digest* "was the American public's principal source of health and medical information, the most important one," said Ken Warner, a University of Michigan researcher who has intensively studied smoking and health.[23]

Norr's article, entitled "Cancer by the Carton," chronicled the surge in lung cancer deaths since the 1930s and noted the cigarettes-are-the-cause conclusions of Wynder, Graham, and other researchers. The article was a face slap to the American public and was soon bolstered by news of additional tobacco-focused studies by Wynder and others. In the fall of 1954, the American Cancer Society's national board of directors announced its unanimous belief that heavy smokers were at greater risk of cancer than nonsmokers. Adult per capita cigarette consumption fell 10 percent from 1952 to 1954—the largest drop since the beginning of the Great Depression.[24]

The cigarette industry fought back using two strategies. One was the increased marketing of filtered cigarettes with advertising that (falsely) suggested that the filters would trap any harmful toxins before they entered smokers' lungs. The other was a public relations counteroffensive arguing that the science on smoking's impact on health was inconclusive, and pledging the tobacco industry would do its own research on the issue. A centerpiece of that counteroffensive was a full-page advertisement entitled "A Frank Statement to Cigarette Smokers," published in four hundred daily newspapers on January 4, 1954. It said, in part: "We accept an interest in people's health as a basic responsibility, paramount to every other consideration in our business. We believe the products we make are not injurious to health."[25]

What did the U.S. surgeon general—the government's chief health communicator—have to say about all this? Very little.

Many doctors at the time didn't think cigarettes were deadly, or were at best indifferent to the idea. Scheele had trained at one of the nation's premier cancer hospitals and was one of the Public Health Service's top cancer experts, so perhaps he should have known better. But he was among many in science who viewed epidemiology as a second-rate science. His thinking: an epidemiological study could use observations and compile statistics to identify disease trends, but only a laboratory study could identify causation, and at that point no lab study had found large quantities of any known human carcinogen in cigarette smoke. Nor had any proved cigarette smoke caused lung cancer in lab animals.[26]

Wynder got a taste of the surgeon general's skepticism when he phoned Scheele one day in June 1950. Still exhilarated by his recent splash in *JAMA*, Wynder had learned the Public Health Service had declined to fund his proposal for a study involving painting tobacco tar on mice and wanted to complain directly to the man in charge. During the call, Scheele said he'd read the Wynder and Graham paper in *JAMA* and admitted serving on the grant review committee that denied Wynder's latest funding request. Scheele said that, regarding a link between smoking and cigarettes, "the same correlation could be drawn to the intake of milk," according to Wynder's account of the exchange. "Since nothing has been proved, there exists no reason why experimental work should be continued along this line," Scheele reportedly added.

Wynder came away from the exchange with the impression that Scheele was "utterly stupid" and did not believe smoking could cause lung cancer.[27]

By 1954, Scheele was willing to allow that there was a statistical correlation between smoking and lung cancer, but remained unconvinced it was a causal relationship. More damning epidemiological studies and more controversy came in the next two years. In the summer of 1956— just before he left office—Scheele finally allowed NIH officials to join the American Cancer Society and the American Heart Association in sponsoring a study group on smoking and health. But whatever they found would be something the next surgeon general would have to deal with.

HEW Are You

Meanwhile, the federal health bureaucracy had changed considerably.

Scheele became surgeon general during Harry Truman's Democratic administration, when the Service was under Oscar Ewing and the Federal Security Administration. In 1950, Truman proposed a federal reorganization that would have turned the FSA into a cabinet-level department of health and human services, with Ewing its head. But congressional Republicans—closely allied with the AMA—shot down the idea. They distrusted Ewing, believing he would use his cabinet position to push national health insurance and expand the bureaucracy.

Dwight Eisenhower revived the proposal after he was elected president in 1952. Ike replaced Ewing with Oveta Culp Hobby, a Houston newspaper publisher and longtime political supporter. Eisenhower and Hobby liked the basics of Truman's earlier plan and submitted a new version to Congress in March 1953. They pitched it differently, winning the AMA over by vowing they had no interest in using the new organization to promote "socialized medicine." Congressional Republicans also embraced the plan. U.S. Senator Joseph R. McCarthy of Wisconsin— the chairman of the Senate Government Operations Committee— thought it would be a good way to get rid of the FSA's "deadwood and debris."[28]

On April 11, 1953, the U.S. Department of Health, Education, and Welfare—HEW, for short—was born. Hobby was named secretary, making her one of the first women to serve in a presidential cabinet. The surgeon general was to still head the Public Health Service, and Eisenhower pledged that Scheele would have direct access to Hobby.

However, he also created a new position right under the secretary, a potential middleman with the title "special assistant for health and medical affairs. The special assistant was something the AMA wanted: a highly placed official who would share the interests of organized medicine and advise the HEW secretary on legislation and health programs, and ideally someone the AMA would help select. The special assistant was to be paid $15,000 a year, less than Hobby's $22,500 but more than the surgeon general's base pay of $14,186.[29] Fifteen grand may have seemed fine to a career Service doctor, but prominent private-practice physicians made much more. Indeed, the amount was so low that it torpedoed the AMA's goals: most interested candidates were either unimpressive to Hobby or too idealistic for the AMA. The first two men to hold the job were physicians from academia who made no attempt to usurp the surgeon general's authority.[30]

Scheele enjoyed a close working relationship with Hobby, who also did little to limit Scheele. She kept the HEW's administrative staff small, and decided not to ask Congress to transfer to her the surgeon general's various legal authorities.[31] Knowing little about federal health programs, she was happy to defer to Scheele on those matters. Ike liked Scheele, too. They had of course met during the war, then again a few years later, when Eisenhower was serving as president of Columbia University and had phoned Scheele to discuss Public Health Service grants to the university. When Ike became the nation's chief executive, he was always friendly to Scheele when they saw each other.[32]

Scheele had good relationships with power brokers in Congress, but was careful regarding Senator McCarthy. McCarthy was elected to the Senate in 1946 but was not well known until February 1950, when he began alleging that Communists, Soviet spies, and their sympathizers had infiltrated the federal government—and that he had a list of some of their names. Ultimately unable to back up his claims, McCarthy was disgraced in 1954 after an ill-advised attack on the U.S. Army. But before then, for roughly four years, he tapped into a growing fear of Soviet Russia and bullied his way to power. He became chairman of the Senate Committee on Government Operations in 1953, giving him power over the creation of HEW.

Most of McCarthy's witch-hunt attacks were aimed at the State Department, the Truman administration, and the army. He never investigated Scheele. Indeed, to Scheele's recollection, McCarthy investigated only one member of the entire Public Health Service—a cancer researcher who aroused suspicion for pulling his shades down at night and having a series of late-night visitors (scientist friends, it turned out).[33]

But to some degree, Scheele was complicit in perpetuating McCarthyism. Scientists who received federal health grants were subject to be reviewed for un-American activities, and the Service sometimes simply cut off researchers if any suspicion arose, even if the questions stemmed from anonymous and unproven allegations. "We were instructed to go and discontinue grants from people without telling them why. . . . They were considered to be security risks. It was very unsavory and we didn't like it," said William H. Stewart, a PHS officer at the National Heart Institute's grants branch in 1953 and 1954 (who would go on to become surgeon general in the mid-1960s).[34] The list of researchers denied NIH grants at this time included some of the most esteemed researchers of the era, including Linus Pauling, the Nobel Prize–winning scientist and McCarthy target who had been speaking out against government loyalty investigations since the late 1940s.[35]

Scheele later called the campaign to root out alleged Communist sympathizers a "silly little business" and said he was glad when White House leaders finally put an end to it.[36] That Scheele himself took no stand against it may be understandable; even Eisenhower initially declined to counter McCarthy. It is lamentable, nevertheless.

The Cutter Incident

While McCarthy was on a tear in the early 1950s, so too was polio. Record-setting outbreaks had occurred in 1949, and 1952 was even worse, with more than 21,000 people paralyzed.[37] It was one of the most dreaded diseases in the public consciousness. Its outbreaks—which usually occurred in late summer—frequently cast a pall over vacations as worried mothers pulled their children from swimming holes or other places where they might catch the virus.

The first U.S. polio epidemic was reported in 1894, when an outbreak in central Vermont killed eighteen children and permanently paralyzed fifty more. By 1916, when more than 27,000 cases were reported in twenty states, it was a full-fledged national heartache.[38] Polio's most famous victim was afflicted in the summer of 1921: Franklin D. Roosevelt—then an athletic thirty-nine-year-old politician from New York—developed the illness while vacationing on an island near the coast of Maine.

In the 1930s, Roosevelt would not only become president but also cofound the National Foundation for Infantile Paralysis, an organization that funded polio research and treatment and that later became known as the March of Dimes. When the organization was created in 1938, the federal government was spending virtually nothing on polio, and the Public Health Service offered little support. The National Foundation—led by Basil O'Connor, who had once been Roosevelt's law partner—in the early 1950s provided pivotal polio vaccine research funding to an ambitious University of Pittsburgh physician named Jonas Salk.

When Salk's vaccine was ready for testing, the National Foundation heavily promoted a national clinical trial involving 1.8 million children. It was the largest trial of a drug or vaccine ever conducted in the world to that time, and the study received breathless, front-page media attention. The results were announced at 10:20 A.M. on April 12, 1955, in a televised press conference at the University of Michigan in front of 150 reporters. As the vaccine was declared a clear success, church bells rang and parents wept with joy.

The National Foundation had already made deals with six manufacturers that would produce the vaccine, and even made plans to distribute it to 7 million first- and second-graders across the country. But only the government had the resources to carry out a comprehensive national vaccination program, and no such campaign could take place until the government licensed the product.[39] Enter Surgeon General Leonard Scheele.

After a hasty review of the vaccine's potency and a final look at the safety data, Scheele approved the vaccine. The approval came the same day as the Michigan announcement, and Scheele was actually tardy about it. His boss, HEW Secretary Hobby, wanted to sign the approval documents in front of photographers at a 4 P.M. press conference, but Scheele begged a little more time to go over everything and the press conference was scratched. Hobby ended up signing at 5:15, saying; "It's a wonderful day for the whole world. It's a history making day."[40]

Six companies were approved to make the vaccine—Cutter Laboratories of Berkeley, California; Eli Lilly Company of Indianapolis; Parke, Davis & Co. of Detroit; Pittman-Moore Company of Zionville, Indiana; Sharp & Dohme of Philadelphia; and Wyeth Laboratories Inc. of Marietta, Pennsylvania.

Almost immediately, there were problems.

Questions quickly arose about when all U.S. children could be immunized. It was already spring—summer polio outbreaks were just a few months away—and each child was supposed to get three shots to be considered fully vaccinated. A large-scale government expenditure was needed, as well as aggressive federal management of the campaign. But Hobby dragged her feet; such a "big government" approach was anathema to the Republican Eisenhower administration. She finally requested $28 million from Congress for the campaign, even though experts estimated that between $100 million and $140 million would be needed to vaccinate all U.S. children.[41] Faced with limited resources and production capacity, Scheele decided that children ages five to nine—the group considered the most vulnerable to polio—would have to be prioritized.

Then a worse dilemma erupted. Scattered reports had begun to surface of polio symptoms in vaccinated children. By April 26—just two weeks after the Michigan proclamation—health officials noticed a pattern of children becoming sick four to ten days after receiving vaccine from one company, Cutter Laboratories.

Federal scientists met around the clock to hash over the problem. Some believed the vaccination program should be suspended immediately until the apparent problem could be sorted out, but others argued there was not enough information to make a sound decision. Scheele was limited in what he could do, anyway. He did not have the legal authority to remove lots from the market, and suspending Cutter's license would be a controversial and lengthy undertaking. On April 27, he called Cutter officials, and they agreed to voluntarily recall unused doses, though 400,000 had already been given.[42] Cutter put out a press release to explain the recall.

Scheele issued his own press statement, too, saying six paralytic polio cases were being studied for their possible link to the product. He quickly added that there was not yet evidence of a relationship between the Cutter vaccine and illnesses—it was possible the unfortunate children had already been infected with poliovirus before they got vaccinated. "But we felt the safest course was to make a study," he said.[43] It was the first of a series of sober, "no reason for anyone to be alarmed" statements from Scheele. In fact, he didn't know if there was reason to be alarmed or not, but was trying to find out. He assigned Public Health Service investigators to look into Cutter's manufacturing process, approved creation of a CDC surveillance unit to look for polio cases in kids who'd recently gotten the shot, and set up a committee of top scientific experts to advise him going forward.

As more reports came in, the news was grim. There was a statistical probability that at least a handful of kids getting each company's vaccine would still get polio, but Cutter was seeing numbers in dramatic excess of predictions. By the first week of May, Cutter-vaccinated children diagnosed with polio numbered thirty-seven—more than twice as many as those from any other manufacturer, including Lilly, which had produced more than eight times as much vaccine.[44]

Investigators soon discovered what was wrong. The Salk vaccine used virus that was killed with formaldehyde, but the Cutter workers weren't doing their job well enough and live virus was getting through. Then, more bad news: one lot of the Wyeth vaccine was linked to twenty-six cases and it also had to be recalled.[45] On May 7 Scheele announced he was suspending the vaccination campaign for several days until an investigation could be completed. The vaccine's supporters called the suspension an outrageous overreaction. Salk, the recently christened national hero, felt any cases of polio in vaccinated kids was merely coincidence. Basil O'Connor went ballistic. "He threatened to have me fired," Scheele later recalled.[46]

Meanwhile, congressional Democrats saw blood in the water from what appeared to be a serious self-inflicted wound by the Republican Eisenhower administration. Senator Hubert Humphrey of Minnesota, a registered pharmacist, accused the Public Health Service of having been too hasty in licensing the vaccine. But most of the ire was directed at Scheele's boss, Secretary Hobby. Technically, *she* was the one who had licensed the vaccines (albeit on the advice of Scheele and his men), and she was the HEW official most berated during congressional hearings over the Cutter incident. Scheele later recalled that more often than not, an angry legislator would say, "It wasn't the Surgeon General. It was that woman over there in the Department of Health, Education and Welfare—Mrs. Hobby. She should be fired."[47]

They wanted her out and they soon got their wish. On May 18, Eisenhower announced Hobby was resigning to care for her ailing seventy-seven-year-old husband. At the press conference, Eisenhower said her leaving had nothing at all to do with the polio vaccination campaign. "I think she has done a magnificent job," he said.[48] The president may have been telling the truth; Hobby would not have been his choice for a scapegoat. She had been one of his earliest and most influential political supporters and he seemed to genuinely like her. But the timing of her husband's illness was certainly convenient, and it seemed like a bone thrown to the vaccination campaign's growing pack of critics.

As Hobby packed her things, the vaccination campaign was beginning to find its feet. Scheele's suspension of vaccination was lifted after only five days, meaning that in mid-May doses were again being released. The government toughened safety testing standards for vaccine production. Reports of illnesses from the Cutter vaccine began to ebb. And by June, the Cutter incident—ultimately blamed for 260 illnesses, including 11 deaths—was considered over. When Congress held hearings on the vaccination campaign in late May and June, the focus had shifted to finding the best way to expand the program.[49]

The nation moved on, but Scheele had clearly erred. The Public Health Service had been lax both in planning the national polio vaccination campaign and in making sure the vaccine was safe. When problems arose, Scheele went on *Face the Nation* and other national TV programs and told everyone the vaccine was all right when he didn't know that was the case. Appearing before the media on almost a daily basis, he delivered messages that were an odd mix of caution about the vaccine and advocacy for vaccination. Many people weren't sure what to think. The *New York Times,* writing about the polio vaccination mess in late May, said, "For five weeks the situation has been characterized by a degree of confusion remarkable even by Washington standards."[50]

Scheele had defenders. Salk, for example, believed Scheele's carefully crafted statements prevented panic and saved the vaccination program. But the surgeon general wasn't honest with the public, and was perhaps too good a friend to vaccine manufacturers. "He endured the Cutter affair without once suggesting that the disaster was a disaster or that any party to it was other than a splendid fellow," the journalist Richard Carter wrote in the 1960s. "When time came to assign blame, he diffused it expertly."[51]

Scheele's Departure

Hobby had taken most of the heat for the Cutter affair, and Scheele seemed to emerge from the mess in good standing. He formed a good working relationship with Hobby's successor, Marion Folsom, a former Eastman Kodak executive who took over in the summer of 1955. Like Hobby, Folsom was largely a hands-off administrator when it came to the Public Health Service. In 1956, Scheele was appointed to his third term, and sworn in on April 16. Two months later, the forty-eight-year-old surgeon general suddenly resigned.

Why? He said he wanted more money. He was leaving his $17,000-a-year government job for a $60,000-a-year executive position at Warner-Lambert Pharmaceutical Company "in the interests of providing more properly for the future of my family," he told reporters.[52] But some in the Public Health Service believed there were other reasons. "I think Scheele was spiritually a casualty of the Salk vaccine," said Warren Palmer Dearing, a longtime Service physician who was a good friend of Scheele's. "He was distressed by it. He kept his own counsel, but I think he was deeply hurt and grieved. He didn't come out looking bad, but he didn't come out looking like a hero."[53]

Scheele would work for Warner-Lambert for twelve years before retiring in 1968. He had an unusual and brief return to federal service in 1962. Needing a pharmaceuticals expert and recognizing Scheele's extensive international health experience, President John F. Kennedy asked him to help in negotiations to get Cuba to free 1,133 captured prisoners following the hapless Bay of Pigs invasion. Scheele traveled to Havana and helped arrange delivery of $60 million worth of baby food and medical supplies in exchange for the captives' release.[54]

When he retired, Scheele moved from New Jersey back to Washington, D.C., where he spent the rest of his life. When he was eighty-five, he came down with pneumonia and died, on January 8, 1993. He was buried in Arlington National Cemetery.

Scheele left the Office of the Surgeon General with lofty status. His successors had it progressively worse.

LEROY BURNEY

A Town Called Burney

Scheele's successor was underwhelming. Leroy Edgar Burney was an unremarkable fifty-year-old—slim, five feet, ten inches with blue eyes and specks of gray in his brown hair. Quiet, amiable, and conservative were the three adjectives most often used to describe him. Reporters trying to make him sound interesting usually failed in the attempt. One journalist wrote that the three great loves of his life were public health, his family, and Indiana. Another noted he liked to swim and read American history.[55]

He was a consensus pick—the Eisenhower administration had asked a few high-ranking, politically appointed health officials to write on paper names of candidates to succeed Scheele, and Burney's was the one name that appeared on every person's submission. He may not have been at the top of anyone's list, but he had two dozen years in public health and was an important soldier in Parran's war on venereal disease. "Dr. Burney's experience eminently qualified him for the post," HEW Secretary Marion Folsom told the *New York Times*.[56]

He seemed to be walking into a good situation. The polio vaccine scarcity problem had been resolved. Congress, stung by Scheele's bolt for private-sector money, had raised the surgeon general's salary to $22,626—a 33 percent increase. What's more, Burney was going to work for Folsom, who had been content to let the Public Health Service take care of itself.

But Burney would leave office after only four years, the first surgeon general not reappointed at least once. He would handle the insult the way he handled everything else—mildly. "I think Dr. Burney was a little bit hurt, miffed, that he was not reappointed," said Luther Terry, the man who succeeded him. "He was not rude or even uncordial, but he wasn't cordial either."[57]

Burney was born on New Year's Eve, 1906, in Burney, Indiana, a muddy village of about three hundred in the state's southeastern corner. The place was named for his Scotch-Irish great-grandfather, a farmer who ended up quite wealthy. Burney's parents were less affluent; his father was a millwright and mechanic, and his mother a housewife. The boy's interest in medicine came from an uncle, Cecil Gardner Harrod, who was the town's doctor. He took young Leroy with him on house calls, initially in a horse and buggy and later in a crank-start Model T.[58]

Later in his childhood, his parents moved to Indianapolis, where he graduated high school in 1924. He attended nearby Butler University for two years, then transferred to Indiana University, where he earned his bachelor of science and medical degrees. During his senior year in medical school, Burney met A.J. McLaughlin, "a very engaging Irishman" who had come to speak to students about careers in the Public Health Service. Intellectually sharp and physically striking in his Service officer's uniform, McLaughlin deeply impressed Burney. After graduating medical school in 1930, Burney interned at the Service's Chicago marine hospital, where McLaughlin worked. He also took the competitive exam to enter the regular corps—and failed. "I am probably the only Surgeon General that didn't pass the first time," Burney later recalled.[59]

McLaughlin helped Burney get a one-year fellowship at Johns Hopkins University's public health school that positioned the young physician for another run at the exam. Burney passed in 1932 and joined the Commissioned Corps; his first assignment was at the marine hospital in Cleveland. That same year he married Mildred Hewins, an Indiana schoolteacher he had met on a blind date. The Presbyterian couple had two children.[60]

Burney moved through a progression of assignments. After Cleveland, he was sent to the venereal disease clinic in Hot Springs, Arkansas. Then came postings in New York City; Springfield, Missouri; and Chicago. In 1936, he was named assistant to Raymond Vonderlehr, chief of the venereal disease program under Parran. (Earlier, Vonderlehr had been the first on-site director of the Tuskegee Syphilis Experiment.) During his stint in Arkansas, Burney had worked for another Tuskegee Study leader, Oliver C. Wenger, who had strongly supported the decision not to inform the study's participants about the care that wasn't provided. (Burney believed in the Tuskegee Experiment his whole life, and allowed it to continue when he was surgeon general.)

After a number of other assignments, the Public Health Service loaned Burney to the state of Indiana, where he served as state health commissioner for nine years. Burney loved the job. He succeeded in getting a variety of public health bills through the state legislature and enjoyed a teaching position at the Indiana University School of Medicine (his academic salary was paid for by the pharmaceutical company Eli Lilly). He had many connections, including a friendship with *Indianapolis Star* columnist Maurice Early, who frequently wrote about what Burney was up to. When Scheele called him to Washington in 1954 to serve as assistant chief in the Service's Bureau of State Services, Burney initially didn't want to go.[61]

Two years later, after Scheele's resignation, Burney was known well enough in Washington to win the surgeon general job. Eisenhower installed Burney through a recess appointment. The Indiana doctor was sworn in on August 8, 1956.[62]

Asian Flu and Arthur Flemming

In February 1957, report of a new flu virus—dubbed the "Asian strain"—began to trickle in from China. It quickly spread and by April and May, U.S. military bases in Japan and Korea were suffering outbreaks, and U.S. officials began preparing for the flu to hit the United States. Flu epidemics had been striking the nation every few years, but they were always driven by a familiar flu bug. This Asian strain was something different, what scientists called a true antigenic shift (as was the 1918 Spanish influenza strain)—and something the flu vaccines developed in the 1940s were not geared for.

The first cases within the United States were reported in June. Just as Rupert Blue had done most of the federal government's talking during the 1918 Spanish flu pandemic, Burney was the point man in 1957. In August, Burney became a constant presence in the media, calmly explaining that a new flu vaccine was being developed and that he had asked six manufacturers to turn out doses as fast as possible, in an effort to vaccinate Americans before the virus became widespread. "This is the first time in history that a country has been able to take such preliminary steps in advance of a possible epidemic of influenza," he told reporters.[63]

But in a turn of events that would largely be repeated in the swine flu pandemic of 2009, the slow pace of vaccine production became an issue. The virus was isolated by May, but it took time to make enough doses to cover the U.S. population. The virus had to be grown in millions of fertilized eggs, then killed and purified before being put into syringes—a process that could take at least three months. Even working seven days a week, the six manufacturers produced no more than 8 million doses by mid-September. Burney recommended—but did not mandate—that shots should be prioritized for certain high-risk patients, for doctors and other health care workers, and for people who worked in the transportation, communications, and utilities industries. He also had the CDC set up a new monitoring system to track the flu's progress. The result was the National Health Survey, involving weekly interviews of a nationally representative sample of two thousand people. Now known as the National Health Interview Survey, it remains an important source of national health trend data.

Burney did a pretty good job as the government's lead spokesman on the unfolding epidemic. Rupert Blue's calming messages in 1918 had proved absurd as it became clear that the Spanish flu was much deadlier than Blue had stated. But Burney was pretty much on the money. He correctly predicted the pandemic would envelop the United States in the autumn of 1957. He accurately warned that a second wave of cases could occur in the winter. He even prodded a reluctant President Eisenhower to get a shot in late August, at the outset of the vaccination campaign, and helped persuade 7 million Americans to get vaccinated in the early autumn.[64]

Burney also settled a problem that seems to erupt in the media every time a new flu pandemic comes along: what to call the virus. The traditional practice is to name it after the place where it was first identified, but reporters were using a variety of monikers, including Asiatic, Far Eastern, Oriental, and—simply—"foreign." The *New York Times* deemed the debate settled after a call to Burney's office elicited this statement: "The Surgeon General says it's Asian."[65]

Despite all that, the program was a failure in one crucial respect. The vaccine was judged 50 to 70 percent effective in various tests and no doubt prevented some illnesses, softened others, and saved lives. But not enough of it was prepared in time for the first wave, and the public didn't buy Burney's prediction about a second wave. After a surge of relatively mild illnesses peaked around Halloween, many Americans assumed the worst was over. Vaccinations fell so dramatically that by December the manufacturers—voluntary partners in the campaign—cut production. When a deadly second wave of Asian flu arrived in early 1958, many were not vaccinated. Modern-day health officials remember Burney's campaign as one that fell short in heading off the second wave. "We didn't want a false sense of complacency, which is what happened in 1957," said Anne Schuchat, the CDC official who was the government's most-used spokesperson during the swine flu pandemic of 2009.[66]

The final toll: the Asian flu caused about a quarter of the U.S. population to get sick. It was also blamed for nearly 70,000 U.S. deaths—nothing like the 1918–19 pandemic, but terrible by today's standards.

As the Asian flu pandemic played out, Burney was dealing with new challenges in the vaccine campaign against polio. The Cutter incident was over, but now there was a different problem—a debate over whether to continue using the Salk vaccine or to switch to an alternative developed by Albert Sabin.

Sabin was a University of Cincinnati virologist who had immigrated to the United States from Poland as a teenager. He began working on polio in the 1930s, and proved that the virus entered through the mouth and digestive system and then invaded nerve tissue (it was previously believed to enter through the nose and attack through the respiratory system). He developed a vaccine using a different approach. Whereas Salk killed polio virus and put it in an injection, Sabin developed a system for attenuating—weakening, but not killing—polio virus and putting it in drops added to a sugar cube or teaspooned into a child's mouth, or both. He believed it was the best way to confer long-term immunity.

Sabin and Salk became intense rivals. Salk's vaccine had distinct advantages. It was assumed to be safer. It was faster out of the gate, ready for its large-scale U.S. trial in 1954, when Sabin's vaccine was still in development. And it had the full support of Basil O'Connor.

O'Connor's March of Dimes had given Sabin more than $1 million to develop his vaccine. But the organization spent more on Salk and, by the late 1950s, was completely in his corner—even as multiple problems with the Salk vaccine became evident. The Cutter incident could be attributed to manufacturing snafus, but even when the shots were made correctly, it soon became clear that three, or even four, shots were necessary to guarantee protection. After an initial decline in polio cases, illness reports were up in 1958 and then again in 1959. (Salk blamed it on manufacturers failing to meet potency standards.) O'Connor and Salk pressured Burney to stay the course, arguing that introducing another vaccine would taint scientists' ability to see how well Salk's vaccine was working.[67]

In 1958, the surgeon general held a special meeting with top health leaders to discuss ways to increase uptake of the Salk vaccine. Swayed by O'Connor and Salk, Burney did not support Sabin's bid to run a large trial in the United States, and Sabin was forced to do his study in the Soviet Union.

The Sabin trial, involving millions of children, was a huge success. In 1960, Sabin and his supporters went to Burney for approval to bring the attenuated vaccine onto the U.S. market. Sabin had gathered important backers by then, including some major pharmaceutical companies. In August 1960, Burney defied O'Connor and approved the Sabin version for trial manufacture, a first step toward licensure. The next year, 1961, would be the last that only the Salk vaccine was given in the United States.[68] The Sabin vaccine would become the nation's primary polio vaccine until around 2000, when an improved version of the Salk vaccine became the new standard.

As he contended with O'Connor, Burney also had to deal with headaches within HEW. One was James Shannon, the former Scheele protégé who had become the powerful director of the NIH. Burney was his boss, but Shannon was becoming quasi-independent. (When it came to medical research, Shannon was considered a more important voice in congressional hearings than Burney.)[69]

The other was Arthur S. Flemming, who became HEW secretary in 1958. Flemming—a university administrator with a long history of advising the government—got the job after Marion Folsom suffered a small stroke and resigned. Folsom had allowed Burney a free hand in running the Public Health Service. Flemming was more of a micromanager, and someone who believed he should be the HEW's lead voice on at least some health matters.[70] He led the Eisenhower administration's drafting of a plan to provide a comprehensive voluntary health plan for the elderly (the kind of thing Parran might have handled a dozen years earlier). And he was the government's primary spokesman during the Great Cranberry Crisis of 1959.

The crisis unfolded at a press conference seventeen days before Thanksgiving. Flemming announced that government testing had found two batches of cranberries from Oregon and Washington that were tainted with aminotriazole, a toxic weed killer that in large amounts has caused thyroid cancer in lab rats. The government hadn't yet worked out how to sort out contaminated cranberries from the others, he said, so consumers should simply avoid buying cranberries until further notice.

The advisory caused quite a row. Cranberry growers hissed at Flemming in the press, accusing him of making a capricious decision that jeopardized their business, and they managed to win shows of support from a list of big names. Agriculture Secretary Ezra Benson publicly ate a bowl of cranberries. Vice President Richard Nixon downed four helpings of cranberry sauce. Presidential candidate John F. Kennedy made a show of drinking cranberry juice. By Thanksgiving a testing system had been developed, and Flemming said the public could again buy them safely. He even allowed a *New York Herald Tribune* photographer to take pictures of him and his wife eating them—a photo that went out on the wire and ran in newspapers around the world.[71]

Flemming actually fancied himself to be good with the press, but he wasn't driven only by love of the limelight. Eisenhower assigned Flemming to work on the elderly health plan, deeming it the responsibility of a cabinet officer. Likewise, the cranberry flap was an HEW secretary responsibility: the HEW secretary had been vested with responsibility for handling this cranberry kind of matter by the Delaney clause of the Food Additives Amendment of 1958, which deemed as unsafe any additive found to induce cancer in man or animal.[72]

But the net effect was that during a high-profile flap over a public health concern, the HEW secretary was the government presence behind the podium, not the surgeon general. And Burney's authority dissipated a little more.

The surgeon general did make a splash, however, on the issue of cigarettes.

Two Statements

Burney is often credited as the first federal official to identify smoking as a cause of lung cancer. Cumming had decried the effect of smoking on women, of course, but his concern had more to do with morals than science. Parran had been silent on the issue, as had Scheele. And no Treasury Department or FSA or HEW administrators had raised any health alarms about cigarettes in all those years. So it was Burney, a pipe smoker who also liked cigars, who became the first to sound a specific health alarm.

But it took some prodding. Just before Scheele left office in the summer of 1956, he allowed NIH officials to join the American Cancer Society and the American Heart Association in a study on smoking and health. In March 1957, the *Atlanta Constitution* newspaper got hold of a draft of the group's report, which called smoking cigarettes a health hazard. In June, the British Health Ministry warned its citizens that heavy smoking was accompanied by a higher risk of lung cancer. It was time—really, it was past time—for the U.S. surgeon general to say something.

Burney issued a 660-word statement to the press on July 12, 1957, saying, "It is clear there is an increasing and consistent body of evidence that excessive cigarette smoking is one of the causative factors in lung cancer." (Excessive smoking was defined as two or more packs a day.) Michael Shimkin of the National Cancer Institute and Ernst Wynder of Washington University had persuaded Burney to make the statement; his political bosses had nothing to do with it. "When I discussed my plans and the supporting data with Secretary Folsom, his response was that it was my decision to make and all he and the White House wanted was a copy of the press release," Burney later recalled.[73]

The statement was sent to the press, to the American Medical Association, and to public health officers of all the states. It got front-page coverage in major newspapers, and helped lead to widespread knowledge of the dangers of smoking.[74] In a national survey later that month, nearly 80 percent of Americans said they were aware of recent reports of the dangers of smoking (George Gallup called it a phenomenal figure in the annals of polling). But knowing and believing are two different things. Smokers remained swayed by the tobacco industry's argument that Burney was talking only about statistical associations and there was no scientific consensus that smoking caused cancer.[75]

It didn't help that the Burney refused to press the issue. Less than two weeks after making his statement, he and National Cancer Institute director John Heller were called before a congressional hearing run by Representative John Blatnik, a Minnesota Democrat who distrusted tobacco advertising. When they were asked what they were doing to warn the public about smoking's hazards, they said it was not their role to lead a national education campaign or put warning labels on cigarettes. "The States are sovereign in matters of health" and should handle such communications, Burney said. The Public Health Service planned but didn't issue a pamphlet to physicians about smoking and health; Service officials couldn't agree to what extent it should blame smoking for lung cancer.[76]

Burney certainly hadn't hurt the tobacco companies. They had been marching together in a public relations strategy developed by Hill & Knowlton, a public relations firm they collectively hired in 1953. The companies made a show of caring about smokers while arguing there was no scientific consensus that smoking was dangerous. Burney—cautious and conservative about the studies, and unwilling to push for federal action—did not dispel the tobacco companies' argument that the science was unsettled. Burney's 1957 statement amounted to little more than a brief splash in the newspapers. Tobacco sales continued to shoot up, setting a new record in 1958.[77]

Burney soon realized he had to do something more. When a Public Health Service information officer suggested he write an article for the *Journal of the American Medical Association,* he agreed. (However, though he was listed as sole author, Burney had relatively little involvement in creating the 5,000-word article. As would become the pattern with future surgeon general's reports, the real work was done by Service officers who wrote, edited, and critiqued the manuscript.)[78] The *JAMA* article, published in the November 28, 1959, issue, was stronger than the 1957 statement. Nodding to even more recent research, it said smoking was the main reason for the national increase in lung cancer, and that nonsmokers have lower risks of lung cancer than all smokers—not just heavy smokers. It also dismissed tobacco companies' claims that the filters in filtered cigarettes were protecting smokers from carcinogens.[79]

But Burney still wasn't saying the government was going to do anything about it. The Public Health Service issued a low-key press release that signaled governmental ambivalence about the article's significance. Tobacco industry officials helped minimize it, calling it a warmed-over rehash of old statistics that failed to give enough weight to contradictory scientific evidence.[80] As a result, the press did not play it as prominently as the 1957 statement. The *New York Times* put a story about Burney's article on page 31. (In the same edition, a photo of Flemming's wife serving cranberry sauce was displayed on the front page.)[81]

Two weeks later, Burney was further undermined by *JAMA*'s new editor. John Talbott was a prickly Buffalo researcher with a conservative bent who had taken over the job just a month before Burney's piece was published. He felt Burney's article needed a follow-up editorial, and the one he wrote was harsh. "A number of authorities who have examined the same evidence cited by Dr. Burney do not agree with his conclusions. . . . Neither the opponents nor the proponents of the smoking theory have sufficient evidence to warrant the assumption of an all-or-none authoritative position," it said.[82]

Burney was shocked by the editorial, and worried that it would be interpreted as the position of the American Medical Association. He was also stung by a response published in *JAMA* a short time later by Joseph Berkson, a Mayo Clinic scientist who would eventually become known as a de facto spokesman for the tobacco industry. Berkson wrote that Burney's article misinterpreted research and "is characterized by an imprecision of language and thought that renders inaccurate almost every important point it deals with."[83]

The smoking efforts aside, Burney believed he'd been doing a good job. He was considered a trailblazer in the arena of radiologic health, warning of the lung cancer dangers to uranium miners and creating the nation's first education programs for management of atomic radiation. So it was a jarring disappointment when he lost his job.

Burney's Departure

John F. Kennedy was elected president in November 1960. Burney had been part of Eisenhower's Republican administration, but had reason to believe he'd remain in the job. Surgeons general were traditionally considered apolitical professionals who carried on through White House transitions. Eisenhower had kept Scheele on; Herbert Hoover had reappointed Hugh Cumming; Woodrow Wilson had retained Rupert Blue; and so forth. But Burney's four-year term happened to end right at the beginning of the Kennedy administration. While the new president was selecting a new HEW secretary and other administration officials, it seemed natural to pick a new surgeon general, too.

Years later, Burney reflected that it was probably for the best. He said he probably would not have liked working for Kennedy's new HEW secretary, Abraham Ribicoff, or for Ribicoff's powerful assistant, Wilbur Cohen. Cohen had helped craft the Social Security program in the 1930s and was returning to federal service to push for dramatic new changes in national health policy. "I'm a moderate and not a social activist," Burney said. Cohen, meanwhile, loathed the prospect of trying to shake things up with such a restrained surgeon general in place. "On Burney, I was adamant," Cohen said years later. "Burney was a competent man but a reactionary. . . . No, Burney was the one man I told Ribicoff that absolutely couldn't be Surgeon General. I'd accept almost anyone else."[84]

Burney's last day in office was January 29, 1961. He retired and then worked for years as a vice president for health science at Philadelphia's Temple University. But he continued to count himself as a member of the Service's old guard, and to defend his legacy and that of his mentors, including the Tuskegee Experiment. In a 1988 interview, Burney blasted the government worker who finally leaked the story to the press, and argued that people who criticized the study did not understand the scientific impulse behind it. "One is reminded of the aphorism, 'Idealism increases in direct proportion to one's distance from the problem,'" he said. "I do not believe there was any substance or justification at all to the outcry."[85]

Burney died in the summer of 1998 at a hospital in Park Ridge, Illinois, at the age of ninety-one. He was buried in his native Indiana, at Crown Hill Cemetery in Indianapolis. Ironically, the first surgeon general to issue a substantial warning about smoking was buried near the mausoleum of Thomas R. Marshall, a U.S. vice president under Woodrow Wilson who famously said, "What this country needs is a really good five-cent cigar!"[86]

It's appropriate that the two are buried near each other. Marshall was a "Progressive with the brakes on" whose hesitation to take strong action would later have tragic repercussions.[87] Burney—and, for that matter, Scheele before him—left similar legacies. They were national leaders who made important contributions, but (like Marshall) failed to assert their power at critical junctures, and that failure had implications for the surgeons general themselves as power would slip away at an accelerating rate.

CHAPTER 6

"They Are Giving the Public Health Service Away!"

Life for surgeons general had been pretty good in the 1950s. As the new decade began, there was reason to believe that would continue. President John F. Kennedy, elected in 1960, appointed two HEW secretaries— Abraham Ribicoff and, later, Anthony Celebrezze. Both had other things to do than monkey with the surgeon general. The department was growing larger and harder to manage and was saddled with controversial issues ranging from Social Security reform to school desegregation. (HEW was sometimes called "the Department of Headaches," the *New York Times* noted at the time.)[1]

But though the secretary was occupied with other things, there was a more meddlesome HEW official whom the new surgeon general would have to deal with. He was Wilbur Cohen, the HEW's bouncy and very determined assistant secretary for legislation. Cohen was the number 3 man in the department, the administrator with the most Washington experience, and the one with the biggest dreams. And he intended to whittle away the surgeon general's authority.

Cohen was responsible for persuading Congress to enact the president's health, education, and welfare legislative proposals, and for getting the department to implement them. The men who had held Cohen's job during the Eisenhower administration had little experience or ambition when it came to changing social policy. Cohen, however, fully realized the position's potential. As a young man in the 1930s, he had been a behind-the-scenes tactician in creating Social Security. He later spent several years as an academic at the University of Michigan, mulling over his liberal ideas for social reform. When Kennedy appointed him to HEW in 1961, Cohen was still only forty-seven, energetic—and ready to shake things up.

Health was very much on Cohen's agenda, and he wanted the Public Health Service to be a change agent. He didn't think Burney was up to the task. Said Cohen; "I think he [Burney] might have supported the Kennedy program but he wouldn't have led it. He wouldn't have been a vigorous, dynamic force for leadership in the health field. The big revolution was coming in health. . . . The one thing I told Secretary Ribicoff is that Burney had to go."[2]

Instead, Kennedy's surgeon general would be Luther Terry, the soft-spoken Alabama physician who would issue a report on smoking that would be seen as one of the most important accomplishments of any surgeon general. Nevertheless, Cohen was disappointed in both Terry and Terry's successor, William Stewart. By the end of the decade, Cohen would give up on the lot of them and would strip the surgeon general position of nearly all its powers.

LUTHER TERRY

Alabama Connections

Luther Leonidas Terry was born September 15, 1911, in Red Level, Alabama, a town of just a few hundred people located about twenty miles south of the state capital. His father and role model, James Terry, was the town's doctor. As a teen, Luther would sometimes drive his father on house calls in the family's Model A Ford. If that wasn't enough to prod young Luther toward a medical career, the boy was also named for a doctor—his father's personal physician, Luther Leonidas Hill. The tie between the Terry and Hill families carried into the next generation. Hill's son, Joseph Lister Hill, went on to become a U.S. senator. Seventeen years older than Luther Terry, Lister Hill would chair the Senate subcommittee handling health issues and be the one who got Terry the surgeon general job.[3]

Young Luther Terry at first aimed only to be a physician. He earned a bachelor's degree at Birmingham Southern University in 1931, then his M.D. at Tulane University in 1935. After that came a hospital internship in Birmingham, a residency in Cleveland, a pathology internship in St. Louis, and a gig as instructor and assistant professor at the

University of Texas in Galveston. His main interest was cardiology, but he had also grown an interest in applying his medical knowledge more broadly to public health.

Terry later described the UT-Galveston of the early 1940s as a toxic workplace. He disliked the faculty infighting and didn't trust his supervisor, and was looking for a way out. He'd been collaborating with staff at a Public Health Service hospital in Fort Worth, and the medical officer in charge there—William Ossenfort—cajoled him into joining the Service by promising a choice of working in New York, Norfolk, or Baltimore. Terry chose Baltimore, and stayed in the Baltimore–Washington, D.C., area throughout his rise through the ranks of the Public Health Service.[4]

He built up a large cardiovascular research unit that would become a principal lab of the NIH's National Heart Institute. More than any previous surgeon general, Terry was a researcher, co-authoring articles in leading medical journals. He became assistant director of the National Heart Institute in 1958 and was enjoying a nice career there when fate (and Lister Hill) intervened.

In early 1961, it became clear that key people in the new Kennedy administration were not interested in reappointing Burney, and that key congressmen were not interested in fighting to keep him. Among those in the latter group was Senator Hill, who had formed a grudge against Burney over information the surgeon general had once shared with certain Republicans in Congress but not with Hill. During the wheeling and dealing involved in new administration appointments, Hill put Terry's name in the hat (without asking Terry if he wanted the job).

Hill was one of the most powerful men in Washington when it came to health legislation and appropriations, and the incoming Kennedy administration was keen to accommodate him. When Hill recommended Terry to Ribicoff, the new HEW secretary, a job interview for Terry was quickly scheduled. During the one-hour interview, Terry said he thought Burney ought to be reappointed. Ribicoff replied, "'Well, I can assure you that Dr. Burney will not be reappointed. Would you be interested?'" Terry later recalled. "I said, 'Yes, of course I would be interested. It would be a great honor and a privilege.'"[5]

Terry also had the support of U.S. Representative John Fogarty of Rhode Island, who controlled public health spending in the House and happened to be a former heart patient of Terry's.[6] On January 15, 1961, Kennedy announced he was nominating Terry for surgeon general.

Silent Spring *and Smoking*

Terry was surgeon general for only about a year when Rachel Carson's watershed book *Silent Spring* began to appear in serialized form in *The New Yorker* magazine. (The book itself was published later that year, 1962.) *Silent Spring* chronicled the effect of pesticides on the environment and called for the government to be more vigilant and aggressive in combating this problem. Becoming a runaway best seller, the book catalyzed an environmental health movement and a push for new and better environmental legislation.

Traditionally, environmental health programs had been a Public Health Service responsibility. The Public Health Service Act of 1912 authorized the surgeon general and his men to investigate water pollution that might be related to disease. The federal Air Pollution Control Act of 1955 and the Water Pollution Control Act of 1956 gave the surgeon general a primary role in identifying and abating foul things in the environment. But by the early 1960s, a growing number of critics felt the Service was lax about regulating polluters and policing newer forms of water pollution, such as chemical spills. In 1961, government attorneys going after industries that had polluted New Jersey's Raritan Bay were frustrated when Service physicians tried to dampen publicity about the case and took other steps to be less confrontational.[7]

That same year—1961, a year before Carson's *Silent Spring* gained the public's attention—Congress shifted responsibility for water pollution control programs from the surgeon general to the HEW secretary. As with other legislation affecting the PHS, Cohen worked out the details. Cohen also was an architect behind the Clean Air Act of 1963, which empowered the HEW secretary (not the surgeon general) to define air quality criteria. These measures were the beginning of a tumble of reassignments and regulation expansions that culminated in the creation of the U.S. Environmental Protection Agency in 1970.[8]

Losing environmental health was a bitter blow to Service veterans who saw those programs as an essential part of the organization's public health mission. Cohen didn't care. He'd come to see Terry's troops as a bunch of footdraggers, not only on environmental issues but also— and more importantly to Cohen—on issues like creating a national health insurance system and planning oversight of how medical services were provided and distributed. Cohen looked for opportunities to shake things up, but gradually, through legislation creating new programs. Even the ambitious Cohen wanted to prevent gear-grinding dissension in the ranks. "If you begin to take control over old things, then the career people think you're interfering with their business," he said years later. "But they do not object when you take control of policy of something new."[9]

Many Service members disliked Cohen, but they were fond of their surgeon general. They soon came to sing his praises even more, for his heroic stand in the battle against smoking.

Terry was playing an assigned role. A coalition of groups had been pushing the issue for years, among them, the American Cancer Society, the American Heart Association, the National Tuberculosis Association, and the American Public Health Association. The groups sent a letter to President Kennedy on June 1, 1961, asking him to appoint a national commission on smoking. Initially, the White House didn't respond, and then told Terry to meet with them. Terry did and told them he agreed it was time for the Public Health Service to update its position on smoking. But nothing substantive happened until May 1962, when Kennedy was put on the spot at a press conference.

Washington Evening Star reporter L. Edgar Prina asked the president for his views on possible links between smoking and certain disease.[10] Kennedy had been dodging the topic; he was juggling conflicts on several fronts, including the ongoing Cold War, the beginning of the Vietnam War, and a fight with an antagonistic FBI director (J. Edgar Hoover) who had declared that he was aware of phone calls between Kennedy and his mob-connected mistress, Judith Exner. He was wary of a new battle with powerful tobacco companies, their advertising firms, and the politicians and constituents from tobacco-growing states. He was also a smoker himself. Backing away from the landmine the reporter had just set at his feet, Kennedy replied: "That matter is sensitive enough, and the stock market is in sufficient difficulty, without my giving you an answer which is not based on complete information, which I don't have." Kennedy promised he would give a more complete response at his next press conference.[11]

He didn't. Instead, Kennedy tossed the matter to Terry, who informed the press two weeks later that a committee of experts appointed by the surgeon general would examine the evidence concerning smoking's alleged damage to health. Terry promised that the committee would produce the most comprehensive report on the topic ever done.

It was a tall order. Simply building the committee was challenging. Terry's staff came up with a list of 150 candidates from a wide range of medical and scientific disciplines. Intending to produce a report impervious to charges of bias, Terry removed from the list the names of any researcher who had taken a public position on the issue or published a study about it. Then, Terry had the list of potential committee members sent to several interested organizations and allowed them to nix—without explanation—any names they found objectionable. Veto power was granted not only to the American Cancer Society and the American Heart Association but also to the Tobacco Institute and the American Medical Association.

Give cigarette manufacturers a say in compiling the roster? The syndicated columnist Drew Pearson likened it to "having big business pick the judges who will try them in an antitrust suit."[12] Meanwhile, Celebrezze— a pack-a-day smoker who had become HEW secretary in August 1962— made it known that he didn't care for the committee to be too ambitious. "I firmly believe that it is not the proper role of the federal government to tell citizens to stop smoking," regardless of what the committee concluded, he said.[13]

By late October, Terry had an unimpeachable lineup, balanced right down to their personal smoking habits. Five of the ten were smokers, with one of them—Louis Fieser, a Harvard professor of organic chemistry— puffing away during the meetings at a rate of four packs a day. (Fieser would be diagnosed with lung cancer about a year after the committee finished its work.)[14]

The committee's task was to help the surgeon general advise Americans about smoking, and to decide—if warranted—what additional steps the government should take to safeguard the public. The group first met in November 1962 and worked through 1963. The members created a process for judging the strength of the link between smoking and various health problems and then, taking the investigation a step further, for determining if smoking was the actual cause. That in itself was a milestone. "How the committee called something causal, rather than a correlation or association, involved setting a series of principles which became the basic principles within epidemiology," said Ken Warner, a tobacco researcher and former dean of the University of Michigan School of Public Health.[15]

The committee's discussions were kept secret, but late in 1963, word began to trickle out that the report would be made public early in 1964. What would it say? Some took it as a clue when, in November 1963, Terry said he had given up cigarettes in favor of pipe smoking.[16]

Terry had a reputation for understatement, but the logistics of the report's January 11, 1964, release were worthy of a master showman.

On that chilly morning, he hosted a press conference remarkable even by Washington standards. It was on a Saturday, to cause minimal impact on the stock market and maximum exposure in Sunday newspapers. He held it in an auditorium at the State Department that was sealed off from the rest of the building. Copies of the 387-page report were delivered by armored car.[17] The two hundred members of the press who attended were given copies when they arrived and granted two hours to read it—and not allowed to leave—before Terry took their questions. Nine "No Smoking" signs were posted on the walls (unusual at the time), though they were ignored by several reporters and government officials, including Terry's nervous press assistant, J. Stewart Hunter. "I must have smoked 15 cigarettes," he confided to one reporter. "We were scared we'd be stormed by 5,000 folks, all clamoring to get in here."[18]

Such a crowd never materialized, but the two hundred journalists proved sufficient for causing a stir. The report dominated the national news with a crystal-clear message that smoking caused lung cancer and was driving up the male cancer death rate. Smoking was also labeled the most important cause of bronchitis in the United States, and an apparent cause of coronary artery disease. What was more, the report said, there was no valid evidence that filters reduced harmful effects.

The committee also called for "appropriate remedial action" by the government to address the problem, but did not recommend specific steps. However, at the press conference, Terry said he would come up with recommendations to send to Celebrezze.[19] Terry also was in contact with the Federal Trade Commission, a federal agency that had earlier been pushed to mandate cigarette warning labels by U.S. Senator Maurine Neuberger of Oregon.

It was a proud day for Terry, but he soon grew disheartened. Although cigarette sales dropped sharply right after the report was released, they bounced back by April. The surgeon general was also disappointed in the American Medical Association, which proved to be an unreliable ally in an education campaign—the AMA put together a pamphlet that said there remained disagreement about the effect of cigarette smoking on health.[20]

Meanwhile, the Federal Trade Commission was swayed by the Terry committee's report and issued a regulation in June 1964 that no cigarette pack or advertisement could henceforth claim that smoking could lead to health or well-being. The FTC also ordered that cigarette packs carry some sort of label warning of the health hazards from smoking.

The regulation originally was set to take effect in January 1965 but was delayed at the request of Congress. In March 1965, an increasingly discouraged Terry pleaded with Congress to support the regulation. But tobacco companies had taken their case to Congress, too. What emerged was the FTC-preempting Federal Cigarette Labeling and Advertising Act of 1965, which required cigarette packs to carry the following milquetoast warning labels: "Caution: Cigarette Smoking May Be Hazardous to Your Health." (The wording about a "Surgeon General's Warning" was not added until 1969.) But significantly for Terry and his successors, the law also required the FTC to report annually to Congress on cigarette labeling and promotion, and HEW officials to report each year on the health consequences of smoking. That last duty was delegated to the surgeon general.

Weak as it was, the law was an advance in what was becoming a full-blown public health war against tobacco. Terry's legacy was established, and even Cohen praised the surgeon general's persistent handling of the whole tobacco affair. "The smoking report gave more political trouble than almost everything else, because you immediately alienated the North Carolina and Kentucky congressmen and senators, and this created a difficult problem," Cohen said. "But the fact of the matter is Terry should get a lot of credit, because here was a professional question and he was competent in that area, and he followed it through."[21]

Those sentiments were not, however, enough to keep Terry in office.

Terry's Departure

Kennedy was assassinated in November 1963, making Vice President Lyndon Johnson the nation's chief executive. Johnson held the office after winning the 1964 election. Terry had seemed to be in good standing with Johnson, and so it was no surprise when, in February 1965, the president announced Terry would be reappointed.[22] But his second term would not last long.

Cohen had grown unhappy with Terry. He thought the surgeon general was preoccupied with the talented but ambitious NIH director, Jim Shannon, to the exclusion of the items on Cohen's agenda. Terry's angst about NIH was understandable. With powerful and direct support from such power players as the Laskers and congressional leaders, the NIH had become nearly autonomous. For a few years, Shannon's bosses at HEW had virtually no say in the NIH budget, though the reins started to grow a little tighter in 1962 when members of the House Committee on Government Operations voiced concerns that NIH had been growing too quickly and had failed to adequately supervise how grantees were spending research dollars. Shannon was sensitive to congressional criticism, but felt he could ignore Terry.[23]

Terry, meanwhile, had given the impression that he would like to ignore Cohen and Cohen's prioritization of the nascent Medicare program. The surgeon general had done some interagency task force work on creating the Medicare system, but it was a grudging, arm's-length involvement. "He was perfectly happy to let me and others fight that battle . . . ," Cohen said years later, "while he handled—which was the major matter within his administration—how to balance the interests of the NIH with the rest of the PHS. That was the big problem that Luther Terry had, which he didn't successfully handle."[24]

Cohen was stewing about this at a time when he was gaining even more power. In July 1965, HEW Secretary Celebrezze resigned to accept a federal judgeship. He was immediately replaced by John W. Gardner, a Republican wunderkind who headed the Carnegie Corporation, one of the nation's largest philanthropies. Although Gardner's forte was education, Johnson expected him to also implement the federal Medicare and Medicaid health insurance programs passed by Congress the same week Gardner was appointed. To do that, Gardner had decided to promote and lean heavily on Cohen.

Cohen wanted a new, more dependable surgeon general. The change was announced by President Johnson at an August 9, 1965, press conference at the NIH campus. The event was to showcase Johnson's signing of a $280 million health research bill. But the president jarred many in the thousand-person audience with a "by the way" that the fifty-three-year-old surgeon general would be retiring at the end of September.[25] Johnson promised that there would be an extensive search for "the most adventurous and most imaginative doctor in the country" to be Terry's successor. "I don't know where he is, but we're going to start looking for him," the president said.[26]

Terry left to become vice president for medical affairs at the University of Pennsylvania and spent the next two decades of his life as a leader of the anti-smoking movement. He was elected to the executive board of the National Interagency Council on Smoking and Health, a coalition of eighteen government and nongovernment health and educational organizations. He co-authored a sixty-four-page children's book on the dangers of smoking (*To Smoke or Not to Smoke*) that was published in 1969, and worked for a ban on radio and television cigarette advertisements that took effect in 1971.

He died of congestive heart failure at a Philadelphia hospital on March 29, 1985. He was seventy-three. He was buried in Arlington National Cemetery.

Terry's watch was a pivotal time in the nation's health. Environmental issues exploded into the national consciousness with the publication of Rachel Carson's *Silent Spring*. The government licensed measles vaccines, and Terry led an immunization campaign against that disease while continuing a national push against polio. At times he was an out-front leader on health issues, including a seat belt safety campaign and a push to ask NBC to telecast a drama about a schoolboy who contracts a venereal disease.

Much of that work has been forgotten by the general public, but his enduring legacy is the advisory committee's report on smoking, known since as the Terry report (though he wrote only the introduction). It proved a turning point in the general public's thinking about whether smoking was dangerous. And it set the stage for warning labels, cigarette advertising restrictions, public education campaigns, and a slew of other measures that contributed to a steady decline in U.S. smoking that began in the early 1970s and continued for decades afterward.

At Terry's funeral, one tribute was offered by Joseph Califano, who served as a tobacco-fighting HEW secretary years after Terry left government service.[27] "The United States has known no finer Surgeon General," he said. "He saved as many lives as any Salk, Pasteur or Curie. He is as much a medical giant." Califano closed by saying, "He deserves a peaceful journey with the Lord. In the no-smoking section, of course."

WILLIAM STEWART

His Father's Footsteps

When President Johnson set about finding a successor to the popular Luther Terry, he promised to search for "the most adventurous and most imaginative doctor in the country." Those worried about the deteriorating state of the Public Health Service no doubt agreed: it would take such a dynamic individual—along with some significant assistance—to restore the strength of the Service and the full authority of the surgeon general.

What they got was Bill Stewart.

William Huffman Stewart was born May 19, 1921, in Minneapolis. He was the son of a pediatrician, Chester Arthur Stewart of Hannibal, Missouri, who had moved north with his family to teach and do public health research at the University of Minnesota. Bill Stewart would later say that his first brush with public health came at the age of eight when he joined his dad on a trip to an Indian reservation to treat a young Native American girl.[28]

He followed his father into medicine, beginning his college career in 1939 at the University of Minnesota as a pre-med student. When his dad got a teaching job at Louisiana State University, Bill followed him to Baton Rouge, finishing his undergraduate studies. (The woman who became his wife, Glendora Ford White, also graduated from LSU.) He earned his medical degree through an accelerated program at LSU designed to produce more doctors for World War II, though he graduated in 1945, just as the war was ending. Commissioned as a first lieutenant in the U.S. Army, Stewart cycled through an internship at a public hospital in Philadelphia, a military hospital in San Antonio, and a VA hospital in Minneapolis. He left the army in 1947, after twenty-one months of duty. When the Korean War broke out, he was ordered back into the military.

Stewart did not want another hitch in the army. He heard that the Public Health Service's Communicable Disease Center in Atlanta was creating an Epidemic Intelligence Service (EIS), and transfers between the uniformed military service and the uniformed Commissioned Corps were possible. The doctor starting up the CDC program, Alexander Langmuir, wanted some pediatricians in his first EIS class, and Stewart fit the bill.[29]

EIS was a corps of newly minted public health investigators who could respond to emerging outbreaks—if invited in by states, of course. It was born out of a Cold War concern about biological warfare, but actually echoed work the Commissioned Corps had done in earlier decades against epidemics of yellow fever, cholera, and plague. As those scourges waned, epidemiology and disease response had become decentralized in the Public Health Service. The CDC's ambitious early leaders wanted to assume much of that responsibility.[30] Young Dr. Stewart was part of their first class.

The work was not glamorous. After six weeks of academic training in Atlanta, Stewart spent most of the next two years at a CDC field station in Thomasville, Georgia, that focused on diarrheal diseases. He helped run a lab that processed more than seven hundred fecal specimens a week.[31]

As his EIS stint was ending, Stewart was persuaded to stay in the Service by James Watt, an NIH infectious disease specialist who had helped get the EIS program going. Watt become director of the NIH's Heart Institute in 1952, and for a time guided Stewart's career up the ranks of the Heart Institute. In April 1957, Stewart got another boost when Surgeon General Burney recruited him to his staff. (Over the next several years, Stewart managed a number of Service projects, including—in the early 1960s—work on the delivery of health services and on how insurance paid for them. He became a resident expert on matters related to national health insurance, and thus a favorite of Wilbur Cohen.) Stewart became the new head of the National Heart Institute on August 1, 1965, and had been in that job only about two months when he was named Terry's successor.

His appointment was something of a relief within the Public Health Service. Johnson's vow to find a uniquely dynamic individual to be the next surgeon general raised the possibility that Terry's successor might be some outsider, like a high-profile hotshot from academia or—worse—some political crony of Johnson's who happened to have "M.D." after his name.[32] Such an appointment seemed very possible, given the other changes happening in HEW. That worst case didn't happen in 1965, though it would not be long before U.S. presidents stopped caring whether a surgeon general appointee had spent time in the Service that he was being put in charge of.

Whether Stewart was dynamic is debatable, but he was certainly bright, and had experience in the powerful NIH as well as other key offices. He looked right for the job, as well—brown-eyed and six foot, three, with a 220-pound frame kept in shape with exercise and hiking. He was likable and fond of camping trips and rocking chairs (he owned four of them). At age forty-four, Stewart seemed to have both the gravitas and the energy to fill the role well.

As surgeon general, he took oversight of 150 federal programs, 38,000 people, and an annual budget of more than $2 billion. But his charge, though still substantial, was dwindling. Environmental programs had begun to migrate to other governmental agencies. The NIH had become a semiautonomous juggernaut, only tenuously under the surgeon general's supervision. The Public Health Service hospitals, which once numbered in the dozens and were a training ground and career ladder for the Commissioned Corps, had dwindled to twelve. Stewart had to deal with an increasingly fluid job description and, of course, the issue of smoking.

Smoking

When Stewart took over, job number 1—at least from a public perspective—was smoking. Luther Terry's report had ensured that.

Stewart didn't have much of a reputation in the smoking arena. His scientific publications focused more on cholesterol and lipids than tobacco. He also was a pipe smoker, and remained one while surgeon general.[33] But he understood that waging war against tobacco was now part of his job. Within six months, he presented estimates that if all Americans were nonsmokers, there would be 12 million fewer cases of chronic disease in the United States. Stewart became a regular voice in newspaper pages and on television talk shows, expressing dismay that so many people had continued to smoke since the Terry report and that half the nation's teenagers were regular smokers by the time they were eighteen.[34]

He fought the tobacco industry, and he did it in person. On *The Today Show* in August 1967, Stewart engaged in a volley with the Tobacco Institute's Harvard-accented spokesman, Clarence Cook Little. The industry's argument, that day and every day, was, "This is only a statistical association. You can't prove anything with epidemiology only. More scientific work has to be done." After Stewart told the show's audience there was clear proof that smoking causes lung cancer, Little replied; "I don't mean to challenge the right of people to have these opinions, but what we know about the causes of lung cancer really is a molehill, and what we don't know, a mountain. I think the plea that the tobacco industry makes, and that those of us who are scientists . . . is . . . be patient."[35]

Stewart's most substantial response came two weeks later when HEW officials released their first annual report on the consequences of smoking (which had been mandated by the Federal Cigarette Labeling and Advertising Act of 1965). The surgeon general wrote the introduction and HEW staffers wrote the rest of the 199-page document. It said that since the 1964 Terry report, about two thousand scientific articles had been published on the health effects of smoking, and *none* contradicted any of Terry's main points. The report also pushed a stronger message about smoking's contribution to heart disease.

But the report didn't make the waves Terry's had. There was no drop in cigarette consumption, not even a short-lived one. In fact, the largest cigarette manufacturers—the R. J. Reynolds Tobacco Co., Philip Morris Inc., and the American Tobacco Co.—reported record sales and earnings for that quarter and for the first nine months of the year. Stewart issued additional reports on smoking and health in 1968 and 1969, though they were more in the way of updates to the 1967 report than stand-alone documents. The surgeon general was building a case, but he was not turning heads. The documents received little public attention.

The tobacco forces seemed to be winning, and the usually affable Stewart was irked. In late August 1967, he told Congress that the tobacco industry's marketing of longer cigarettes was "unconscionable." In November, he announced the formation of a federal task force to explore ways to discourage the nation from smoking.[36]

Some believe that both Stewart and President Johnson were less committed to battling tobacco than Terry and Kennedy were.[37] But in fact Terry got a fair amount of recognition at the time for becoming increasingly confrontational with the tobacco industry. Luther had involved cigarette makers in the creation of the study committee and had been careful not to vilify the industry. But Stewart, over the industry's objections, approved a study that ranked cigarettes according to their tar content. He also said it was "indefensible" for cigarette manufacturers to advertise their products "in a context of happiness, vigor, success and well-being without even a hint appearing anywhere that the product may also lead to disease and death."[38]

As Stewart soldiered on with limited effect, other federal officials had a bigger impact. Leading the pack was the Federal Communications Commission, which in June 1967 ordered that radio and television stations provide free air time for public service announcements about the health hazards of smoking. (The PSAs were to appear at a ratio of at least one anti-smoking TV spot for every three cigarette commercials.) The order was based on the "fairness doctrine" of allowing opposing points of view, customarily used for political issues but invoked in this case to allow a medical rebuttal to cigarette advertising.

The ads fostered by the FCC decision would sway how the public thought about smoking. A popular American Heart Association spot entitled "Like Father, Like Son" showed a young boy copying his father's behaviors during a Saturday spent together and then reaching for his dad's pack of cigarettes. Even more striking was an American Cancer Society spot featuring Bill Talman, the actor who played the regular opposing counsel on *Perry Mason*. Talman, speaking directly to the camera, revealed he was dying of lung cancer and entreated the viewer not to smoke. Jarring at the time, the spots were credited with a 7 percent decline in per capita cigarette consumption from 1967 to 1970.[39] (Consumption dropped by 15 percent immediately after Terry's report, but was down at that level for only three months. Cigarette sales picked up again, and by the end of 1964, consumption was down only 3.5 percent.)

In 1970, Congress passed a law banning TV cigarette advertising, but it actually undid some of the good done by the FCC. The advertising ban was followed by a 4 percent *increase* in per capita tobacco consumption.[40] The experience taught a valuable lesson to the public health community—that counteradvertising could be extremely effective—and it was a basis for the American Legacy Foundation's anti-tobacco "Truth" campaign, which aired thirty years later.

Another advance involved warning labels. The Cigarette Labeling and Advertising Act of 1965 required cigarette packs to carry warning labels that said, "Caution: Cigarette Smoking May Be Hazardous To Your Health." Stewart, health advocates, and officials at the FTC argued that these warnings failed to convey the mortal danger that people were exposing themselves to. Congress, circumventing tougher language proposed by the FTC, passed the Public Health Cigarette Smoking Act of 1969 to change the warning. There was still no mention of death or cancer or heart disease, but a source of medical and moral authority was added to theoretically give it more punch. The new labels were mandated to read, "Warning: The Surgeon General Has Determined that Cigarette Smoking is Dangerous to Your Health." Thus was born the "Surgeon General's Warning," which became boilerplate on tobacco packaging for more than forty years.

Whether adding "Surgeon General" was much of a deterrent is open to debate. Some have argued that, if anything, it may have weakened the message because it didn't simply state as a fact that something was deadly dangerous but rather seemed to suggest such a thing needed attribution. (Indeed, there's some evidence tobacco companies prefer the surgeon general warnings.)[41] "By saying 'the Surgeon General has determined,' that suggests a bureaucrat in Washington has made this opinion and nobody else is really sure," said John Banzhaf III, a George Washington University professor of public interest law who, as a young attorney in the 1960s, argued a case that caused the FCC to open the gates for "Fairness Doctrine era" anti-tobacco TV spots.[42]

Medicare

Stewart became surgeon general in large part because of his interest and expertise in health services administration and health insurance payment systems. Such topics had been anathema to his predecessors, who

knew well the story that Thomas Parran had been pilloried for supporting President Truman's ill-fated health reform proposals. But Stewart
was in place at a unique time in American politics, during an unusual
alignment of the political stars that allowed the creation of the kind of
national health insurance that had been unattainable in the past.

Medicare is a health insurance program that pays medical bills of the
elderly and disabled and is financed through payroll taxes. Cohen
championed its creation, negotiating directly with congressional leaders, answering their questions, allaying their concerns, and rebutting
their arguments. He was not always successful; one version of the proposal was defeated during the Kennedy administration. But after
Kennedy's assassination, a wave of public support lifted the fallen president's legislative goals. Medicare also benefited from a rare constellation of political leaders with talent for getting things through Congress,
including Lyndon Johnson and U.S. Representative Wilbur Mills, an
Arkansas Democrat who led the important House Ways and Means
Committee. Congress passed Medicare in the summer of 1965, and the
law went into effect in the summer of 1966, along with Medicaid, a
health insurance program for the poor.

Of course, the battle wasn't over. For decades, the AMA had argued
that any form of national health insurance was an intrusion into the
doctor-patient relationship (not to mention a government control on
their potential income). AMA leaders had opposed Cohen's nomination. They opposed Medicare. And delegates to the AMA's 1966 convention urged all doctors to ignore Medicare and continue to directly
bill their patients.[43]

Doctors weren't the only obstacles. As HEW officials attempted to
implement Medicare, they also had to square off against another force
in the health care system—U.S. hospitals. Stewart was tapped to lead
this particular battle.

Medicare's impact on hospitals was going to be huge. At the time the
Medicare law was passed, more than a third of hospital care was
devoted to patients sixty-five and over. That meant collectively a giant
chunk of U.S. hospitals' income would now come from the new program. A wrinkle in this financial changeover involved Title VI of the
Civil Rights Act of 1964, which banned racial discrimination in any
federal assistance program. Medicare was such a program, so hospitals
receiving Medicare money would therefore not be allowed to turn away
or discriminate against any patients. The Johnson administration had
not emphasized that detail to legislators during the precarious negotia-

tions that went into getting the Medicare bill passed. But after President Johnson signed the Medicare bill into law on July 30, 1965, HEW officials moved into action. In September, James Quigley—the HEW assistant secretary responsible for civil rights activities—told a packed room at an American Hospital Association meeting that hospitals would have to comply with Title VI if they expected Medicare money.[44] About six months later, the government went public with the effort, with Stewart as the official point man.

In early March 1966, Stewart told reporters that the Public Health Service had sent letters to all the nation's general hospitals warning that discrimination and segregation would not be tolerated at Medicare-participating hospitals. He also told them that the Service had set up a special Office of Equal Health Opportunity, with a staff of one hundred, most of them based in regional offices, charged with investigating complaints of discrimination. As hospitals were surveyed and inspected, federal health officials met with influential newspaper editors in Tennessee, Georgia, and Florida to emphasize the gravity of the situation. "Where the discrimination persists, the hospital will be excluded from any new Federal assistance programs," Stewart told the *New York Times,* adding that his staff would pursue court orders to desegregate certain hospitals, if necessary.[45]

Would hospitals comply? That question proved to be a nail-biter. In April 1966, preliminary data suggested only about half of U.S. hospitals were complying with Title VI, and only a quarter in the South were. In early June, with Medicare's launch less than a month away, more than one thousand hospitals still had not given the government any assurance they would meet Medicare's requirement, again with most of them in Dixie. Stewart and 360 of his Public Health Service officers blanketed the South in a late-in-the-game push to get hospitals to desegregate in time to be part of the new health insurance program. In some cases, they dispelled simple confusion over the new rules, clarifying, for example, that not every room had to be desegregated, or that the hospital did not have to maintain a patient census that always reflected the demographics of the hospital's service area. In other cases, they dealt with stubborn racism and had to make blunt arguments about the financial hits and other potential repercussions hospitals would face if they didn't get on board. In a few instances they dealt with shenanigans, as at Americus Sumter Hospital in Georgia, where black employees reportedly were ordered to lay in beds and pose as patients when federal inspectors came through.[46] Philip R. Lee, at the time the special assistant secretary for health and scientific affairs at HEW, got a taste of what Stewart was encountering during a visit to Atlanta's Georgia Baptist Hospital. "A cardiologist said, 'Dr. Lee, if I put a nigger in a room with one of my patients, it will kill the white patient.' That's the kind of attitude they had," Lee said.[47]

But HEW was aggressive, and Stewart's credentials as the nation's doctor were uniquely persuasive. "It's one thing for a Social Security person to say, 'You have to be desegregated or we're not going to pay you.' It's another for a doctor to say, 'You have to desegregate because it's best for the patient,'" Lee explained. On July 1, 1966—the first day of Medicare's implementation—Stewart could tell reporters at a Washington, D.C., press conference that 94 percent of the nation's general hospitals were in compliance with the civil rights rules and quality standards.[48]

Within the federal health bureaucracy, some believe Stewart's work on the desegregation of hospitals counts him as one of the most influential surgeons general of the past fifty years.[49] But his efforts aside, key HEW leaders came away from the desegregation campaign with a low opinion of the rest of the Public Health Service.

The Service was responsible for the Hill-Burton program, created in the late 1940s under Surgeon General Thomas Parran to provide postwar construction and expansion funds for medical centers. But the Service had never policed hospitals receiving Hill-Burton funds as to racial discrimination. In the early 1960s, the U.S. Department of Justice had taken up the cause of hospital desegregation in a lawsuit brought by black dentist George Simkins Jr. when a Greensboro, North Carolina, hospital—Moses H. Cone Memorial—had denied admission to a patient with an abscessed molar. The DOJ saw it as a federal matter because the hospital had received federal Hill-Burton money. The government won the case in November 1963, but still the Service did not respond. Part of the problem was the provincialism of the Service staff who administered the Hill-Burton program and had been certifying hospitals for funding for decades. They worked in local offices and lived in the communities where hospital desegregation was routine. And a significant number of them believed, despite the *Simkins* decision, that Hill-Burton did not specifically outlaw segregation once a patient was admitted.[50]

So there had been reason for hospital administrators in the South to at first question how serious HEW was about denying them Medicare funding because of racial discrimination. Even during the big Medicare push, some Service staffers who had been working in the South were reluctant to be confrontational. Indeed, Lee and his deputy, George Silver, had grown so worried that they set up an emergency backup plan under which elderly patients could temporarily go to federal medical centers. They feared the Service simply couldn't be counted on to make the changes required in the new wave of Great Society legislation. The Service, Silver said, "was sort of an anachronistic animal, anti-Semitic, anti-black, had to be dragged kicking and screaming into the 20th century."[51]

Reorganizations

Cohen and other top HEW officials had already developed a low opinion of the seemingly inbred Commissioned Corps officers leading the Public Health Service, and the foot-dragging on Medicare reinforced that assessment. Many Service officers were disease investigators acculturated during the VD campaigns of the 1930s and 1940s, and they simply did not see themselves as suited to running a national health insurance program—what some of them called being in "the check-writing business." And of course there was the long-standing wariness of crossing swords with the AMA. "The bitterness of this 30-year fight with the AMA made a lot of people not want to tackle it," recalled Warren Dearing, who served in the PHS from 1934 until 1961.[52] More than that, some Service doctors identified with the AMA. "They didn't want to be thought of like government employees who couldn't make it in the world of private practice. There was a lot of attention to try to maintain a very positive identity with the American Medical Association," said Paul Ehrlich, a Service physician serving in Washington at the time.[53]

Johnson administration officials had watched the Service pass up opportunities to lead the government's efforts in health insurance, environmental regulation, automobile safety, family planning, and other initiatives important to advocates, Congress, and the public. It was not simply a matter of the PHS's unwillingness to respond; in some cases it was unable to do so, lacking leaders with expertise in some of the emerging areas of public health concern. Stewart acknowledged the perceived lack of forward thinking. "The Commissioned Corps was more identified with the way things were," he said, "and not the way things were going to be."[54]

Cohen wanted an overhaul. He had begun exploring ideas for departmental reorganization as early as 1961, his first year at HEW. He pushed harder when John Gardner took over as HEW secretary in 1965 and Cohen was elevated to undersecretary. Gardner was a brainy leadership guru who agreed with Cohen about a shake-up. He tipped his hand the day he announced Stewart's appointment as surgeon general. Gardner said of the PHS, "It stands at a critical point in its history. It will either take a leap forward, or it will be mired in its own internal conflicts and history will pass it by."[55]

On April 25, 1966—just seven months after Stewart was first nominated—Gardner issued a directive transferring all of the surgeon general's statutory powers to himself. This gave Gardner, not Stewart, the authority to reorganize the Public Health Service.[56] President Johnson told reporters a change was needed because more than fifty new programs had been placed under the Service since 1950, its budget had increased by nearly 900 percent, and the old organizational structure had become "clearly obsolete" for managing all that.[57]

Under the reorganization, the top positions in the Service no longer had to be filled by officers of the Commissioned Corps. The Service's traditional structure of four bureaus was changed to five, and the director of the new Bureau of Health Manpower was immediately recruited through the civil service—the first PHS bureau chief to be a civil servant. "It was no longer an organization built around a professional staff, headed by a professional career individual with relative statutory invulnerability, but was now an organization much more subject to changing personalities and to partisan political influence," wrote Albert Snoke, a national leader in health-care administration, in 1969.[58]

Stewart remained in charge of the Service by virtue of powers delegated to him by Gardner. He had long been a team player at HEW, in both the Kennedy and Johnson administrations, and was entrusted to continue overseeing the Service. He had much the same authority as Terry had had and for a time was optimistic he could maintain that state of affairs, but soon found himself at odds with his fretful bosses. Stewart asked for patience, and on at least one occasion refused to dismiss a commissioned officer whom Gardner wanted out. "His style was to bring people in the Corps along, not just order them," Silver said. He recalled that Stewart liked to say, "You don't always pull a tree up by its roots to see whether it's growing."[59]

The situation lasted only fifteen months. The fall 1966 national elections had produced a swingback, with some liberals losing their seats on Capitol Hill. Congress could no longer be counted on to approve the Johnson administration's health proposals or to maintain support for programs already under way. Meanwhile, HEW was becoming a loose collection of warring agencies, and the Public Health Service's top brass—who couldn't even control the NIH—were part of that problem. Gardner grew unwilling to wait for Service officers to come around.

In 1967, Gardner quietly decided to take oversight of the Service away from Stewart and give it to Phil Lee.[60] But Gardner wasn't in office long enough to see that baton toss. He resigned in February 1968, following a dispute with President Johnson over whether to raise taxes (as Gardner wanted) or make more cuts in the HEW budget (which Johnson wanted). So the reorganization that formally stripped Stewart of his power was carried out by the next HEW secretary—Wilbur Cohen.

Cohen executed the change in March 1968, less than two weeks after Gardner's departure. Stewart was away on a trip to Africa, supporting a CDC-led global smallpox eradication program.[61] "He kept getting phone calls from his deputy . . . saying 'Bill, you have got to come home! They are giving the Public Health Service away!'" recalled David Sencer, the CDC administrator at the time. (Stewart did not immediately return, Sencer said, adding, "Whether his being there would have made a difference or not, he wasn't there to put up a fight.")[62]

Lee was put in charge of the Public Health Service and the Food and Drug Administration. That meant that for the first time, the nation's top public health official was a political appointee, not a career professional. Stewart's powers and staff were scattered to others in HEW.

What was left for the surgeon general to do? Well, he remained the ceremonial head of the Commissioned Corps, which accounted for about 20 percent of the Public Health Service in the 1960s. He became Lee's deputy, meaning he was involved in running the day-to-day operation of the Service (though with virtually no staff or line authority). It also was understood at the time that the surgeon general, a career professional somewhat free of politics, would still be an important spokesman on health issues. "They would leave the Surgeon General free to make pronouncements, whether they were politically popular or not," recalled John Kelso, a Public Health Service veteran. But it was small consolation to Stewart. "I didn't like the idea of having to have a spokesman who had no authority to do anything," Stewart later said.[63]

Stewart's next year in office was one of frequent frustration and occasional apathy. He had spent years dealing with the impatience and criticism of his political bosses at HEW, and now he was denounced by members of the Commissioned Corps for not trying harder to retain control of the Service. "He sort of let things roll over him and didn't take any kind of strong leadership position. I'm sure he would not agree with that characterization, but at least that is what many people said," said Paul Ehrlich, a Commissioned Corps officer who would become acting surgeon general in the 1970s.[64]

The surgeon general's loss of power was barely noted by the press, though one *Washington Post* reporter did briefly marvel at the significance of the change in "overall command of the formerly untouchable Public Health Service."[65]

Stewart's Resignation

In late 1968, the United States was hit by a pandemic of "Hong Kong Flu"—named for the city where the first outbreak was identified earlier that year. It was a different strain from the viruses behind the 1957 and 1918 pandemics and one that turned out not to be as deadly. But there was still uncertainty as it unfolded. Stewart was a leading government spokesman, urging that limited doses of vaccine be used for the highest-risk patients. But he didn't own the stage. The CDC began to emerge in the press as a primary quoted source on the flu, signaling a shift in the government's release of national disease outbreak information.[66]

At about the time the virus hit the United States, Richard Nixon was elected president. The Johnson appointees in the top tiers of HEW were swept out of office, meaning Stewart—with a four-year term—outlasted Wilbur Cohen and the others who had taken his administrative powers away. Stewart remained in office when Nixon's man, Robert Finch, became HEW secretary.

But there was not much point in sticking around. Stewart had less than a year left in his term. Nixon, known for his partisan politics, was not going to reappoint Johnson's surgeon general. Even if he did, Stewart would remain emasculated; Finch was keeping the surgeon general as a deputy to the assistant secretary for health and scientific affairs. In May 1969, Nixon announced that Stewart would be resigning, effective August 1, to become chancellor of the Louisiana State University Medical Center in New Orleans.[67]

Stewart, just forty-eight years old when he resigned, spent the next twenty-five years at LSU in various posts, including as a professor of pediatrics and public health. From 1974 to 1977, he served as head of Louisiana's state health department. He retired in 1986. He died of kidney failure on the evening of April 23, 2008, at Ochsner Medical Center in New Orleans. He was eighty-six.

Stewart was a caring administrator who propelled the war against smoking and helped lead the desegregation of U.S. hospitals. He advocated for noise to be considered a pollutant, warned about the dangers of air pollution, and urged consumers to voice their ire at the "glass curtain" separating the poor from quality care. "He was a civil servant in the best sense of the word, and he was very much devoted to public health," said Russell Klein, a Louisiana State University medical school official who knew Stewart, speaking to a *New Orleans Times-Picayune* reporter after Stewart's death.[68]

Stewart is also remembered as the castrated surgeon general who lost administrative powers that were never to return. But that didn't mean Stewart's successors would become invisible. Not if Jesse Steinfeld had anything to say about it.

CHAPTER 7

Bossed Around

Richard Nixon's surgeon general was going to face a new kind of challenge—competition from his immediate boss.

In the Johnson years, Assistant Secretary of Health and Scientific Affairs Phil Lee took over the surgeon general's place on the organization chart, but was not much for the media spotlight. He was content to let Stewart remain the government's expert voice on federal public health matters.

Lee's replacement was not as happy to stand behind the curtain. Roger Egeberg, once General Douglas MacArthur's personal physician, was a tall military veteran with a take-no-guff attitude—which he sometimes emphasized by wearing a yellow BULLSHIT button on his lapel. He was also a good public speaker, and clearly enjoyed it. Indeed, when he was first considered as Lee's successor, Egeberg asked if he could also be surgeon general. He was told that was not possible, because of a requirement at the time that the surgeon general had to be younger than sixty-five, and Egeberg was just over that age limit. When his bid failed, Egeberg pledged he wouldn't try to take over the surgeon general's bully pulpit. "The Surgeon General was our representative all over the world, and he had gained a great deal of respect over the years. I certainly didn't think any administration should or could step in and destroy something that was as important and useful as that," he said in a 1988 interview.[1]

So he said. But Egeberg saw himself as the nation's chief health officer and number one doctor, despite a common and lingering perception that the surgeon general was the nation's doctor—a role the new surgeon general, the cantankerous Jesse Steinfeld, was interested in playing. Steinfeld and Egeberg would clash repeatedly in the early 1970s. Later in the decade, Steinfeld's successor—the courtly Julius Richmond—would find himself pushed out of the limelight by an even higher-ranking official: HEW Secretary Joseph Califano.

It was a tough era for the Office of the Surgeon General, but the men who occupied it helped change the nation's health in important ways. Steinfeld, in particular, also made some powerful enemies. He was such a vexation for the Nixon administration that the post went unfilled for three years after he left office. "The last thing we wanted was a Surgeon General to deal with; we had problems enough without having a Surgeon General," said Charles Edwards, a high-level health official in the Nixon administration.[2]

JESSE STEINFELD
The Center of Things

Jesse Leonard Steinfeld was born January 6, 1927, in West Aliquippa, a town in western Pennsylvania about twenty miles from Pittsburgh. His parents were Jewish immigrants from Austria-Hungary who met in Pennsylvania. His father, a prizefighter and jack-of-all-trades, was a heavy smoker who died of a heart attack in his early forties, when Jesse was only five. From an early age, Jesse's mother pushed him to become a doctor.[3]

A precocious student, Steinfeld skipped grades and finished high school at age sixteen. Then he attended the University of Pittsburgh, a suburban teenager commuting from home into the Steel City each morning via a bus and two streetcars. He graduated from Pitt in just two years, thanks to extra credit and a burning ambition to become a physician. He completed medical school at Cleveland's Western Reserve University in 1949 at age twenty-two.[4]

He didn't smoke, not as a youth and not later, setting him apart from virtually all the doctors and many of the nurses who worked around him during his next several jobs, which included a residency at the Veterans Administration Hospital in Long Beach, California. "I have vivid memories of the nurses and doctors lighting cigarettes and holding them to the mouths of men who had lost fingers and toes—some of whom even had tracheotomies. This wasn't so unusual in those days," Steinfeld once recalled.[5]

Steinfeld enlisted in the Public Health Service a short time after medical school, when the Korean War started. He was among a number of smart young doctors who joined the PHS for the same reason. "The major attraction was to avoid the Army, Korea, or being shot at. So we had our choice, generally—people who were very high in their class and interested in research," he recalled.[6] He was in the Commissioned Corps, but his experience was different from that of earlier surgeons general. There were no years of being a quarantine officer or mucking around the marine hospital system. The studious Steinfeld was interested in more rapidly evolving fields. He spent a year in a fellowship at the Atomic Energy Commission, learning research techniques and how to use isotopes. Then he re-enlisted with the Service and was assigned to the National Cancer Institute. There, he and his colleagues experimented with chemotherapy and other new treatments on desperate, late-stage cancer patients.

He left the NCI—and the Service—in 1959, to spend most of the 1960s at the University of Southern California, where he eventually became a full professor. In 1968, Steinfeld returned to the NCI for a job as deputy director. He was in line to become the NCI's director; the man who had the top job at NCI, Ken Endicott, was expected to take over the NIH when Jim Shannon retired. But when Endicott didn't get the promotion, Steinfeld decided to return to the Los Angeles area to start a cancer hospital. That was about the time Richard Nixon, of California, was elected president. Steinfeld was a Democrat, but had made some connections with Nixon's cabal while treating a high-ranking Nixon campaign official for cancer.[7] Those associations would be important when Nixon's men were in office and scrambling to make appointments at HEW.

One initial challenge was filling the position of assistant secretary for health and scientific affairs. Nixon's new HEW secretary, Robert Finch, wanted to give the job to John H. Knowles, the admired general director of Boston's Massachusetts General Hospital. Knowles was an innovative administrator, but the AMA didn't like him; Knowles thought doctor's fees were too high and had advocated for comprehensive national health insurance. AMA leaders fought the Knowles selection for months, and it began to hurt Finch's ability to run the department. Finally, Nixon told Finch to pick someone else. So Finch—like Nixon, a California politician—turned to Roger Egeberg, the wise-cracking dean of USC's medical school. Egeberg, a Democrat but seen as loyal to Nixon, was approved.

Egeberg knew Steinfeld from USC, where they had worked together. "I'd been at meetings at USC, where he'd been teaching, and I had liked the way he looked for facts. And I liked the way he often went against the grain," Egeberg recalled.[8] Steinfeld agreed to spend a few weeks in Washington to help Egeberg and his colleagues at HEW sort through their new challenges and set priorities. He was quickly involved in meetings with Finch and other top officials, and had an influential voice in discussions of water fluoridation and other important topics. Steinfeld enjoyed it. "It was kind of exciting. I mean, I had never been at the center of things," Steinfeld said.[9] At about that time, HEW officials had a meeting at Camp David to discuss the structure of the department and whether to do away with the reorganized Public Health Service and the defanged surgeon general. After the meeting, Steinfeld recalled, "Bob Finch came to me and said, 'Would you stay here if we appointed you Surgeon General and we kept the Public Health Service?'"[10]

Steinfeld agreed, but on one condition: he insisted on some degree of line authority. He was granted a second title, principal deputy assistant secretary for health and scientific affairs. It was a guarantee of some degree of administrative power to prop up the higher-sounding but powerless title of surgeon general. Steinfeld was confirmed by the Senate on December 18, 1969.

Up the Organization

Steinfeld piped up right away. In early January 1970, just a few weeks after being confirmed, the surgeon general was in the newspapers for telling Congress that he believed the United States was moving toward a national health insurance program and the federal government should prod doctors to lower their fees.[11] The comments were not made out of school; Egeberg, his boss, was pushing for pretty much the same thing. But according to some HEW officials, it soon began to irk Egeberg that Congress and the public seemed to prefer to hear from the surgeon general. There may have been a surgeon general–demoting reorganization within HEW, but the rest of the country acted as though it hadn't gotten the memo. As Paul Ehrlich recalled:

> "Whenever there was some testimony that had to be given, the congressional committee would always ask for the Surgeon General, not for the Assistant Secretary. That used to just rankle the Assistant Secretary and the people around him. They would frequently go back to the committee and say, "The surgeon general is not the spokesman on this issue. The Assistant Secretary

is. If you want somebody, the Assistant Secretary will come." And that used to antagonize some of the people in Congress, because they didn't want some Assistant Secretary testifying; they wanted the Surgeon General. That just added fuel to the fire of the Assistant Secretary not being identified as the senior line officer, and the Surgeon General being his deputy."[12]

Egeberg did draw press attention, however. He criticized the criminal legal penalties for using marijuana, saying they were too severe. He also became a louder and louder critic of the Nixon administration, complaining to reporters that HEW Secretary Finch was not following his counsel and that President Nixon's advisers ignored him. Meanwhile, others were bashing Egeberg. In June 1970, *Time* magazine published an article entitled "Sickness at HEW" that described a department torn by struggles between the Nixon administration's budget cutters and HEW staffers with more Democratic ideals. The indecisive Finch—"Secretary Flinch," one senator called him—was on his way out, but Egeberg was also singled out for a series of top-level firings at the FDA and other disruptive personnel changes. Some labeled Egeberg incompetent. The June 18, 1970, issue of *Washington Sounds,* the newsletter of the National Association of Hearing and Speech Agencies, commented on problems at HEW: "Morale is sagging. A lack of leadership from Dr. Roger O. Egeberg, who has not yet mastered the complexities of his health empire, has caused more than one official of an operating program to throw up his hands in despair trying to get decisions out of the front office."[13]

Part of the problem: Egeberg's position was not well defined. The assistant secretary for health and scientific affairs was the titular head of the Public Health Service, but budget management, personnel management, and other functions were actually placed under other HEW officials. Leaders of PHS agencies like the FDA and NIH found it expedient to go around Egeberg on a variety of matters. Adding to the melee was Steinfeld, who spoke and acted as if he had more power than he actually had. Egeberg began to believe that Steinfeld was intercepting duties and keeping important information from him. Said Egeberg: "He became imbued with the idea that I was the enemy of the Public Health Service. . . . He went, I think, beyond what any other person would have done in his efforts to discredit me and keep me in the dark about things. You know, I finally had to go to his secretaries and say, 'I'm going to try to get you people transferred if you don't give the mail that comes to me, to me!'"[14] "By the time I got there, the two men were literally no longer speaking to each other," said Merlin DuVal, who was appointed to replace Egeberg in 1971.[15]

Egeberg was moved out, to become a special assistant for health policy to the HEW secretary. Next up was DuVal, a University of Arizona medical school dean. DuVal changed his title from assistant secretary for health and scientific affairs to the simpler assistant secretary for health, and asserted more control over the NIH and other HEW agencies.

Steinfeld, meanwhile, rolled on. He became an oft-quoted federal health official even before the Senate confirmed him, starting with some rancor over cyclamate, an artificial sweetener that in the 1960s was commonly used in soft drinks like Tab and Fresca. Some studies indicated it caused or contributed to cancer in rats, and in October 1969, HEW Secretary Finch told reporters that cyclamate was no longer considered safe in foods. At the press conference he was supported by Steinfeld, who cooled anxiety levels when he told reporters and an alarmed public that there was no evidence cyclamate had caused cancers in people. The surgeon general handled the matter beautifully, said David Sencer, director of the CDC at the time. Steinfeld was "courageous" in handling "one of the first times the Public Health Service had taken a strong stand on an environmental issue or a toxic substance issue."[16]

Next up was marijuana. In January 1970, Steinfeld was widely quoted during a battle in the District of Columbia over a proposal to reduce criminal penalties for smoking marijuana. Yes, he said, marijuana use must be controlled, and its long-term health effects needed more study. But penalties like one or more years in jail for a first-time conviction of puffing a marijuana cigarette were so harsh that "many of our jurors do not invoke them at all," he said.[17]

In the fall of 1970, the surgeon general turned heads with a national campaign against lead poisoning that hinged on a new way of looking at the health threat. Previously, children were considered to have lead poisoning only if they had blood lead levels of 60 micrograms per deciliter or above. Most children at that standard suffered convulsions, coma, and lasting neurological damage. Steinfeld issued guidelines that lowered the standard to 40, thereby expanding the number of children with lead poisoning to as many as 400,000. In so doing, he issued an important call for screening young children to detect peril before the most severe symptoms set in.[18] Since his breakthrough push, the standard has been repeatedly lowered. As of this writing, the government standard is 5 micrograms per deciliter.

Around the same time, Steinfeld became the government's most listened-to voice on the controversy over a chemical in laundry detergents called NTA (nitrilotriacetatic acid). Detergent makers had turned to NTA after being criticized for using environment-polluting phosphate, and in 1970 NTA was used in 5 percent of the laundry detergents on the market, including popular products like Cheer and Gain. But in December 1970, Steinfeld said rodent test data had shown that NTA had contributed to alarmingly high rates of birth defects in rodents. As with cyclamate, there was no evidence NTA had harmed people, Steinfeld said during a press conference. But already embattled manufacturers— at the government's urging—had agreed to stop using it. Howard Morgens, president of Proctor and Gamble, the maker of Cheer, told reporters that he was absolutely sure NTA was safe for people but that it was unwise to fight Steinfeld on the matter. "Once the Surgeon General has made the statement he has, public confidence in products containing NTA is bound to be adversely affected," he said.[19]

Steinfeld was partly occupied in those days with a push to make the conquest of cancer a national goal. Months later, in March 1971, he— not Egeberg—was selected to present the administration's testimony at a special Senate subcommittee hearing on proposals to escalate the medical war against cancer, the nation's most feared disease. Steinfeld convincingly argued against proposals that would create a new authority outside HEW and the Public Health Service to manage the government's cancer efforts.[20]

He was also fighting the administration's efforts to do away with the Commissioned Corps and what was left of the marine hospital system. Assorted Washington officials increasingly questioned the need for the Corps, an organization-within-an-organization, and some were irritated that doctors could satisfy their military obligations by spending time in the PHS. It was a continuation of an earlier battle. There had been some talk of eliminating the Commissioned Corps in the 1950s, around the time Corps members were made eligible for certain Social Security wage credits and other benefits traditionally reserved for military veterans. In the 1960s, Wilbur Cohen and other Johnson administration officials had marginalized the Corps within HEW.[21] Now the Nixon administration—trying to build a reputation for economizing the federal bureaucracy—decided it had no more use for the Corps and its hospitals.

In June 1970, Nixon appointed a Boston Brahmin attorney named Elliot Richardson to replace Finch as secretary. Richardson, pressured by his political bosses to do something about the Corps, appointed former HEW Undersecretary John A. Perkins to lead a committee that would report on the Corps's future. The Perkins report came out in 1971, recommending the Corps be disbanded. It noted Nixon was planning to end the military draft (he did, in 1973), a move that would likely reduce the interest of doctors in joining the Commissioned Corps. The report also said HEW should do away with the Corps's chief, the surgeon general.[22] In November 1971, Richardson announced he would implement the report's recommendations.

Steinfeld fought the proposal, talking to his powerful allies in Congress. One was U.S. Representative Paul Rogers, a Democrat from West Palm Beach, Florida, who chaired the House Subcommittee on Health. First elected in the 1950s, Rogers had come to be known as "Mr. Health"—he had succeeded Hill and Fogarty as the legislator with the most influence on health matters. Rogers liked the Public Health Service, its hospitals, and its surgeon general. Holding sway over the HEW budget, he discounted the Perkins report. Richardson backed down. The Corps and its leader were saved.[23]

The general public took little notice of this important battle within the federal health bureaucracy. But Steinfeld's war on smoking was another matter.

Steinfeld may have been the first surgeon general who was not a smoker.[24] He had been convinced smoking was potentially harmful at least since his medical training, well before Terry's 1964 report. When he became surgeon general in 1969, he inherited an office with more than a dozen ashtrays scattered about, and promptly had them all removed. In what was a somewhat unusual action at the time, he also posted a sign that said "Thank You for Not Smoking." He made it a policy to ban visits from tobacco industry lobbyists. And he began preparing his campaign.

He made a report to Congress in February 1971 on smoking and health, the kind that surgeons general had been submitting on a mostly annual basis for several years. The 488-page report expanded on the perils of cigarette smoking and drew new attention to cancer dangers from pipes and cigars. It also mentioned, almost in passing, some small studies in which animals passively exposed to cigarette smoke had developed health problems. In particular, a study was noted in which hamsters had developed premalignant and malignant changes in their larynx.[25]

The report drew interest, partly because of a bomb Steinfeld set off a few weeks before. On January 11, 1971, at an interagency meeting to mark the seventh anniversary of the release of the Terry report, Steinfeld ended a speech by suggesting that smoking should be banned from most public places. That would include restaurants, theaters, airplanes, trains, and buses. "Evidence is accumulating that the nonsmoker may have untoward effects from the pollution his smoking neighbor forces upon him," he said. "It is time that we interpret the Bill of Rights for the nonsmoker as well as the smoker."[26]

It was quite a statement. Some consumer advocates, like Ralph Nader, had already petitioned the government to ban smoking on planes and buses. But this was different: a top federal health official flatly stating that smokers were poisoning the people around them. It gave instant credibility to the many people who had claimed to be sickened by the smoking of others but had been marginalized as fussy complainers. Letters of applause began appearing on newspaper editorial pages, like one from Madilyn Reynolds of Lanham, Maryland. She wrote: "Being an asthmatic, allergic to tobacco smoke, daily life outside of my home is a nightmare of trying to breathe in public places. I have been driven by smokers from the checkout line at the grocery, the pediatrician's office, airplanes, buses, restaurants, even movie theaters where the secret smoker cannot wait until the show is over. Onward Jesse Steinfeld, onward Ralph Nader—at last someone's on my side."[27]

Steinfeld again emphasized the dangers of smoking to nonsmokers in a 1972 surgeon general's report. One of his primary aims with that document, he later said, was to create social pressures on smokers to get them to quit.[28] But as he pushed this message, Steinfeld was venturing out on a limb. His warnings about the dangers of secondhand smoke had little scientific basis. Only a few small animal studies had shown harm from passive smoking. More comprehensive and rigorous studies involving humans were years away. Past surgeons general had been cautious in their statements about smoking until the medical evidence was nearly overwhelming, but here was a surgeon general speaking not as a coolheaded reflector of scientific consensus but as an agenda-pushing advocate.

It worked. Just two weeks after Steinfeld's speech of January 11, 1971, smoking was banned on the Staten Island Ferry by a transportation official who said the surgeon general's words had persuaded him to act.[29] Steinfeld stoked a nascent nonsmokers' rights movement in the country that boomed in the years that followed. He sent a memo to HEW Secretary Richardson in July 1971, pushing the department to set an example and establish no-smoking areas in all HEW building cafeterias and institute a no-smoking policy in all conference rooms and auditoriums. He also plunged into local fights over smoking policies, as in

October 1971 when he wrote to the president of the Montgomery County, Maryland, Board of Education, urging him to re-establish a no-smoking rule for the school system.[30]

The tobacco industry condemned Steinfeld and began painting him as a science-ignoring propagandist. But according to Steinfeld, industry leaders also tried to quietly win him over. At one party, he found himself in conversation with Jack Mills, senior vice president of the Tobacco Institute. Alluding to Steinfeld's struggle to preserve the Commissioned Corps and the Office of the Surgeon General, Mills said the Tobacco Institute would be pleased to use its influence to take a position against the Perkins report, if Steinfeld thought it would be helpful. Steinfeld declined, and became convinced the tobacco industry reacted by trying to get him fired.[31]

Steinfeld's Final Year

As 1972 began, Steinfeld found himself facing a new set of adversaries—the television networks.

It was not a fight of Steinfeld's choosing. Some U.S. senators, including Connecticut's Thomas Dodd and Rhode Island's John Pastore, had become concerned in the 1960s about television violence and pressed HEW officials to study the issue. TV had become the dominant medium in the United States, and children were watching two hours of television a day on average. As they watched, they witnessed significant numbers of (mostly fictional) robberies, shootings, kidnappings, and other acts of violence. Even Saturday morning cartoons featured more and more fistfights, explosions, and other forms of mayhem. Pastore, the chairman of the Senate Subcommittee on Communications, wanted to know; Was all this TV violence having an effect on children? Was it making them more likely to ape what they saw on television and be violent themselves?

In March 1969, Pastore got William Stewart—then in his final months as surgeon general—to commit to studying the issue. HEW officials set up a scientific advisory committee akin to the kind that had produced the 1964 smoking report. And just as Luther Terry had allowed cigarette companies to veto potential members of the committee, HEW allowed network executives to veto potential members of this study committee. Actually, it was worse than Terry's model. Terry had also allowed the American Cancer Society and other health advocacy groups to have an equal say on the composition of the smoking committee, whereas only the networks were granted such input in the creation of the TV committee. Of the twelve names that made the committee's final roster, five had ties to the TV industry, including two who were network executives.[32]

Steinfeld had inherited the situation, but it was his name that would be stamped on the cover of the committee's report. By the second week of January 1972, the document and twenty-three supporting studies were completed. They reported a preliminary and tentative finding that viewing violence on TV could lead to aggressive behavior, but only in children predisposed to being aggressive, and only in certain situations. In mid-January, Steinfeld found himself defending it, telling reporters that "this study is not a whitewash" and that it "shows for the first time a causal connection between violence shown on television and subsequent behavior by children."[33] Characteristically, he soon went one step further. In a hearing convened by Pastore in March, Steinfeld said the data required some sort of government action to restrict violence on television. He did not spell out exactly what kind of action, but his words gave impetus to proposals for a possible ratings system.[34]

The White House was not pleased. Administration officials had ordered Steinfeld not to testify about the TV report to Congress, though he had to after receiving a subpoena to appear.[35] On Valentine's Day, NBC's national nightly news broadcast reported that top HEW officials had told Steinfeld to look for another job and even drafted an announcement stripping the surgeon general of his authority if he did not resign. "The campaign to dump Steinfeld has taken some petty forms," reporter Ron Nessen said. Nessen then referred to a series of meetings between U.S. and Soviet health officials that had culminated the previous week in a groundbreaking pact to collaborate on cancer, heart disease, and environmental health research. A leader in the effort, Steinfeld had met with Soviet officials in Geneva the year before, but was left out of the press conference announcing the final agreement. Steinfeld was also notably excluded from the government's response to the Tuskegee Syphilis Experiment, which had been made public by reporters in July. DuVal did most of the talking for the government on that matter, even though original responsibility for the study resided with the Office of the Surgeon General.[36]

(The rancor between Steinfeld and HEW ultimately gave rise to urban legends that have been passed around by the men and women who succeeded him as surgeon general. One says that when Steinfeld refused to quit, "they took away his office, took his secretaries, they took away his parking. He wandered around with no place to sit except chairs in the hall," said C. Everett Koop, who served as surgeon general in the 1980s and in an interview years later spoke admiringly of Steinfeld's backbone. But the tales are exaggerated. The administration didn't take away his office or his secretary. "I didn't lose any [privileges]. I just was not consulted," Steinfeld said.)[37]

Coincidentally, the same week Nessen's report aired, Steinfeld appeared on *The Mike Douglas Show.* John Lennon and Yoko Ono were guest cohosts for a week on the popular, usually noncontroversial daytime TV talk show. The former Beatle and his warbling wife were granted free reign to select other guests and came up with a list of iconoclasts that included yippie activist Jerry Rubin and Black Panthers Party chairman Bobby Seale. They also invited Steinfeld, and asked him about the recent television violence report. Steinfeld, in a dark suit, spoke like a calm, authoritative member of the establishment. He encouraged Lennon, a chain smoker, to quit cigarettes. After Rubin bitterly lamented social oppression in the United States, and Lennon lamented youth apathy in doing something about it, Steinfeld interrupted. "I want to say something," he began. "My parents came over here and got married in this country. They came to escape oppression in Eastern Europe. I did manage with scholarships to go to college and medical school. I became a professor and I became Surgeon General and I can't think of any other country where that would have happened," Steinfeld said, drawing applause from the audience and grimaces from Rubin and Lennon. Some friends and colleagues later called Steinfeld to congratulate his performance, one of them saying he "made Jerry Rubin look like a schnook."[38]

Steinfeld faced a conflict later that year over an effort to place more doctors in rural areas and urban ghettos where medical services were sparse. The idea was to make a deal with medical students in which they would agree to work in such areas for a few years after graduation in exchange for scholarships and loan repayment. The program was called the National Health Service Corps, and the legislators behind it originally wanted to put the surgeon general in charge. Steinfeld quietly embraced the program as a way to revitalize his office and the Public Health Service. But more senior HEW officials were against any legislation that would give the surgeon general new life, and insisted to the bills' sponsors that authority over the program be placed with the HEW secretary.

During a November 25, 1972, congressional hearing over the shaping of the program, Steinfeld was a witness for the administration and was ordered to parrot HEW talking points. He did so, but there were moments when the strain was apparent. One came when Rogers asked how long Public Health Service physicians served; specifically, was it true that they served "subject to the pleasure of the Surgeon General?" Steinfeld replied, "Subject to the needs of the Public Health Service. I don't get too many pleasures in this job."[39]

He had reason to be glum. Less than three weeks earlier, with Nixon having won reelection as president in a landslide victory, the secretary's office called Steinfeld to say that all the presidential appointees at HEW were being called to a meeting. The Nixon administration was asking for the resignations of all his top appointed officials, a move viewed as something of a postelection formality.[40] As surgeon general, Steinfeld knew that he had certain statutory protections and could not be fired without cause. He also realized the president could—and probably would—choose not to reappoint him to another four-year term, and was prepared for that fate. But Steinfeld still had another year left on his term. He believed his postelection resignation would not be accepted, because he needed only about one more year of service until he qualified for government retirement benefits. "Usually they were very nice to people who have another year or two to go to retirement," he said.[41]

Steinfeld talked to Richardson and said he planned to seek an academic position and probably would leave office the following summer. "He said, 'Well, that's fine Jesse. I think that's appropriate. I don't think you're in tune with the philosophy of this administration,'" Steinfeld later recalled. Steinfeld also noted he was expected to start a one-year term as president of the Association of Military Surgeons of the United States, an organization of government doctors, at an upcoming meeting in San Antonio. Richardson said to go ahead to the meeting and accept the title, since he would be surgeon general well into the next year. He made the trip, but while in Texas got a call from the HEW's chief of personnel, informing him that Nixon was announcing Steinfeld's resignation the next day.[42] Steinfeld's last day as surgeon general was January 30, 1973.

Though not remembered as a particularly dynamic speaker—even at his best he was more blunt than inspirational—Steinfeld must be counted as one of the most evangelistic surgeons general to hold the office. He was a firm believer in the dangers of secondhand smoke and helped initiate a movement toward public smoking bans. In 1973, the Civil Aeronautics Board required domestic airline flights to have separate smoking and nonsmoking sections. In 1974, the Interstate Commerce Commission said smoking on interstate buses must be confined to the last several rows. That same year, Connecticut became the first state to restrict smoking in restaurants.

Steinfeld became convinced that the tobacco industry successfully lobbied the White House for his dismissal, and has said repeatedly that somewhere there is a smoking gun that proves it—specifically, a letter to Nixon from David S. Peoples, president of the R. J. Reynolds Tobacco Company, in which Peoples demands that Steinfeld be fired. Steinfeld even claimed to have a copy. But he has never produced such a document, nor has one matching that exact description been unearthed from any governmental or presidential library or from any archive of tobacco industry documents.[43]

Bitter after he left office, Steinfeld remained a high-profile commentator on health issues. At a September 1973 press conference, he endorsed a health reform proposal by congressional Democrats and lambasted the Nixon administration for never being serious about health reform. He also said the National Health Service Corps program suffered from a lack of leadership and had spent only a fraction of the $50 million authorized for it by Congress.[44]

As he continued to speak out after leaving office, Steinfeld held a series of academic positions. From 1973 to 1974, he was director of the Mayo Clinic Comprehensive Cancer Center and a professor at the Mayo Medical School. From 1974 to 1976, he was a professor at the University of California–Irvine and chief of medicine at the Veterans Administration Hospital in Long Beach, California. From 1976 to 1983, he was dean and professor at the Medical College of Virginia. From 1983 until his retirement in 1987, Steinfeld served as president of the Medical College of Georgia. In recent years he has lived in a retirement community in Pomona, California.

After Steinfeld

After Steinfeld, the Nixon administration didn't want another surgeon general. But there were Commissioned Corps duties—some of them ceremonial—that required a surgeon general, so HEW appointed Paul Ehrlich to serve as acting surgeon general. Ehrlich, a Minnesota native, had first joined the Public Health Service in 1957. He was director of the Public Health Service's Office of International Health and had been a de facto assistant to Steinfeld.

In those days of limbo, Representative Paul Rogers protected the Office of the Surgeon General. Rogers told HEW officials that any

attempt to eliminate the position would have to go through his committee and he was simply never going to support it because he thought the
job was too important.[45] Rogers also helped derail a renewed cost-saving
effort by HEW in 1973 to close the remaining Public Health Service
hospitals. Earlier, Rogers had been among those who had fought a
Nixon proposal to create an even larger federal Department of Human
Resources and stick HEW in it. Rogers actually wanted to go the other
direction, pulling public health out of HEW and making it a stand-alone
federal Department of Health.[46]

Ehrlich was acting surgeon general during the resignation of Richard
Nixon and the swearing-in of Gerald Ford as the new president. He
enjoyed great support from a dynamic new assistant secretary for
health—Theodore Cooper, a veteran of the Commissioned Corps, who
thought that Ehrlich should be officially made surgeon general. "He felt
it was important for the federal government to have a professional
health person who could speak without political baggage, that is, to
speak objectively about certain health issues," Ehrlich recalled. But the
higher-ups told Ehrlich nobody was going to propose that Ford nominate a new surgeon general.[47]

Ehrlich was pretty much invisible during the infamous swine flu scare
of 1976. It started when a flu virus linked to swine was detected in soldiers
at Fort Dix, New Jersey, including one who died. Health officials feared
the new bug might be something like the Spanish flu that killed millions
around the world in 1918 and 1919. HEW leaders convinced President
Ford to launch a national vaccination campaign to prevent widespread
illnesses and death. In past flu pandemics it had been the surgeons general
who guided the government's response and handled much of the communication with reporters and the public, but this time Ehrlich sat on the
periphery. CDC director David Sencer drove response plans, and Cooper
handled most of the talking in the push to get the public to get vaccinated
and the vaccine makers to speed production. More than 40 million Americans got swine flu shots that year, but an epidemic never materialized.
Instead, the government began to receive dozens of reports of a paralyzing
condition called Guillain-Barré syndrome that was blamed on the vaccine.

The campaign was suspended in December 1976, during the lame-
duck months of the Ford administration, after Jimmy Carter had been
elected the next president. The swine flu vaccination campaign was seen
by many in the public as a debacle. Early the next year, Carter's new
HEW secretary used the swine flu episode as an excuse to clean house,
jettisoning Sencer and replacing Cooper.

JULIUS RICHMOND

When Julius Richmond was appointed surgeon general in 1977, Victor Cohn got suspicious. Cohn, the esteemed medical reporter for the *Washington Post,* began peppering federal health officials with questions about the simultaneous appointment of Richmond to two positions—surgeon general and assistant secretary for health. The journalist was "thinking of all kinds of ulterior motives," Richmond later recalled.

Richmond phoned Cohn to explain that the dual appointment was his idea, and the reason for it stemmed from his wish to combine a position of historical prestige and visibility (surgeon general) with a less recognized job with more administrative power (assistant secretary for health).[48] Richmond recognized the sorry state the Office of the Surgeon General was in. The position had been off the public stage for four years while a temporary and powerless replacement had been filling in. He wanted to accomplish some things, and didn't believe the distinguished title of surgeon general would confer enough power.

The gambit paid off. Richmond became one of the more powerful and accomplished surgeons general of the bully pulpit era (that is, the post-Stewart period, when the surgeon general's main role was as health educator). He helped create the *Healthy People* report, which for the first time set national goals for health improvement and encouraged personal responsibility for illness prevention. He also became a globe-trotting health diplomat and was an important domestic spokesman on issues ranging from cigarette smoking to toxic shock syndrome. And though he did not particularly enjoy public speaking or dealing with the press, he could still get his point across. On May 31, 1977, Cohn's story about Richmond's selection appeared in the *Post,* describing a choice that promised a powerful new presence in HEW. "He is a gentle, soft-spoken man with a velvet glove, his friends say. But inside the velvet glove is a steel hand," Cohn wrote.[49]

"A Well-Developed Social Conscience"

Julius Benjamin Richmond was born September 26, 1916, in Chicago. Like Steinfeld he was raised by Jewish immigrant parents—Russian Jews, in Richmond's case.

The family came to know the people of Hull House, a Chicago residence that had been turned into a social settlement where immigrants received help in learning English and were provided food, a library, and even a salon for debate. Hull House's social reformers and child advocates made a lasting impression on young Julius, as did the death of his mother, Anna, when he was ten. He decided to become a physician.[50]

After his mother died, Richmond spent three years at Allendale, a boarding school for dependent boys, which he later described as a nurturing environment. He was back in Chicago at age thirteen, graduated high school, and then at seventeen, traveled downstate to attend the University of Illinois at Urbana. He took an unusually heavy course load, but also was involved in demonstrations protesting segregated housing at the university. Richmond returned to Chicago for medical school, an internship at Cook County Hospital, and two pediatric residencies.[51]

Most of his education occurred during the Great Depression, and he developed an intense interest in creating programs that addressed societal health problems. "I seemed to have a well-developed social conscience," Richmond once said. During World War II, he was inducted into the Army Air Corps and served from 1942 until 1946 as a flight surgeon with the Flying Training Command. His duties included examinations of Air Force cadets—a group he expected to be in better physical and mental condition than most other recruits, but that had a surprising amount of psychological and social problems. From that experience, Richmond developed an interest in the development of young children. "If these young people represented the cream of the crop, then there were earlier experiences that should have—and perhaps could have—been better, and should have created an atmosphere of greater competence," Richmond said.[52]

After the war, Richmond took a series of teaching and research jobs, first at the University of Illinois, then at the State University of New York at Syracuse College of Medicine, where he became dean in 1965. He often juggled multiple responsibilities, but increasingly focused his research on how a child's cognitive abilities developed, and how poverty threatened that development as early as the toddler years. His work came to the attention of Sargent Shriver, who created the Peace Corps during the Kennedy administration and became head of a new federal agency, the Office of Economic Opportunity, under President Johnson. Shriver wanted Richmond to head a new program to be called Head Start, which would provide comprehensive education, health, nutrition, and parent involvement services to low-income children and their families.

Richmond served as Head Start's director for about two years, helping to develop a grant program that provided grant funding to local institutions and embed the program in communities. But he deserves only partial credit for bringing the program out of the gate. Richmond suffered an attack of tuberculosis and another official, Jule Sugarman, took over much of the Head Start work during Richmond's illness.

Richmond returned to Syracuse in 1967, and then moved to Boston in 1971. That was a year of tragedy and change for Richmond—Dale, the youngest of his three sons, was killed in a street mugging in Chicago. He reacted to his son's death by working even harder. He became a professor of child psychiatry and human development at Harvard, chief of psychiatry at Boston Children's Hospital, and director of the Judge Baker Guidance Center. When a Harvard dean asked him if he would also chair the university's department of preventive and social medicine, he told Richmond, "You've always held more than one job, so this will be sort of in character."[53]

He Was "the Science"

Jimmy Carter, elected president in November 1976, picked an aggressive political veteran named Joseph Califano to lead HEW. Califano was a short, activist, Brooklyn-bred attorney with a historical willingness to blaze away at powerful entities, including the government itself. In the 1960s, he was President Johnson's senior domestic policy aide. In the early 1970s, he was a Washington lawyer who represented the *Washington Post* as it faced the threat of a legal injunction if it published portions of the Pentagon Papers—the leaked top-secret federal report documenting the government's internal planning and policymaking regarding the Vietnam War.

As he began to build his HEW staff, Califano looked for a dynamic physician with strong credentials to lead the department's Public Health Service programs. He initially pursued a big name from Massachusetts General Hospital, Charles Sanders, but Sanders turned him down because the position didn't pay enough. "Money. Straight-out money" was the reason, recalled Hale Champion, Califano's undersecretary. "He would have taken the job if somehow we could have found a way for him to get another $50,000. . . . He was willing to make a sacrifice, but not that big a sacrifice at that time."[54]

Califano then turned to Christopher Fordham, the dean of the University of North Carolina School of Medicine. He agreed and began working with Califano in Washington. But Fordham quit after only a few weeks—a decision widely attributed to Califano's penchant for meddling. "I think Califano, as he has a tendency to do, was just getting too much involved in what Fordham and others felt were the duties of the Assistant Secretary," said Ehrlich, the acting surgeon general who remained with HEW in the early days of the Carter administration. But there was also some unhappiness by the administration with Fordham, who wanted to install a UNC colleague as director of the CDC and seemed "intent on building his dominion" within HEW, as one department official put it.[55]

Next up was the sixty-year-old Richmond. In the spring of 1977, Richmond—"Julie," to his friends—said he would take the job if he could also be surgeon general. Richmond believed that having separate individuals in the two jobs would create operational problems, as well as confusion for outsiders who still perceived authority in the Office of the Surgeon General. Califano went along. "I think that he saw it as an expediency," Richmond recalled in an interview. "He said, 'Well, if that's what it takes to get you, why not?'"[56]

Whether combining the two positions was actually Richmond's idea is a matter of debate. Richmond may have been the first to mention it in his conversations with Califano, but the idea had already been discussed within HEW. It likely originated with Peter Bell, who assisted Califano in making appointments and later became deputy undersecretary. Bell said as much, adding that the idea was to extend an "honorific" title to Richmond that would sweeten the offer and carry some weight in dealings with the Commissioned Corps on personnel matters and with the public when it came to the next smoking reports.[57] Whoever came up with the idea, it made Califano happy. Said Richmond: "Califano said to me one day, 'You know, that was a great idea . . . everywhere I go, when I refer to you as Assistant Secretary, nobody knows quite what that means—they wonder if you take shorthand or something. But when I say the Surgeon General suggested this, that or the other thing, everybody thinks they know.' So he felt that had sort of simplified his life."[58]

But working for Califano wasn't easy. The feisty HEW secretary recruited a team of young people—he called them special assistants, while others called them spies—who were placed throughout HEW and brought Califano intelligence. He also tended to deal directly with the directors of the CDC, FDA, and other public health agencies. The assistant secretary for health and his counterparts "were to some degree ineffectual, because the policy decisions were made in Joe's office. If there were any major operating problems or decisions or crises, Califano or Champion or one of Califano's special assistants would pick up the phone and deal directly with the people responsible," said Charles

Miller, who became a deputy to Richmond in 1978.[59] Richmond disliked the meddling. "I thought that his management style was too activist; that he would often dip into dealing with people in the agencies without letting me know," Richmond once recalled. "I could always confront him with it, and he'd always vow that he wouldn't do it again. But I knew and he knew he would do it again."[60]

Califano's activism extended to speaking for HEW on matters of public health, with Richmond as his straight man/second banana. Newspaper and wire service articles from the period followed a similar structure: first, a lead about HEW drawing attention to an important health issue, such as a campaign to eliminate measles or an investigation into workplace illnesses associated with beryllium; next, the punchiest quote in the story, delivered by Califano; then Richmond introduced—identified as the official who will implement the program or oversee the task force. "He was 'the science,' if you will," Califano said years later. "While Julius wasn't out front, I think part of the bully pulpit is the guy that turns the electricity on so that you can speak into the microphone. And Julius Richmond certainly gave me plenty of electricity," he added.[61]

Richmond didn't complain, because he wasn't particularly fond of speaking to the press or public. "I didn't find it enjoyable," Richmond said years later. He did only a few press interviews each month and made public speeches only about once a week. He acknowledged it made him one of the less visible surgeons general of the past few decades, but said he would do it when he thought it was important.[62]

The Califano-Richmond relationship is perhaps best illustrated by the HEW campaign against smoking. Past HEW secretaries had been content to let their surgeons general handle smoking reports and speeches, but Califano had a personal interest in tobacco. For years he had been a chimney, at times smoking four packs a day. But he gave it up in the summer of 1975 when his son, turning eleven, said the birthday present he most desired was that his father quit. As HEW secretary, Califano called cigarette smoking "Public Health Enemy No. 1."[63]

In January 1978, the fourteenth anniversary of the Terry report, Califano outlined the hardest-hitting anti-cigarette program ever proposed by a Cabinet-level official: he planned to ban smoking on all commercial airline flights, prohibit smoking in federal buildings, and increase the federal excise tax on cigarettes, set at 8 cents a pack for the previous twenty-seven years. He made it personal and the media reported it that way. The headline in the *Washington Star* read "Califano Declares War on Smoking." It was soon followed by a political cartoon in the same newspaper, depicting a lady principal confronting a group of smoking elementary schoolboys and saying, "No I'm not going to tell your parents! I'm going to do worse than that—I'm going to turn you in to Joe Califano!"[64] Califano, not Richmond, had become the successor to Jesse Steinfeld—the nagging nanny government health official who attacked tobacco companies and scolded people not to smoke.

But Califano knew he needed a credibility assist. Following the launch of his anti-smoking campaign, he asked Richmond to assemble a fifteenth-anniversary report that would provide strong ammunition for the crusade. (His instructions essentially were "OK, Julie, you get the science," Califano said.) Richmond put together a doorstop report twelve hundred pages long that some inside the government referred to as "the big blue whale." "It was with real intent that 15th anniversary report is not a short summary, but it physically is a very thick volume that's very heavy to carry around. Because I wanted particularly the journalists to see what had developed" in terms of research demonstrating the harmful effects of tobacco, Richmond said.[65]

The report was political dynamite. Among those agitated about its release was U.S. Senator Jesse Helms—the powerful, pro-tobacco politician from the tobacco-producing state of North Carolina—who in 1978 had criticized Califano's crusade for "demonstrating callous disregard for economic realities, particularly for the economy of North Carolina." Days before the report's scheduled January 11, 1979, release, Helms asked for an advance copy. Califano declined. Helms issued a blistering complaint to the media, alleging HEW was trying to gain an unfair advantage in the war of public opinion. On January 10, Helms's allies in the tobacco industry also attempted a preemptive strike, by attacking the federal war on smoking as a "publicity stunt" staged by Califano, who they said displayed the zeal of a reformed sinner and preferred "propaganda barrages" to responsible investigation.[66] (Califano was indeed zealous, and Richmond reined him in on a few points. For example, Califano wanted the report to declare smoking addictive, but Richmond declined, saying at that point there was not sufficient scientific data to make such an unequivocal declaration.[67])

The White House was not enthusiastic about Califano's push. President Carter's father had died of lung cancer, and he was a nonsmoker who was sensitive to the issue. But Carter, a former Georgia governor, also owed his narrow victory in the 1976 election to a near-sweep of the South, and he was extremely wary of alienating traditional tobacco-producing southern states like North Carolina, Virginia, and Kentucky.

The White House decided to distance itself from Califano's crusade without disavowing it.

Then, in July 1979, came a reckoning. Preparing for the 1980 election, Carter decided to shake up his Cabinet and oust five department heads who had been viewed as too disloyal or too independent or who didn't get along with key White House personnel like Chief of Staff Hamilton Jordan, Carter's most trusted aide.[68] Califano was among the five, and his forced resignation drew applause from the North Carolina congressional delegation and condemnation from consumer advocates. (Ralph Nader said ousting Califano was like "firing Mickey Mantle because he couldn't get along with the bat boy.") Although Califano acknowledged a testy relationship with Jordan and some others on Carter's staff, the dismissal was seen by many—both then and afterward—as largely due to Califano's activism on tobacco, and Carter's nervousness about losing tobacco states in the 1980 election.[69]

Califano was replaced by Patricia Harris, a prominent African American Democrat who was secretary of housing and urban development before the cabinet shake-up. Months later, HEW was split into two agencies—the Department of Education and the Department of Health and Human Services. Harris was named head of the latter, and became Richmond's new boss.

Healthy People

While the pugilistic Califano was on the outs with the White House, the lower-key, lower-ranking Richmond had much better standing. It helped that he had formed a good friendship with the first lady, Rosalynn Carter.

They had met in 1977. Richmond had been appointed to the President's Commission on Mental Health; Mrs. Carter was the group's enthusiastic honorary chairperson. They also worked together on a campaign aimed at persuading all fifty states to require vaccinations for school attendance. (The effort succeeded.) Mrs. Carter liked Richmond, and she and her husband sent him warm notes and letters on several occasions, including when Richmond's wife, Rhee, became ill with cancer in 1977. And Richmond was the first person she asked to accompany her on a visit to Thailand in November 1979 to support an international relief effort for Cambodian refugees who had fled their country following a Vietnamese invasion. Mrs. Carter grew even fonder of Richmond during the trip, after he helped her through a difficult moment. In a refugee camp, she came upon a woman lying on a mat on the ground who had just given birth. An aide worker told Mrs. Carter the women was dying and wouldn't last much longer. The first lady froze, grasping for the right thing to do or say but unable to come up with anything. It was at that moment that Richmond whispered in her ear, "Tell her that she has a beautiful baby."[70]

The Carter administration frequently used the tactful Richmond as a public health ambassador. The surgeon general went to Cuba in 1977 as part of a groundbreaking exchange of medical personnel. He went to the USSR in 1978 as part of an early step toward lifting a moratorium on visits by U.S. officials to the Soviet Union. The same year, Richmond met with Egyptian president Anwar Sadat to talk about food and nutrition concerns. But not everyone appreciated his travels. Hale Champion, the HEW undersecretary to Califano, wasn't crazy about Richmond as an administrator and felt his trips were part of the problem. "Things would happen, and you'd look for Julius and he was in Budapest or some place," recalled Champion, who said he pushed for a deputy administrator for Richmond who would be a more constant presence.[71]

But Richmond was on hand to help the administration respond to a March 29, 1979, accident at the Three Mile Island Nuclear Generating Station near Harrisburg, Pennsylvania. The incident involving loss of coolant was brought under control but led to the authorized release of 40,000 gallons of radioactive waste water into the Susquehanna River, as well as the evacuation of pregnant women and children. For several days, it was a harrowing crisis. State and federal health officials scrambled to understand the extent of the radiation release as people living nearby anguished that they might develop cancer. As readings came in, Pennsylvania health officials claimed that only low levels of radioiodine had been released. Concerns persisted and erupted in Congress, and the following week it was Richmond who told legislators during a televised hearing that the general population was in no significant danger. But he also recommended that plant workers be issued potassium iodide pills as a precaution against damaging exposure to radiation. The work was intense, with Richmond writing a key memorandum on how the federal government thought the situation should be handled. "It was the only time he didn't come home at night," recalled Richmond's son, Barry, years later.[72]

The situation was resolved without turning into the disaster that Americans initially feared. In interviews years later, Richmond would contrast Three Mile Island with the AIDS crisis encountered in the

1980s by his successor, C. Everett Koop. AIDS was not resolved, and Koop became a national leader in addressing the epidemic. "People ask, 'How come I hear so much about Dr. Koop, and I didn't hear so much about you?'" Richmond said. "I say 'Well, that's good, because we didn't have a crisis.'"[73]

But one thing Richmond did *is* well remembered, at least in the public health community. In July 1979, he released *Healthy People: The Surgeon General's Report on Health Promotion and Disease Prevention*. The report set five objectives for reducing infant mortality and improving other health measures, and helped light a fire under federal, state, and county health officials to make more progress. In fact, the *Healthy People* report became something of a turning point in the way Americans think about their health. Unsanitary conditions and terrible infections were no longer the largest threat—unhealthy behaviors were. The report called on Americans to cut their intake of alcohol, salt, sugar, and saturated fats. Califano said the report represented a medical consensus as important as Terry's report on smoking and health. *Healthy People* has been imitated by states and other nations, and is updated every ten years to insure its continued importance—subsequent reports set a more specific and growing list of goals for 1990, 2000, 2010, and 2020. Interest groups jockeyed to add goals to each iteration, the most recent of which expanded the number to more than one thousand. Public health officials continually talk about the goals and the work of meeting them. "It is something we think about all the time," said Lance Rodewald, a former CDC vaccination expert.[74]

How much credit Richmond deserves for the report is a subject of debate.

The idea wasn't exactly new. *Healthy People* was preceded by a 1974 report issued by Marc Lalonde, Canada's minister of national health and welfare. A path-blazing document, the Lalonde report kickstarted the emerging field of health promotion, and argued that health was influenced by socioeconomic factors and not just the issues addressed by traditional medical and public health practice. It also listed seventy-four "possible courses of action" for improving health in Canada, some of which called for subsequently setting specific goals to reduce morbidity and mortality. Some have called the surgeon general's report a U.S. response to the Lalonde report and similar efforts going on internationally, a conclusion that some of the *Healthy People* report's creators do not contest, though they note their report went further and actually set concrete goals for ten years in the future.[75]

But did Richmond play a primary role in shaping the U.S. document? The truth seems to lie in a thicket of semantics. Richmond, in interviews, said his desire to set a health promotion platform for the nation is what triggered the work on the first *Healthy People* report. Califano said it really started when he asked the department to come up with a way to measure progress in health. Others have given credit for the goal system and other innovations to CDC director William Foege, who was responsible for goal setting in an earlier, epic campaign against smallpox in India. Kudos also have gone to Michael McGinnis, the young HHS official who had been part of the India campaign and was assigned the task of putting the *Healthy People* report together.

The consensus opinion: McGinnis was the true creator of the report, and the specific goal setting that followed. In an interview, McGinnis said as much, and that Richmond was "not a hands-on kind of guy" when it came to putting together a report. The decision to make it an ongoing project, with goals measured and reset every ten years, came from a conversation between Foege and McGinnis. Another key contributor was a CDC staffer named Dennis Tolsma, who came up with the name "Healthy People." But Richmond championed the project, helping to make sure adequate resources were available for McGinnis and others to do their work. Foege said there's no reason to take credit from Richmond. "If it was not his idea, it certainly came on his watch," he said.[76]

Important as it is considered in retrospect, the *Healthy People* report got very limited play in the press at the time. The *Washington Post* buried the story on page A28, and the reporter covering it—Victor Cohn—noted it suffered from a lack of advance publicity. It was simply released, along with a written statement by Califano, "with no fanfare whatsoever, despite its ambitious goals," Cohn observed.[77] Years later, McGinnis acknowledged it was rushed out because Califano was in his final days as HEW secretary and badly wanted to be involved in presenting it to the public.[78]

Richmond's Departure

In the 1980 election, Carter was beaten badly by Republican Ronald Reagan. As it took over the executive branch in early 1981, the new Reagan administration showed the door to Carter appointees at the Department of Health and Human Services. As assistant secretary for health, Richmond was a political appointee who had to clean out his desk immediately. But as surgeon general, Richmond was entitled to stay in office for his entire four-year term—that is, until the summer. Richmond decided to officially stay on for a few months, but used leave time and was largely absent as the Reagan appointees moved in.[79]

Richmond returned to Harvard, where he was a professor of health policy. His wife died in 1985, and he later remarried. Richmond also served as an expert testifying in two trials in which the plaintiffs claimed secondhand smoke was the cause of their health problems. He retired from his Harvard post in 1988, but held emeritus status and continued to write books and to influence public health. He died of cancer at his home in Chestnut Hill, Massachusetts, on Sunday, July 27, 2008. He was ninety-one.

The following October, a memorial service was held at the Harvard Club in Boston. Rosalynn Carter spoke. Also among the nearly two hundred in attendance were two of his successors as surgeon general— C. Everett Koop and David Satcher. They and others in attendance praised Richmond for his wisdom and accomplishments, and for being a gentle soul who quietly stood out in a political milieu full of harsher personalities. By also holding the assistant secretary for health position, he gained administrative power and resources that most of the surgeons general of the past forty years have lacked.

"I think Julius was the underrated Surgeon General," said Satcher, who became surgeon general in the late 1990s. "When you look at what he did, the things he launched in this country, I think he was one of the most productive."[80]

Richmond and his predecessor, Jesse Steinfeld, were each successes of a kind. They both managed to keep the Office of the Surgeon General relevant and influential to the public health. But their good deeds would quickly be eclipsed by a doctor who would take the job a step further and make its holder a public health icon.

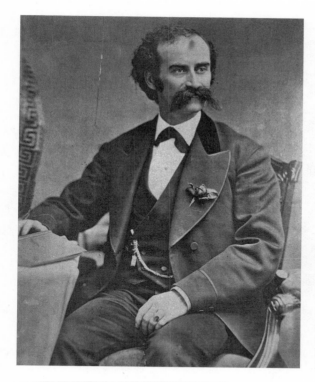

FIGURE 1. John M. Woodworth, the first U.S. surgeon general (photograph undated). His title at the time was supervising surgeon of the Marine Hospital Service. Courtesy of the National Library of Medicine.

FIGURE 2. John B. Hamilton, Woodworth's successor (photograph undated). Here he is dressed in the Marine Hospital Service uniform, complete with sword. Courtesy of the National Library of Medicine.

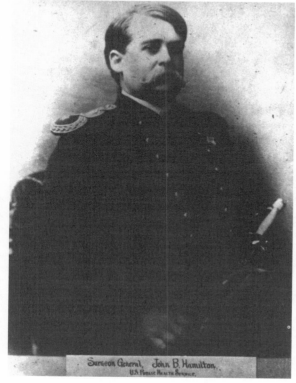

Surgeon General, John B. Hamilton,
U.S. Public Health Service.

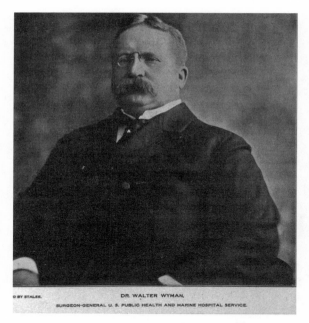

FIGURE 3. Walter Wyman, the third surgeon general, in a photograph published in a 1906 souvenir album. Courtesy of the National Library of Medicine.

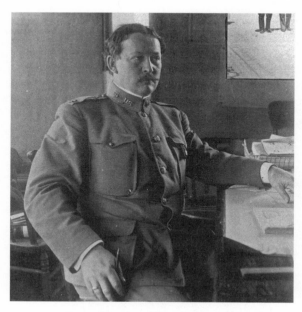

FIGURE 4. Rupert Blue, in uniform, in 1909, during the San Francisco plague campaign. He would later be named U.S. surgeon general and face the double challenge of World War I and the Spanish flu pandemic. Courtesy of the National Library of Medicine.

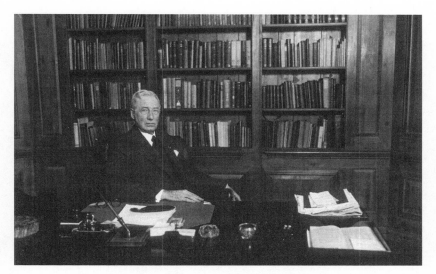

FIGURE 5. Hugh Cumming (photograph undated), who held the office through the 1920s and early 1930s. Courtesy of the National Library of Medicine.

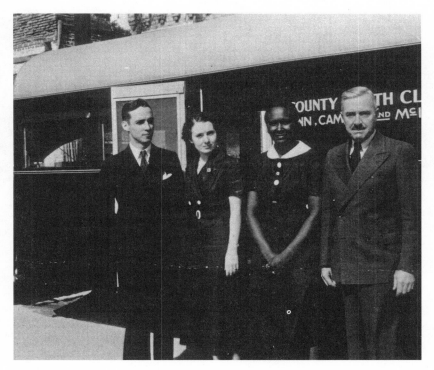

FIGURE 6. Surgeon General Thomas Parran (*far right*) in front of a mobile syphilis trailer in Brunswick, Georgia, in 1939. At far left is a young Leroy Burney, who would become surgeon general nearly a decade after Parran left office. Courtesy of the National Library of Medicine.

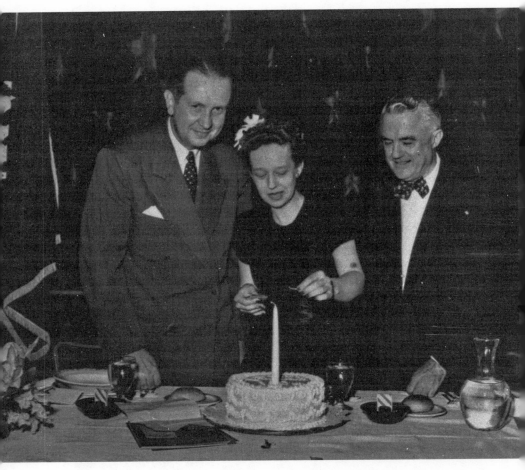

FIGURE 7. Leonard Scheele (*at left*), the seventh surgeon general, at a social event (photograph undated). Next to him are Gladys Dearing and FSA administrator Oscar Ewing. Courtesy of the National Library of Medicine.

FIGURE 8. *(opposite, top)* Surgeon General Luther Terry (*at podium*) at the January 1964 press conference in which he released the landmark report on the health risks of smoking. Courtesy of the National Library of Medicine.

FIGURE 9. *(opposite)* Surgeon General William Stewart (*far left*) walking at the NIH campus in 1967. To the right of Stewart are President Lyndon Johnson and NIH director James Shannon. The younger man behind and just to the right of Shannon is Philip Lee, who would assume the bulk of the surgeon general's administrative powers in a 1968 reorganization. Courtesy of the National Library of Medicine.

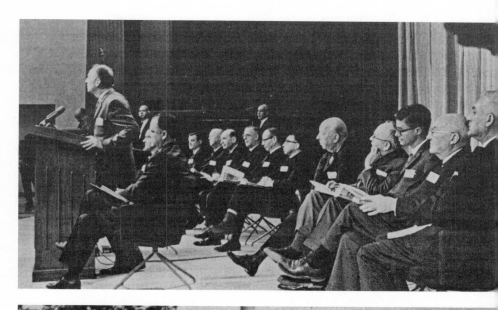

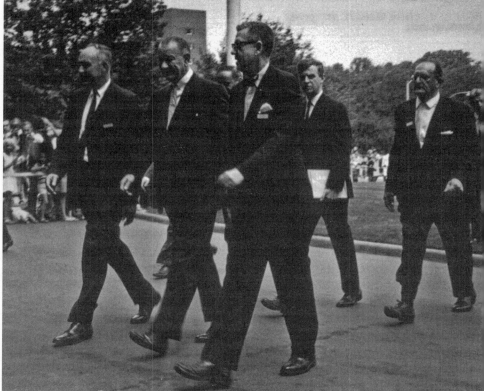

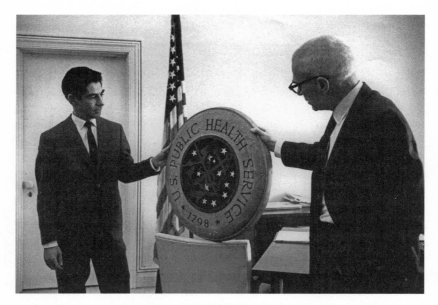

FIGURE 10. Surgeon General Jesse Steinfeld (*left*), with the U.S. Public Health Service emblem. Courtesy of the National Library of Medicine.

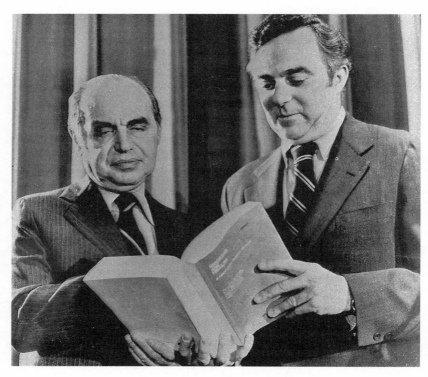

FIGURE 11. Surgeon General Julius Richmond (*left*), holding a smoking report with HEW Secretary Joseph Califano in January 1979. AP Photo/Harvey Georges.

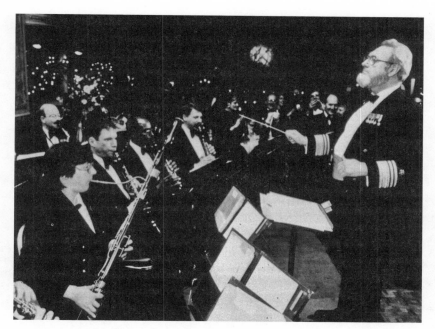

FIGURE 12. Surgeon General C. Everett Koop (*right*) conducting the Coast Guard band. Courtesy of the National Library of Medicine.

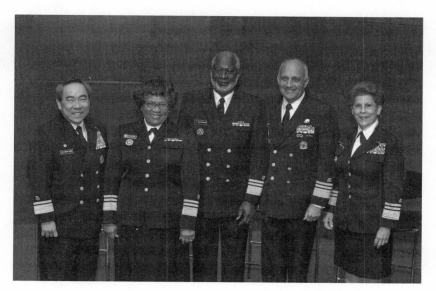

FIGURE 13. The surgeons general of the 1990s and the early 2000s, assembled for a group photo (*left to right*): Kenneth Moritsugu, who served as acting surgeon general twice; the outspoken Joycelyn Elders; the professorial David Satcher; the embattled Richard Carmona; and the eventually dishonored Antonia Novello. Courtesy *Winter Park Magazine*.

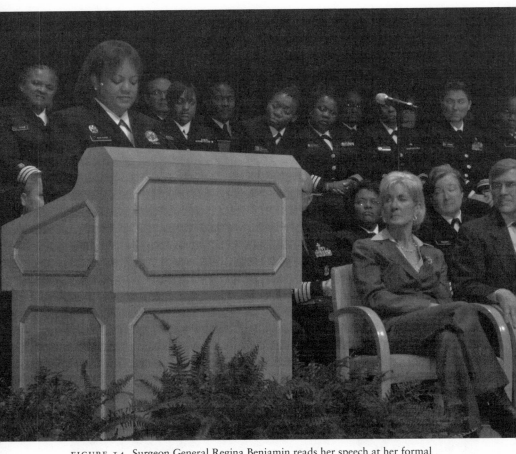

FIGURE 14. Surgeon General Regina Benjamin reads her speech at her formal swearing-in ceremony in January 2010. Sitting to the immediate right is HHS Secretary Kathleen Sebelius. Author's photo.

PART THREE

Struggle, 1981–2001

CHAPTER 8

Resurrection

"Senator No." That was the nickname for Jesse Helms, a powerful North Carolina politician famous for his opposition to civil rights, gay rights, disability rights, feminism, and affirmative action. But as 1981 began, the famously sour Helms was downright giddy.

Fellow Republican Ronald Reagan had been elected president in November, and all of Carter's HHS political appointments were packing up and moving out. The anti-smoking crusader Joseph Califano was already gone, and his scientific sidekick Julius Richmond was preparing to head back to Harvard. The new HHS secretary, Richard Schweiker, was a conservative who supported a constitutional amendment prohibiting abortion, and there had already been repercussions for federal health policy. What's more, the suddenly influential (and conservative) Heritage Foundation had issued a blueprint for changing business at the Public Health Service that would close PHS hospitals and turn into block grant programs the PHS services dealing with drug abuse, mental health, and other problems.

All of this was pleasing to Helms, but then came the cherry on top—news that President Reagan had decided to name C. Everett Koop as the new surgeon general.

Koop was a social conservative's dream. He was a booming personality at six feet, one and 205 pounds, a distinguished pediatric surgeon, an evangelical Presbyterian, and a candid doubter of the theory of evolution. More important, he was a leader in the national campaign against abortion who only a year before had completed a lecture tour in which he said abortion would lead to Nazi-like practices like euthanasia of the elderly. Liberal groups, public health organizations, and prominent journalists were appalled that Koop might become the nation's doctor. Surgeons general traditionally played a "voice of science" role that undermined conservative policy initiatives (and hurt Helm's tobacco-producing constituents), but Koop was shaping up to be the kind of surgeon general Helms could be proud of.

Ah, but Helms's elation would soon turn to dismay. Koop shocked nearly everyone by holstering his personal beliefs and taking a science-first approach to public health concerns. He almost immediately began condemning cigarettes, becoming a more vocal foe of Big Tobacco than even Califano. Koop became the administration's spokesman on AIDS, and pointedly rebutted conservatives' contention that it was a gay disease that resulted from—as Helms once put it—"disgusting" and "unnatural" homosexual behavior.[1] Koop even laid down his sword on the issue of abortion: when Reagan requested a report on the long-term effects of abortions on women, Koop said he was not able to produce such a report on the grounds that there was no reliable evidence on that question. He elevated the job to heights of visibility and influence not seen since the days of Thomas Parran, and in the process became a hero to liberals, a luminary to moderates, and an acrid shock to social conservatives. (It was during Koop's reign that journalists began to refer to the surgeon general as "the nation's doctor."[2])

After a few years of the new surgeon general, Helms grew so embittered that he tried to sic the inspector general on Koop, over an allegation that Koop had timed release of a report on nicotine addiction to cause maximum damage to cigarette manufacturers. "It was a ludicrous charge, and I think he knew it," Koop would later recall. "But I never heard from him again."[3]

"CRABS IN A BARREL"

Koop, as surgeon general, is commonly remembered as a commanding presence in a uniform and mustacheless beard. Various wags likened him to a Dutch sea captain, an Amish farmer, an Old Testament prophet, and one of the founders of the Smith Brothers cough drop company. The beard suited his sometimes stern, finger-pointing manner. He was an earnest, serious personality who had been that way much of his life.

Charles Everett Koop was born in Brooklyn, New York, on October 14, 1916, a descendant of Dutch settlers. He was an only child who grew interested in medicine as a young boy, impressed by Justice Gage Wright, an imposing, neatly pressed homeopathic physician who made house calls carrying a bag filled with hundreds of corked glass vials. "When he entered the house my family spoke more softly, as though a normal sound would break the spell," Koop wrote in his autobiography.[4] Young Koop settled on surgery early on, and as a boy worked to develop his dexterity by tying knots one-handed. Later, as a tall four-teen-year-old, he masqueraded as a medical student to sneak into oper-ating-theater galleries to watch doctors work at Manhattan's Columbia Presbyterian Medical Center. After a while, he did surgeries at home on rabbits and stray cats.[5]

Koop grew into a beefy young man, and joined the football team when he first arrived at Dartmouth College. He quit the team after a scrimmage concussion left him with double-vision and an enduring headache, and a doctor treating him said football could leave him too injured to be a great surgeon. Besides good advice, at Dartmouth Koop also gained the lifelong nickname "Chick" (as in "Chicken Coop") and met Betty Flanagan, the woman who would become his first wife. He graduated in 1937.

The next stop was Cornell Medical School, followed by an internship at Philadelphia Hospital. It was then that a University of Pennsylvania surgery professor—an intimidating bear of a man named I. S. Ravdin—invited him to do a five-year residency. Ravdin helped get Koop declared as essential to Penn and thus excused from military service in World War II.[6] At Ravdin's urging, Koop became a specialist in pediatric sur-gery and was soon named surgeon-in-chief at Children's Hospital. At the time, surgeons operated mainly on adults and commonly wrote off children with complicated medical conditions—especially congenital ones. Koop was, by his own count, just the sixth U.S. doctor to special-ize in pediatric surgery. Over the next three decades, Koop built up the program at Children's to great size and acclaim. By the time he left the hospital, it had eight divisions of surgical specialties, and Koop had earned a reputation as one of the fathers of pediatric surgery.

Koop's imperious persona, modeled on his domineering mentors, was a perfect fit for his chosen profession. "You know, I've never met a surgeon who didn't have a strong ego," said Edward Brandt, who would become Koop's supervisor years later at HHS. "As a matter of fact, I think it is probably essential to going in the operating room and picking up a knife and start cutting on people. If you don't believe you are right, it would be pretty hard to do that." Years later, Georges Benjamin of the American Public Health Association made a similar assessment. "Everyone who goes into surgical training doesn't end up as a surgeon, and so it's crabs in a barrel. And so that means he's tough," Benjamin said.[7]

Koop drew national attention in November 1953 when the *Saturday Evening Post* chronicled his groundbreaking surgical treatment of hydrocephalus (also known as "water on the brain"). But his greatest surgical fame involved separations of Siamese twins.

In October 1957, newspapers across the country announced Koop's successful operation on nine-day-old Pamela and Patricia Schatz, Siamese twins who had been joined at the pelvis. It had been harrowing—the heart of Patricia, the smaller child, had stopped beating and had to be massaged back to a normal rhythm. In September 1974, national media chronicled his successful separation of thirteen-month-old Clara and Altagracia Rodriguez after a ten-and-a-half-hour operation. (*People* magazine noted the Rodriguez family regarded Koop and his fellow physicians as gods who had performed a miracle.) In 1977, the *Philadelphia Inquirer* told the Pulitzer-nominated story of one of Koop's most mind-racking challenges—performing a surgery to separate fragile newborn twins who shared a fused heart, knowing that he would have to kill one of the sisters in the process.[8]

Adding to his renown was his unusual mustacheless beard, described by one reporter as "Lincolnesque." He first tried it in the 1960s, at the end of a three-week archaeology trip with one of his sons. Neither man shaved during the three weeks and at the end, Koop decided to shave his mustache but keep the beard, and his son did vice versa. Koop retained it for a good reason, he once said, with a slight grin. "It hides two double chins."[9]

Koop also favored a bow tie and large silver-rimmed classes, giving him the appearance of a Mennonite farmer trying to impersonate a college professor. He further stood out from many of his colleagues by developing a strong religious streak, which intensified after a co-worker at Children's Hospital suggested he attend a Presbyterian church in Philadelphia that featured a minister known for taking an intellectual approach to Christianity.[10]

As he was becoming famous for his surgical skills and eccentricity, Koop suffered a personal tragedy. In April 1968, Koop's twenty-year-old son, David, died from a fall while climbing Cannon Mountain in

New Hampshire. Koop got a phone call with the news on a Sunday evening when some of the family had gathered to watch the TV show *Mission Impossible*. He immediately gathered his family at the family piano and they prayed together, with Koop saying, "Lord, we know you made no mistakes here. This is obviously the day that you wanted to take my son home. We trust you." The family already had a strong Christian faith, but David's death "took us 10 steps deeper into it," said Koop's son Norman, who became a pastor.[11]

Koop's religious beliefs and strong feelings about children eventually led him to crusade against abortion. He began speaking about it after the U.S. Supreme Court's 1973 *Roe v. Wade* decision, which he feared would lead to a dramatic jump in the number of abortions. In 1975, Koop met prominent theologian Harold O.J. Brown, and they discussed ways to recruit more Protestants into an anti-abortion movement. In 1976, in the course of just two days, Koop wrote a 120-page book laying out his concerns: *The Right to Live, the Right to Die*. During those years, as his reputation as an evangelical Christian grew, he also became friends with the Reverend Billy Graham.[12]

Then, in 1977, came a chance meeting in Toronto with an old friend, the theologian and author Francis Schaeffer (an influential figure of the Christian Right). The two had a lengthy discussion about abortion, and decided to collaborate on a book and a five-part film that would become infamous during Koop's nomination for surgeon general.

The project was titled *Whatever Happened to the Human Race?* It was a Schaeffer family production, written and directed by the theologian's son, featuring Schaeffer's grandchildren in several scenes and spotlighting Schaeffer as he talked about morality and philosophy. Koop's role in the film was akin to Richmond's role in Califano's anti-smoking crusade: he was "the science." In the film's first installment, Koop discussed at what point a fetus can recoil from pain and the like. He then bluntly described the sordid details of methods of abortion. His narration took place while the camera panned over a thousand baby dolls floating on the crystalline Dead Sea. The scene ended with Koop—still talking—standing on a small rock in the water. He noted that the location in Israel is reputed to be the setting of Sodom, the Biblical city remembered for its impenitent sin. "Sodom was the most humanly corrupt city on Earth, a place of evil and death," Koop said. "Sodom comes readily to mind when one contemplates the evils of abortion and the death of moral law."[13] Koop went on a twenty-city speaking tour with Schaeffer in 1979 to support the film.

By 1980, as Reagan was running for office, Koop was winding down his medical practice and was open to something new. That fall, he listened with mild interest when some conservatives called to gauge his interest in being surgeon general if Reagan won the election. (Among the callers was Carl Anderson, an aide to Jesse Helms who was also a Roman Catholic strongly against abortion.) Koop's wife, Betty, urged him to do it. The morning after Election Day, Koop decided he wanted the job. In his characteristic aggressive manner, he contacted several people about it, including then–U.S. Senator Richard Schweiker of Pennsylvania, who was said to be the leading choice to become secretary of health and human services. But Koop's was not the only name in play. The powerful American Medical Association was uncomfortable with Koop, and pushed instead for Edward Brandt Jr., the respected vice chancellor of health affairs for the University of Texas.

Julius Richmond—still the surgeon general—advised Schweiker to keep the jobs of surgeon general and assistant secretary for health united in one person. But Schweiker, trying to satisfy multiple constituencies, ultimately decided to separate the roles. He named Brandt the ASH and Koop the surgeon general. Brandt was in place, fully confirmed, within a few months. But Koop became embroiled in a yearlong political battle that was the fiercest ever seen over a surgeon general nominee.

FIRE AND SMOKE

In February 1981, the Reagan administration named Koop as a deputy to Brandt, giving Koop a paycheck while the process began to win Senate confirmation for him to become surgeon general. Koop started in March, but had no real responsibilities, only orders from Schweiker to keep his head down during the confirmation process.

He tried, but it didn't matter. The line of people opposing his nomination already wrapped around the block. The AMA urged the Reagan administration to choose someone else. Planned Parenthood and the National Organization for Women, both pro-choice, took early, vocal stands against him. The American Public Health Association—which hadn't opposed the appointment of a surgeon general in a century—opposed Koop, saying he had no public health experience. Groups as disparate as the National Gay Health Coalition and the United Mine Workers expressed their concerns. The *New York Times* used the phrase "Dr. Unqualified" to headline an editorial lambasting him. Even Schweiker voiced misgivings, but bowed to the wishes of the White House.[14]

In addition to the lined-up opposition was a more immediate challenge. Koop was sixty-four and a half, too old for the job, legally speaking. The Public Health Service Act of 1944, enacted during the Parran era, said no surgeon general nominee could be older than sixty-four. Koop's supporters called the old rule a technicality and an instance of age discrimination, and Helms quickly and quietly tried to change the law through an amendment tacked on to an unrelated bill (one that banned surcharges on credit card purchases). It was a sneaky move that leading Democrats in Congress noticed, resented, and fought. "Why should a private bill for Dr. Koop be handled in such a surreptitious manner?" complained Representative Henry Waxman, a California Democrat who chaired the House Subcommittee on Health.[15]

Meanwhile, Koop was in a grueling limbo. He had left his surgical career and board positions with pro-life groups for a job with no power, no budget, and no voice. The respected Brandt quickly established himself as a tough administrator capable of talking to the press and public about public health matters, so it was becoming unclear how much Koop would be used even if he were confirmed. And at HHS, Koop was isolated both by his own ignorance of how the department worked and by PHS veterans who deemed him unfit for such a historically important, science-based office.

In his autobiography, Koop recalled how lonely he was at that time. "One day I decided to have lunch in the Humphrey Building cafeteria," he wrote, referring to the HHS's Brutalist headquarters. "As I walked into the dining room itself, I heard someone say, 'Here he comes.' By the time I reached my intended table at the far end of the room, the usual hum and clutter had subsided and a hush had fallen over the entire room. As I walked to my seat, I was absolutely astounded to see how many forks were poised in midair between plate and mouth as this unbelievable two-headed monster, the most unqualified surgeon general appointee in history, prepared to eat his lunch."[16]

But as he met with HHS officials, they found him personable and gradually grew sympathetic. "Those of us who knew Dr. Koop during those days sort of marveled at the fact that he stayed here in town, because of the enormous attacks upon him," said Edward Martin, a Public Health Service veteran who later would become Koop's chief of staff. Koop said those days in limbo proved pivotal to his later success. He established rapport with key officials at the FDA, the CDC, and elsewhere in the department. "Out of those tough months I made a number of very important friends in HHS who believed in me, believed

I was being given a raw deal, who did think I was credible, who did think I was able, who did think when I had an idea and the ability to do something with it, I would be successful," Koop said. (He would later call on those friends to lend him staff and funding for the surgeon general workshops and reports that helped make him famous.)[17]

By the end of August 1981, Congress had passed two amendments to remove the age limitation and any other legalities that might stand in Koop's way. A bigger turning point came in October when he appeared before a Senate Labor and Human Resources Committee. He criticized the Reagan administration for not trying to curb promotion of baby formula in developing countries.[18] He further surprised his detractors by pledging that if he became surgeon general, he would zip it regarding his own views on abortion. "It's not my intent to use any government post as a pulpit for ideology," he said. Later that month, the committee voted 11 to 5 to recommend that the full Senate confirm Koop. The Senate confirmed him in November, by a vote of 68 to 24.[19] On January 21, 1982, Koop finally was sworn in as surgeon general.

His first press conference was held a month later, to present the latest surgeon general report on smoking. The report fingered pipes and cigars as causes of at least four types of cancer, and broadened the list of cancers attributable to tobacco use. Koop's role was an assigned bit part. This was yet another installment in the nearly annual series of surgeon general reports on smoking, and, as with the others, the work and writing that went into the report was done years in advance by other experts. The surgeon general merely put a face on it, writing a short introductory note to the report and presenting the findings. At the press conference, Brandt was the initial speaker, with the surgeon general finishing up.

But Koop knew the smoking reports had become something of a raison d'être for the Office of the Surgeon General, and he carefully prepared for that press conference. "I think I saw smoking as the most visible thing my predecessors had done, and if I wanted to have some kind of platform from whence to jump to other things, I better do that one well," he said.[20]

He dominated. Oddly imposing in a dark suit and bow tie, he gave clear and unsparing answers to reporters' questions. He dismissed arguments by the Tobacco Institute that a scientific conclusion on causation could not yet be reached. He called smoking the nation's most pressing public health concern. Among those Koop impressed was Donald Shopland, a longtime government expert on smoking who had been involved in the surgeon general smoking reports for decades. "He had read that thing cover to cover," Shopland later recalled. "If you ever saw a press conference where someone really knew their shit, that was the press conference."[21]

Koop's performance was also a hit with the media. The *New York Times* and the *Washington Post* gave the press conference front-page treatment, and Koop detected an immediate shift in how he was written about. "I began to be quoted as an authority. And the press from that time on were on my side until I left Washington," he said. "I made the snowballs and they threw 'em."[22]

Koop found himself somewhat out of step with the Reagan administration, however, regarding the topic of smoking. The Office of the U.S. Trade Representative pushed to open foreign markets to American tobacco. Federal Trade Commission chair James C. Miller III told the press he didn't have time to read the results of a five-year FTC investigation into cigarette advertising abuses and had no interest in strengthening health warnings. "If people want to smoke, that's their business," Miller said.[23] But Koop bluntly and consistently talked about the need for stronger warnings against tobacco—and through the rest of the decade, he would be the only person in the Reagan administration to consistently take such a stand.

Every year, Koop came out with a new report on the dangers of tobacco. He took up Steinfeld's warnings about secondhand smoke and equated the addictive properties of cigarettes with those of heroin. He said cigarette company executives were morally corrupt. He gave speeches to medical associations, high schools, and numerous other groups, hammering away with his message and then going down into the crowds afterward to hand out buttons that said: "The Surgeon General personally asked me to quit smoking." In May 1984, at the annual meeting of the American Lung Association, Koop called for a smoke-free society by 2000.

The U.S. tobacco industry reacted accordingly. Edward Horrigan, chairman of R. J. Reynolds Tobacco, wrote Reagan two months later to complain about "the increasingly shrill preachments" of Koop, which he called "the most radical anti-tobacco posturing since the days of Joseph Califano."[24]

Tobacco officials worried because Koop was widely considered to be effective. Smoking rates dropped from 38 percent in 1981 to 27 percent in 1989, according to Gallup poll information. That was the largest drop seen since Gallup started regular polling on smoking in the early

1940s. Of course, the decline can't be attributed solely—or even mainly—to Koop. "To give him credit for the steep decline in the 1980s is to ignore everything that went on before," notes Ken Warner, an esteemed University of Michigan tobacco researcher (who counts himself as one of Koop's fans). That said, Koop's aggressive and unrelenting campaign against tobacco kept the issue high in the public mind. "On tobacco, he was the gold standard" for surgeons general, says the University of Alabama's Alan Blum.[25]

THE UNIFORM AND BABY DOE

Koop used tobacco as a springboard to other topics. Some were perhaps predictable, like his lectures against marijuana. Others were a bit more surprising: he was ahead of his time in placing significant focus on youth violence, and raised eyebrows in the fall of 1982 when he blamed the video game industry for contributing to the problem. The National Coin Machine Institute, which represented the cigarette machine and video game industries, called Koop's words "one of the most irresponsible and unthinking statements we have ever heard from an official of the federal government" and said it could "cast serious doubt on every action and statement emanating from the office of the Surgeon General."[26] As Koop knocked heads, controversy-loving reporters increasingly turned into admirers and increasingly sought him out.

He made another media splash when he became a leading figure in the Baby Doe story. "Baby Doe" was a boy born in Bloomington, Indiana, in April 1982. Blue at birth, the child was diagnosed as having Down syndrome and was also unable to eat normally because his esophagus was not attached to the stomach. The obstetrician who delivered the child said he would probably die of pneumonia in a few days. The parents went along with medical orders to sedate their son and deny him food, water, and medical aid. However, other physicians argued that the boy should be referred to an Indianapolis hospital for surgery. A fierce battle broke out among the medical staff about the right course of action. The situation rapidly escalated, hitting the media and the courts, with other families trying to adopt the boy. The baby died of starvation six days after his birth.[27]

Reporters called Koop—the renowned pediatric surgeon, pro-lifer, and now credible surgeon general—for comment. He initially declined, but it wasn't long before he became the government's lead spokesman on the matter.

Jesse Helms and a small group of other conservative congressmen pushed Schweiker to take action. President Reagan, also moved by the story of Baby Doe, instructed his HHS secretary to develop regulations to prevent doctors from stepping away from care and allowing infants born with birth defects to die. HHS did, and the regulations took effect in March 1983. They were immediately challenged in federal court by the American Academy of Pediatrics and the National Association of Children's Hospitals and Related Institutions, which argued that some babies have no real chance of survival and prolonging their lives was inhumane. The Reagan administration needed top health officials to explain and defend the rules, but had trouble finding anyone to fill the role. Brandt, the assistant secretary for health, had opposed the rules as overbearing and refused to defend them publicly. Schweiker wasn't around to defend them; he left office the month they went into effect, for a job as president of the American Council of Life Insurance. His replacement was Margaret Heckler, a former Massachusetts congresswoman who had opposed federal funding for abortions but was unfamiliar with clinical issues and somewhat averse to controversy. She chose Koop to do the talking.[28]

In a hastily called press conference in March 1983, Koop defended the rules as necessary. But federal judges invalidated them, sending HHS back to the drawing board. Koop agreed to help lead the effort, but said this time he wanted more control. "I went to Margaret Heckler and said, 'If you think I should continue to take this flack, I think it is only fair that I write the next set of regulations, so that at least any flack I take is deserved,'" Koop recalled.[29] The surgeon general wrote a new set of regulations, which also were struck down in court. But he also gathered the American Academy of Pediatrics and other groups together to forge a consensus document, which led Congress to expand the definition of child abuse to include the withholding of fluids and nutrition—a victory of sorts—which Reagan signed into law in October 1984.

Koop's handling of Baby Doe and other issues won him respect inside and outside HHS, and he increasingly gained visibility as power vacuums began to appear at the end of Reagan's first term. Brandt and others left HHS, creating an environment where temporary replacements were holding a number of key jobs. Among them was James Mason, the CDC director, who agreed to also be the acting assistant secretary for health in 1984—a role he would keep until 1986. Mason was busy running the Public Health Service, and happy to let the surgeon general continue in the bully pulpit. "I don't see my big ability as public speaking and it's not something I particularly enjoy doing," Mason said.[30]

Koop, now an important face at HHS, was reappointed by Reagan in October 1985. It meant four more years, and made him the first surgeon general to serve more than one term since Leonard Scheele in the 1950s.

That same year Koop got a new boss: Otis Bowen, appointed in 1985 to replace Margaret Heckler as HHS secretary. He had a résumé that made him unusually qualified (for an HHS secretary) to speak on health issues—"Doc" Bowen was a physician and former army medic as well as former governor of Indiana. But he recognized Koop's tremendous credibility with the media and was content to designate Koop the department's spokesman on certain controversial health topics. "When we wanted to explore an idea or had something that we wanted to get a fair shake, Chick talked about it for us. Chick operated within the Public Health Service, but I gave him broad discretion on what he did," Bowen later recalled in his autobiography.[31]

By the time Bowen took office, Koop was already working on something else—a bid to restore luster to the Commissioned Corps. Two things happened at the very beginning of Koop's time in Washington that sparked the effort.

First, in 1981—while Koop was still just a candidate for surgeon general—President Reagan ordered the closing of the last eight Public Health Service hospitals for seamen, and his Office of Management and Budget (OMB) began pushing for additional cuts to the Service and for the curtailing and eventual dismantling of the Corps. In June 1982, Representative Henry Waxman held a hearing to protest the actions. Ed Brandt, still very much in charge of the Service at that point, spoke at Waxman's hearing—with the kind of neutral, just-the-facts restraint required of a political appointee in such a situation. The OMB persisted, and pushed a proposal to strip Brandt of his power to manage and supervise the Service. That effort failed, but the Service was under attack and Brandt was barely holding the line.[32]

Second, Koop received a confidential letter in February 1982, less than a month after he was sworn in. It was from Luther Terry. He noted Koop came into office under a "relatively dark cloud," opposed by many in the Public Health Service, including Corps personnel. Terry also observed that Koop had no history with the Service and was no doubt seen as an uninformed interloper. Of course, Julius Richmond hadn't had any such experience, either, when he became surgeon general five years earlier, but Richmond worked hard to reverse that deficiency by focusing on science, celebrating Service tradition, and working hard to gain credibility with officers. Terry lobbied Koop to do the same. "I think that you should make a concerted effort to save the PHS as a proud team," Terry wrote.[33]

Koop took the advice to heart. By the fall of 1982, he had put away his trademark bowties and instead wore the navylike uniform of the Corps. It was a surprising wardrobe change. Uniforms had fallen out of use in the Public Health Service except for ceremonial occasions. In fact, it had been decades since surgeons general had regularly dressed in uniform—they thought of themselves as doctors and public health leaders, not military men, and so dressed the part. For Koop to push a new dress code was incongruous: He was the first surgeon general who lacked prior experience not only with the Corps but also in any unformed service. While other surgeons general had been to war, Koop's only exposure to wearing a uniform was through the Boy Scouts. He was blessed with the dominating bearing of a military commander, but it still took some real chutzpah for Koop to start dressing up each day like a decorated war hero.

But there was a method to his brashness. He believed wearing the surgeon general's navy-modeled, vice-admiral uniform granted him a greater aura of authority, and it was an early step in Koop's attempt to revitalize the Corps.

A century earlier, membership in the Corps had meant passing the most rigorous exams of the day to join an elite national squadron of disease-fighting physicians. Through the decades, however, it had become little more than a second personnel system with some better benefits than Civil Service. The uniform had fallen out of favor at PHS agencies like the NIH and CDC, agencies that by the 1970s and 1980s were full of researchers lacking any military inclination. The Vietnam War hadn't helped, nor had the perception that some of those who had joined the Corps in the late 1960s and early 1970s were mainly trying to avoid service in the real military, giving birth to the derisive description of Corps members as "yellow berets." "The uniform became a symbol of derision. I mean, if I was to have worn my uniform in the '70s through the Humphrey Building or even the Parklawn Building, I think people would have thrown eggs at you," said Paul Ehrlich, the former acting surgeon general, referring to two Washington, D.C.–area buildings where PHS staff were concentrated.[34]

Koop believed the 5,600-person Corps—just a fraction of the people who worked at PHS agencies—had languished. Without action, he reasoned, the OMB would succeed in its long-standing attempt to do away with the Corps. He thought that if Corps members started wearing their uniforms again, it would make them more visible and build a perception they were a vital group of federal personnel. With Bowen's support, Koop assumed formal command authority over the Corps's officers in April 1987. He required people to wear the uniform more often, promoted recruitment to the Corps, and revised mobilization guidelines.[35]

The uniform requirement did not go over well with many PHS researchers and scientists.

"There were a couple of places where we had some very serious problems," recalled Ed Martin, appointed Koop's chief of staff for promoting revitalization. He described a meeting at the CDC with hundreds of officers upset about questions like "What does mobility mean to me?" and "What's this bullshit about wearing a uniform?" and "Here I am, a lab scientist. What do you mean I'm going to be sent to the Indian Health Service?" One CDC officer told a *New York Times* reporter that wearing a uniform probably would interfere with certain kinds of public health work. "Could you imagine going into a ghetto in New York and trying to get people there to talk to you about IV drug abuse?" he asked. Adding to the rancor: some in the Public Health Service were perturbed by a report that Koop had (unsuccessfully) tried to arrange a Christian prayer breakfast at one meeting of the Commissioned Officers Association.[36]

But CDC's leadership stood behind Koop, and Koop was forthright and forceful. "He just said, 'This is the way we're going to do it, and we are not just another personnel system,'" Martin said. Opposition dissolved in six to twelve months within the PHS. And in the late 1980s, OMB officials voiced support for the Corps—the first such statement from that office in four decades.[37]

KOOP AND AIDS

In June 1981, while Koop was still awaiting confirmation, the CDC published the first report of a terrifying new disease that eventually became known as acquired immunodeficiency syndrome, or AIDS.

The illness started with flulike symptoms but progressed to a fatal condition that destroyed the body's immune system and allowed other infections and diseases to run rampant. It was first detected in five gay men in Los Angeles, and the media called it GRID (for gay-related immune deficiency). The name AIDS did not come into standard use until the summer and fall of 1982, after it became clear that other people—including Haitians, hemophiliacs, and some drug addicts—were also getting the illness. There was no treatment. An AIDS diagnosis was a death sentence.

Complicating matters was a persisting and widespread societal belief that it was a disease of homosexual men, not something most heterosexuals had to worry about. If ever there was a situation requiring a powerful and skilled national health educator, the AIDS outbreak was it. Koop saw that responsibility as his. "By Congressional mandate—by public health law—the one thing that is absolutely clear and indisputable is that the surgeon general is to provide information to the public on how they can protect themselves against disease, and what they can do to promote good health," he said years later.[38]

But Brandt did not assign Koop to speak on AIDS. Quite the opposite: when Koop was to appear before the media, HHS public affairs staff told reporters he would not be answering questions on AIDS. "The attitude of the people that handled public affairs for me—who dealt with my speaking engagements and so forth—was almost as though there was some tribal taboo on the very word AIDS passing through my lips," Koop said. Technically, Koop wasn't being muzzled; the job was tasked to others. Koop found his exclusion awkward, but Brandt said it was simply an administrative decision.[39]

Heckler and Brandt were the ones handling questions about AIDS, but not well. They called AIDS the administration's "number one health priority" but would not say why the government wasn't spending more on AIDS research. At a press conference announcing Robert Gallo's discovery of the AIDS virus, Heckler foolishly predicted a vaccine would be available within two years.[40] Heckler hampered Brandt: In May 1984, he had agreed to attend an annual awards dinner held by the Fund for Human Dignity, the fund-raising arm of the National Gay Task Force. Conservative groups heard about the appearance and flooded the White House with telegrams demanding Brandt be fired if he attended. Heckler was worried about the political fallout, and soon after an HHS spokesman announced Brandt would not be going to the dinner because of another meeting.[41]

Brandt left HHS that year; Heckler grew embattled. Her claims that the administration was giving researchers what they needed were challenged by prominent researchers and by some members of Congress. In late 1985, the CDC stopped spending money on AIDS education, buckling to pressure from White House conservatives who believed the government was essentially teaching gay men how to commit sodomy.[42]

President Reagan himself had been silent on the issue of AIDS, prompting growing criticism from the gay community and others. Finally, in February 1986, Reagan asked Koop to prepare a report on AIDS for the American people. The surgeon general spent most of the rest of the year interviewing health officials, researchers, leaders of the gay community, and others. He wrote the report himself—a first, given that surgeon general reports were always written by squadrons of others. He did not submit it for White House clearance.

His frank thirty-six-page report, released in October 1986, was hailed as the government's first major statement on what the nation should do stop the spread of AIDS. It called for Americans to set aside their differences and work together to stop the epidemic. Koop called for condom use and sex education, which he said (in answer to a reporter's question) should start in the third grade. He also opposed compulsory blood testing to identify infected individuals.[43] It was a remarkable statement from a religious conservative, containing the implicit argument that advocating for distribution of condoms in schools was not incompatible with advocating for the protection of unborn fetuses.

The report was a sensation. "This wasn't some tedious call for a blue-ribbon commission or bureaucratic coordination; this was about rubbers and sex education," wrote the journalist Randy Shilts in *And The Band Played On,* his renowned book about the unfolding of the AIDS epidemic. "Uncorrupted by the language of AIDSpeak, Koop was able to talk in a way that made sense; at last, there was a public health official who sounded like a public health official. Not only that, he was able to utter words like 'gay' without flinching. . . . Koop quickly became so in demand for speeches that he was called a 'scientific Bruce Springsteen.'"[44]

It was not as well received at the White House, however, where some officials were in favor of mandatory testing and isolating the infected from the rest of society—something Koop had argued against. Particularly unhappy was Gary Bauer, Reagan's domestic policy advisor and a staunch defender of "family values." James Mason, the official who filled in as assistant secretary for health after Brandt's departure, voiced a common perception about the mindset at 1600 Pennsylvania Avenue. "I hope I'm not misjudging, but it was almost as though it was a vindictiveness toward the gay man and they were hoping that this disease would take them all out," Mason recalled years later.[45] Some Reagan staffers were also irked by Koop's frank talk about condoms. Two White House staffers visited Koop a few months later, asking that he drop the word "condom" from the next edition of the report. Koop didn't believe they had been sent by Reagan himself, but rather by others in the White House, and refused.[46]

Koop said Bauer made it difficult for him to call or meet with the president. But he believed Reagan was not against him. "His staff would call up my staff and say 'My boss didn't like what your boss said.' We had a standard answer; 'When your boss feels that way and talks to my boss, he'll get some action.' Period. He [Reagan] never called about anything like that," Koop said.[47] "He called the bluff," said Anthony Fauci, Koop's good friend and personal physician and one of the government's leading infectious diseases scientists.[48]

Koop was beginning to feel untouchable. The unique nature of the surgeon general's four-year appointment meant he technically could not be fired, not by the president and certainly not by Bauer and his cronies. He confided to reporters that he didn't always walk his talk: he exercised little and favored steaks and two dry martinis at lunch and lobster and coffee ice cream for dinner. He was well aware of his popularity. "I'm a folk hero, and you can't bash a folk hero too hard," he told one reporter at the time.[49]

Conservative leaders made it clear that they thought Koop had become a problem. The activists Phyllis Schlafly and Paul Weyrich decried the idea of teaching high school students about condoms, and said the AIDS issue could be a litmus test for Republican candidates in the upcoming 1988 elections. Politicians were listening. U.S. Representative William Dannemeyer, a conservative Republican from California, said Koop might have to be replaced. And Jack Kemp and Bob Dole were among the presidential contenders who pulled out of their earlier commitments to a testimonial dinner to honor Koop.[50]

But Koop's fan base mushroomed. Democrats, gays, liberals, public health workers, and others became unabashed admirers. U.S. Representative Gerry Studds, a Massachusetts Democrat, had Koop's report mailed to all 268,000 households in his district. Representative Waxman, who had called Koop "scary" during the confirmation proceedings of 1981, now spoke of the surgeon general as "a man of heroic proportions." Waxman was echoed by Richard Dunne, executive director of the Gay Men's Health Crisis in New York. "He's an unlikely hero, but on this issue, he's a hero and he came along when we really needed him," Dunne said.[51]

Koop pushed forward with the campaign as it elevated him to new heights of notoriety. He answered questions about AIDS in a first-of-its-kind HBO special that aired in October 1987. He topped that the following year by engineering the largest public health mailing ever done.

The CDC had planned a mailing of AIDS information to U.S. households but abandoned the plan because it could not get clearance from Reagan administration officials. Koop, accustomed to working around the White House, took over the effort. The result was a pamphlet entitled "Understanding AIDS," which was sent to all 107 million households in the United States in June 1988. The cover carried Koop's photo with a message from the surgeon general: "Some of the issues involved in this brochure may not be things you are used to discussing openly. I can easily understand that. But now you must discuss them. We all must know about AIDS. Read this brochure and talk about it with those you love."[52]

Koop, lacking any real budgetary authority, put the project together by begging funds and assistance from his growing list of allies within the Department of Health and Human Services. Among those who helped was Fauci, the Brooklyn-born director of the National Institute of Allergy and Infectious Diseases. Koop often visited Fauci because the surgeon general's home was on the NIH campus, next to Fauci's office building. From the parking lot, "he had to go through [my building] to get to his house," Fauci recalled. "He'd knock on the door and say 'We gotta talk about AIDS.'" The two had lengthy discussions about what to tell the public about the disease, and Fauci helped Koop get a few hundred thousand dollars through an interagency transfer of funds.[53]

In the first eighteen days after the mailing, more than 100,000 extra calls were made to a special government AIDS hotline, some asking for more explicit instructions on how to use condoms. (The government received only a few hundred complaints.) The mailing was a success, and enshrined the surgeon general in the public mind as the leading government source for health information. A few years later, a survey of a 1,600 adults found that 94 percent had heard of the surgeon general.[54]

KOOP'S DEPARTURE

Koop had become the highest-profile surgeon general of all time, and there was every reason to believe he would get a third term if he wanted it. True, he had many conservative detractors, but he seemed to be on very good terms with Vice President George Bush, who had sought Koop's counsel on AIDS and other issues, sometimes over lunch.[55]

When Bush was elected president in November 1988, Koop assessed the situation and decided to ask for a promotion.

Given his years of experience within HHS and around the capital, Koop believed he was a logical choice to become Bush's HHS secretary. But Bush surprised him by choosing Louis Sullivan, a prominent African American physician from Atlanta who was an old friend of Bush and his wife, Barbara.

Koop quickly grew embittered with the new administration. He phoned Sullivan the day the announcement became official, offering congratulations and advice, but the call wasn't returned. Then a White House staffer told Koop's friend and supportive boss, Otis Bowen, to clean out his desk within three days. Koop found the Bush people rude and concluded he was not wanted. He submitted a letter of resignation to Bush in February 1989, saying he would serve several more months but would finish by the time his term expired that November. In Koop's final months, Sullivan's staff took away the surgeon general's personal assistant (leaving him with two secretaries). They also canceled Koop's executive dining room privileges.[56]

But before he left office, Koop enjoyed a victory lap of sorts with the media and public, as examples of his willingness to speak truth to power accumulated. In January 1989, he disclosed to the press that his office had, at the request of President Reagan, studied the impact of abortion on women's health, but determined there was no conclusive evidence of harmful physical and emotional consequences. Koop remained opposed to abortion, but "we could not prepare a report that could withstand scientific and statistical scrutiny," Koop told a House subcommittee two months later. "On the abortion issue, Koop made it clear he was the nation's doctor, not the nation's chaplain," the syndicated columnists Jack Anderson and Dale Van Atta wrote two months later.[57]

In the late spring of 1989, Koop took on alcohol, recommending new taxes on beer, restrictions on alcoholic beverage advertising, and reduction of the permissible blood-alcohol level for drivers. Even conservative columnist George Will—who found the proposal for raising taxes debatable—praised Koop for his "constructive irritability" and his "splendid legacy."[58]

Koop's term officially ended October 1, 1989, but he continued to be a headliner.

He remained an oft-quoted authority on a range of health issues. In 1992, he called for licensing gun owners as a way to cut homicide rates. In 1994, he helped launch the "Shape Up America!" campaign to encourage Americans to lose weight. In the early 1990s he joined the Clintons in campaigning for health reform, and a few years later joined FDA commissioner David Kessler in pushing for greater government regulation of tobacco products.[59]

Koop's enduring popularity and prestige were such that in 2003— fourteen years after he stepped down as surgeon general—he was a featured guest on *Da Ali G Show,* a satirical HBO program in which the British comedian Sacha Baron Cohen masqueraded as a dim-witted, hip-hop TV interviewer. Cohen introduced Koop as "the main man medicine," meant as (intentionally ungrammatical) high praise. Koop memorably glowered as Cohen asked him a series of bizarre anatomy-related questions like "Does all of us really have bones, or is that what the media want us to believe?" and "Why is all skeletons involved in evil stuff?"[60]

In the years after he left office, Koop increasingly traded on his good name. Among his more successful ventures: He was hired by NBC to do a successful series of health specials for television, wrote an autobiography for Random House, and published another book with ABC medical correspondent Timothy Johnson. Early in the twenty-first century, he was a regular presence on TV, appearing in commercials for Life Alert, a company making medical emergency warning bracelets for the elderly.

Not every venture went well, though. He got a black eye for DrKoop. com, a health information website that Koop cofounded in 1997. It was a terrific idea, tapping into a public hunger for good medical advice that was just a few clicks away, and initially the service was wildly popular. But it ran into trouble after it went public in 1999 and came under investigation for violating federal securities laws. More personally damaging to Koop were criticisms that the site blurred the line between objective information and advertising, and failed to disclose that Koop and others received a commission on products and services sold because of the website. (Koop gave up his commissions following the complaints.) The company went into bankruptcy, and afterward Koop spoke of the whole experience with great bitterness. "I wasn't in management. I was at the board level. But management really ran it into the ground," he said.[61]

Yet Koop is still remembered mainly as one of the greatest surgeons general of the modern era. His legacy included more than a dozen reports and formal communications while he was in office, on topics as varied as AIDS, nutrition, smoking, and sexual abuse of children. He helped move the needle on U.S. smoking rates. He shone a clarifying light on the emerging issue of AIDS to an ignorant public. Improbably, he also transformed the surgeon general into superstar status. Past surgeons general had been widely known—most notably Thomas Parran, who in the 1930s and 1940s was a multimedia presence with a best-selling book and his face on the cover of *Time* magazine. But most of them got onto front pages because of the power they held. Koop had no real power, just ambition and an outsized personality that he used to fill a vacuum of medical authority within the federal government.

Surgeons general have been attacked as meddlesome nannies always trying to tell the public how to behave (e.g., not smoke, exercise, eat less). But Koop's appearance and authoritative manner helped him shrug off such attacks. He was no nanny, but rather a stern, wise, and well-intentioned grandfather that people listened to. Indeed, he was so good at his job that all of his successors suffered in comparison, something that federal health officials freely admit. "We all remember Dr. Koop as the Surgeon General," said Kenneth Moritsugu, who served as acting surgeon general from 2006 to 2007. "Even today, when we talk about the Surgeon General, people always come back at me and say, 'Oh, you mean Dr. Koop!'"[62]

Koop died on February 25, 2013, at his home in Hanover, New Hampshire (the home of his beloved Dartmouth College). He was ninety-six.

His family held a funeral service two weeks later, at a church in nearby Woodstock, Vermont, where Koop's son Norman was pastor. One of the more moving parts of the two-hour service came when Norman Koop led the 350 in attendance in singing "It Is Well with My Soul," a spiritual written in 1873 by a Chicagoan named Horatio Spafford. Norman Koop told the gathered mourners that Spafford wrote the song after a personal tragedy—Spafford's wife and children preceded him on a vacation trip to Europe, and were on a ship that sank off the coast of Ireland. Spafford received a telegraph from his wife that contained only two words: "Saved. Alone." (She had survived but their children had died.)

Norman Koop told the story in an effort to share a message about acceptance and even thankfulness to God in the wake of a loved one's passing, but the story contains an analogy to Koop as surgeon general. Koop lifted the office to new heights, and as he left, it was seemingly safer than it had been in decades. But there would be no successor like him. The happy, swaggering days Koop had enjoyed would not be seen again.

CHAPTER 9

Drawn as Villains

It was perhaps inevitable that there would be a comic book character named the Surgeon General. Crime fighters with quasi-military and quasi-medical names were common sights in newsstand racks, including Captain Marvel and Doctor Strange. Some comic book writer was bound to create a Surgeon General, especially in the wake of the uniformed, larger-than-life C. Everett Koop.

In the spring of 1992, it happened. The Surgeon General debuted in Marvel Comics, showcased in a two-issue story line with two of Marvel's most popular heroes—Spider-Man and Daredevil.

But for those who saw the real surgeon general as a heroic public health figure, two aspects of this character were no doubt surprising: Marvel's Surgeon General was a woman, and she was a villain.

To be specific, she was a crazed female surgeon who picked up men in Manhattan nightclubs and cut out their organs to sell on the black market. Drawn as a sexy redhead in a tight dress while cruising bars, she donned surgical scrubs and mask with a bandolier of assorted knives while fighting superheroes. (Fittingly, she had no real powers.) Dan Chichester, the writer who created the story line, said there was no real-life inspiration for the character. He simply needed to give a name to the knife-wielding villain in a dark tale about a black market for organs, and resorted to what he later called "a bad pun." He recalled being dimly aware that the surgeon general at the time was a woman, but didn't know much about her. He in no way meant to malign any actual surgeon general from that era, he emphasized in an interview.[1]

Many others have, however. Two women held the title of surgeon general in the early 1990s—Antonia Novello and Joycelyn Elders—and both are remembered as troublemakers (though for different reasons). Elders was intensely vilified as a too-frank spokeswoman for masturbation, marijuana legalization, and other politically unpalatable topics. She was the LeRoy Nieman of public health, accused by some health policy tastemakers as being splashy and loud but lacking the subtle skills expected in a respected health leader. Like Nieman, the artist, she was also more popular and better known than those who tsk-tsked her, and retained a fan base that adored her unflinching candor.

Novello, meanwhile, was a disappointment in office who years later became the first former surgeon general to plead guilty to a felony. One farceur called Novello the Leona Helmsley of public health. Others were less colorful, but no less severe. "She was pretty much a zero," said the late David Sencer, former CDC director.[2]

The truncated terms of Novello and Elders would serve as hard lessons for their successors. The dismissal of the unconforming Elders became a warning sign that no surgeon general can expect free reign to say whatever he or she wants. But just as important was the example set by Novello, who accomplished little but hung on for years by being careful never to irritate her political bosses.

ANTONIA NOVELLO
The Pride of Fajardo

Antonia Novello was a minority hire, plain and simple.

Louis Sullivan, the new secretary of health and human services, was a black southerner keenly interested in addressing the health needs of blacks, Hispanics, and other minority populations. For Sullivan, two things about her stood out, "First of all," he said, "she was female and I was interested in having females in my administration. And secondly, she was Hispanic, and I was interested in promoting minorities in significant positions in my administration."[3]

Novello was the only current or former surgeon general to decline to be interviewed for this book. But it's clear from other sources that she reveled in being known as the first woman and first Hispanic to be surgeon general.

She was born Antonia Coello on August 23, 1944, the oldest of the three children. Her birthplace and childhood home was Fajardo, a small, pretty coastal city on the eastern end of the island of Puerto Rico. Her father, Antonio Coello, died when she was eight. Her mother later remarried, wedding an electrician named Ramon Flores.[4]

Her mother—Ana Delia Flores—was the guiding force in Antonia's life. Mrs. Flores was principal of Fajardo's junior high school and, later, of the high school. She also would sometimes substitute-teach for Antonia's classes, and would preselect the teachers in charge of Antonia's education. "She would say, 'Education is the reason by which we exist, and I will make sure that the best teaches you, because public school is a good system.' She made sure of that. All my life I almost felt that my grades were not mine, that my grades were a product of my mother making sure that I was educated by the best," Novello recalled years later.[5]

Some students questioned her academic achievements, suggesting her mother not only placed her with the best teachers but also negotiated top grades for her daughter. These doubts "only motivated me to be better," Novello would later recall. Young Antonia strove to please her critics, describing herself as a cutup who tried her best to make others laugh. She acted in school plays and was the lead soprano in the high school chorus.[6]

Young Antonia was also dealing with a severe medical condition. She was born with congenital megacolon, which left her unable to move her intestines. (As she later described it, "I was born without the cells that make you think you have to go to the bathroom.") She spent two weeks in the hospital every summer as a child, and came to be impressed by her pediatrician and her gastroenterologist and also by a favorite aunt who was a nurse. "I always felt I was going to be a doctor," she said.[7]

She suffered far longer than was necessary. A surgery to correct the condition was first recommended when Antonia was eight, but she didn't get the operation until she was eighteen. When the procedure was finally done, the surgeon was a cardiovascular specialist who was the only doctor at her Puerto Rican hospital willing to try it. She suffered complications until she was twenty, finally resolving the problem through two months of care at the Mayo Clinic in Rochester, Minnesota.[8]

Those operations interrupted her college years. She attended the University of Puerto Rico at Rio Piedras, finally earning her bachelor's degree in 1965. She then attended the University of Puerto Rico School of Medicine at San Juan, where she got her medical degree in 1970, graduating near the top of her class. In San Juan, she met a navy flight surgeon, Joe Novello, and married him the day after her medical school graduation.[9]

Joe and Antonia Novello moved to Michigan in 1970, where she did her internship and residency in pediatrics at the University of Michigan. She specialized in pediatric nephrology after growing interested in the specialty following the death of a favorite aunt (the nurse) from kidney failure. When she finished, she opened her own pediatrics office, but closed it in 1978 to take a job with the National Institutes of Health.[10]

In the early 1980s, Novello took a legislative fellowship that would prove important for her future career. She worked for U.S. Senator Orrin Hatch and helped draft the legislation that would become the National Organ Transplant Act of 1984, a valuable addition to her résumé. (That law banned the sale of human organs, meaning Novello helped outlaw the criminal activity perpetrated by the Surgeon General character in Marvel Comics.) Perhaps just as important, Hatch got to know Novello as a well-spoken "ball of energy," and he later became her main supporter in the Senate during her surgeon general confirmation process.[11]

Novello progressed through a series of jobs at NIH, rising through the ranks to become deputy director of the National Institute of Child Health and Human Development (NICHD). In 1987, she became coordinator for AIDS research at NICHD, a responsibility that gave her visibility as a specialist in pediatric AIDS. Another feather in her cap came from serving as a U.S. delegate to the International Ethics Committee on AIDS in Paris.

She also gained some notoriety, through her husband. Joe Novello had become a popular child psychiatrist who frequently made television and radio appearances in Washington to speak on health topics. And Joe's brother was even more famous: Don Novello, a comedian who played the hip Catholic priest Father Guido Sarducci on the TV show *Saturday Night Live*. The fact that Father Sarducci was a chain-smoker gave Novello some comic material when she later became surgeon general. "For the longest time, we didn't want Donnie to admit he was related to us," she told *People* magazine in 1990.[12]

Still, Novello was at best a dark horse candidate for surgeon general. Speculation had raged for months about who would be named to fill Koop's gigantic shoes, and the names considered most likely included Robert Redfield, a noted researcher at Walter Reed Army Institute of Research, and James H. "Red" Duke, a charismatic Texas trauma surgeon who hosted the PBS television show *Bodywatch*. Also in contention was Mary Guinan, who had played a prominent role in the CDC's response to AIDS in the 1980s and was promoted by the American

Medical Women's Association as the strongest female candidate for the job.[13]

But White House officials wanted a lower-profile surgeon general than Koop, and also one who supported the president's opposition to abortion except to protect a woman's life or in the event of rape or incest. "We don't hire people that don't support our policies. That is a hard and fast rule," said White House spokesman Marlon Fitzwater. That hurt the chances of Guinan, who professed neutrality on the issue but had served on a Planned Parenthood medical advisory board years before. (Guinan may also have fared poorly in her White House interview, which was conducted by the president's personal physician and longtime friend, Burton Lee. Guinan recalled chafing at questions she considered inappropriate, such as "How old are you?" and "How tall are you?")[14]

Novello was Louis Sullivan's idea. He had come across her when he was president of the Morehouse School of Medicine, through his dealings with the NIH. When Sullivan became HHS secretary, he appointed a committee to help him find women and minorities to fill key jobs within the department. The effort led to the appointment of Gwendolyn King as social security commissioner and Gail Wilensky as head of the Health Care Financing Administration, and to the naming of Novello as well. "I had a conscious policy of trying to improve or increase the diversity in the department," Sullivan recalled, "and so that was really one of the driving forces in asking her to become Surgeon General."[15]

Novello said she was as surprised as anyone to be tapped. She asked Sullivan why he picked her, and wondered aloud if it was to fill some kind of minority hiring quota. "And he said, 'I have read your curriculum and I can see that you can do it. I don't need quotas, because I myself am a minority.' That's when I said, 'Okay, let's keep going on the interview.'" Novello came to revel in being considered "a package deal"—a woman, a doctor with AIDS credentials, a minority who embodied the American Dream, and "someone who was kind of conservative, but with common sense."[16]

In November 1989, a month after the official end of Koop's term, the White House formally announced she was Bush's choice to succeed Koop. Novello may not have been as formidable as her predecessor, but she also was not as controversial. Her confirmation went smoothly, and she officially began her term in March 1990, at the age of forty-five. When she was sworn in, she told Bush, "Mr. President, thank you very much for bringing West Side Story to the West Wing," she later recalled.[17]

One of her first official acts was to return to Fajardo, her hometown, where four thousand people filled the seats of a baseball stadium to cheer her as she walked down a makeshift runway, carrying a bouquet of flowers. "I've been in the White House and in the senate of Puerto Rico, but there is no feeling like this one," Novello, in tears, told the crowd. "I am the Surgeon General of the United States, but in this town I'm still Miss Flores' little girl."[18]

Attacking Joe Camel

Like Koop, Novello came late to a new HHS administration. Sullivan had been in place more than a year when Novello started as surgeon general, and James Mason had been assistant secretary for health for about as long. Mason showed no interest in elbowing Novello out of the bully pulpit, but Sullivan did. In the pattern of Joe Califano, he wanted to be primary spokesman on the issue of tobacco.

In 1989, Sullivan pushed R.J. Reynolds to cancel a marketing campaign for Uptown, a new mentholated cigarette brand aimed at black people. He also proposed a smoking ban in all federal buildings, and said he expected recipients of federal health grants to restrict smoking in their offices. In most administrations, the surgeon general led the war on tobacco, but Sullivan informed Novello that would not be the case while he was running the department. "She was not excluded from that," Sullivan later recounted. "She also would speak about smoking at times. But it was understood between us that this was really a major interest of mine."[19] The HHS public affairs staff had the same understanding. Her appearances before the media were cleared through Sullivan's office. "It was very tightly controlled in the speaking area, and Lou Sullivan got the pick of talks and Toni got what was left over," Mason recalled.[20]

But the Bush administration's campaign against smoking had limits. Mason learned that lesson in early 1990 after delivering a forceful keynote address at a World Conference on Tobacco and Health meeting in Australia. Mason said U.S. tobacco companies had been "playing our free-trade laws and export policies like a Stradivarius violin" and that it was "unconscionable" for those firms "to be peddling their poison abroad." He was reading from an old hymnal: Koop had been a strong critic of such practices, publicly arguing that "there is a higher good than the greed market." But when U.S. Representative Henry Waxman called on Mason to repeat his statements at a congressional hearing in May 1990, Mason's appearance was canceled with an HHS letter that deemed it inappropriate for a health official to discuss trade matters. In response, Waxman said the Bush administration was muzzling an anti-tobacco voice.[21]

The Mason incident seemed to have made an impression on the new surgeon general. In September 1990, Novello was asked at a press conference why she hadn't opposed U.S. Trade Representative Clayton Yeutter's efforts to start selling U.S. cigarettes in Thailand and other Asian countries. She replied that she had no comment about that. "For me to talk about it would be almost disrespectful of my [political] party," she said.[22] The statement brought the surgeon general's credibility to a new low. Granted, politics had always been a consideration and had influenced the decision making of Novello's predecessors. But for decades, surgeons general had striven to appear as straight-talking, science-first experts who always put public health over politics. Koop and Steinfeld, especially, took considerable political flak playing that role. Now here was Novello, saying—at a press conference, no less—that regardless of the health dangers posed by smoking, she didn't want to say anything about it that might displease the Bush administration. Her statement was widely interpreted as a foolish moment of candor that offered a glimpse of her true mindset.

For their part, tobacco industry officials had already decided Novello posed no threat. That's the indication, at least, from internal documents from the Washington office of Philip Morris that were printed years later in the *Washington Post*. In an October 18, 1989, memo, Philip Morris lobbyist Jim Dwyer said that, having learned Novello was being considered for surgeon general, he had searched for any speeches, statements, or papers she had made on tobacco and found nothing. "She seems to be a candidate least likely to interfere with our activities and we may well want to discuss possible ways to express support for her appointment," Dwyer wrote.[23] In a March 8, 1990, memo, penned a day before Novello officially started her job, Dwyer wrote that he had discussed Novello with the White House: "We intervened with the White House, OMB and HHS to urge that Dr. Novello take no position on any pending anti-tobacco legislation. We stressed to her handlers and to interested parties that we were interested in making sure she focused on non-tobacco health problems. We were successful in that both our objectives were met."[24]

Indeed, much of Novello's time in office was spent on other issues (she did issue one report on smoking, which dealt with cultural issues behind smoking). But ironically, she is probably best remembered for her attack on Joe Camel.

Camel cigarettes had been sold since 1913, but by the late 1980s they accounted for just 3 percent of the market and were favored mainly by rural smokers and older, factory-worker types. In 1988, R. J. Reynolds decided to pep up Camel sales by rolling out a new advertising campaign featuring a cartoon character named Joe Camel. Joe was a cool camel, cigarette dangling from his mouth, sometimes with adoring women at his elbows. (Some observers noted that he had a long, rounded-off face that bore a remarkable resemblance to a penis). R. J. Reynolds devised a Joe Camel marketing campaign featuring "Camel Cash" coupons on cigarette packages that could be redeemed for items like T-shirts, posters, and neon signs. Health advocates complained the campaign was clearly aimed at teenagers, and in 1991 an anti-smoking organization called the Coalition on Smoking or Health petitioned the Federal Trade Commission to halt the ad campaign.[25]

By that time, Joe Camel was perhaps the most recognized figure in tobacco marketing, even eclipsing the long-successful "Marlboro Man" cowboy figure. In 1991, the *Journal of the American Medical Association* published a series of articles demonstrating Joe Camel's resonance with kids. One found the proportion of adolescent smokers who smoked Camels rose from less than 1 percent to 33 percent in just three years. Another study—a small survey done in Georgia preschools—found that 30 percent of three-year-olds knew Joe Camel represented a type of cigarette, and that kind of brand recognition was as strong in many young children as was the knowledge that Mickey Mouse represented the Disney Channel.[26]

Novello considered herself a champion for children's health, but going after cigarette manufacturers represented a walk through a minefield, what with Sullivan's primacy on smoking issues and other political considerations in the Bush administration. Still, this seemed an acceptable fight for this surgeon general. In her first year on the job, Novello had gained attention for pushing beer makers and other manufacturers of alcoholic beverages to stop any advertising that could be seen as targeting underage drinkers. The Joe Camel campaign was another iteration of her battle against the marketing of harmful adult products to kids.

In March 1992, Novello joined with the American Medical Association to ask R. J. Reynolds to withdraw its cartoon campaign, arguing that Joe Camel was a crass effort to encourage underage smoking. She punctuated her case by leading a two-mile "Dump the Hump" parade in Chicago, joined by more than two hundred children and AMA physicians. It was said to be the first time a surgeon general had called for a halt to a continuing ad campaign for an existing cigarette brand, and the campaign received a flurry of national media coverage. This was clearly unusual—a public entreaty from a government official who had no authority to do anything about the ads if the company declined. Novello acknowledged as much at a news conference by pointedly emphasizing the AMA's backing of the appeal. "Calling for the voluntary withdrawal of a successful advertising campaign is not a traditional role of organized medicine," she told reporters. "Yet it is the only responsible position that physicians must take regarding these advertisements."[27]

Her effort was ineffective. R. J. Reynolds had bowed to Sullivan on the marketing of the Uptown cigarettes, but this time the company flatly refused, issuing a statement that advertising did not determine whether a young person started smoking. The FTC declined to halt Joe Camel marketing, and the company kept with the campaign. Its market share in the twenty-four-and-under crowd rose from 4.4 percent to 7.9 percent.[28] As with her push against youth-focused alcohol advertising, the problem persisted during Novello's watch.

R. J. Reynolds did drop the campaign five years later, saying simply it was time to try a new marketing approach. Some credit Novello for starting a drumbeat that may have ultimately led the company to nix Joe Camel. But others labeled the attacks on a cartoon character as a lame effort that diverted energy from more substantive issues like increased cigarette taxes, tougher trade restrictions, or even an outright ban on smokes. "Of all the half-hearted measures to come along lately, this joint government/AMA proposal to ban Old Joe Camel ranks up there with metal bars on park benches and cab drivers wearing jackets and ties," wrote the novelist Emily Prager, in a March 1992 newspaper editorial.[29]

Novello and the Bully Pulpit

Louis Sullivan was interested in public speaking, and not only about tobacco. He made key appearances on AIDS, led the charge for better food labeling, stumped on racial disparity issues, and took credit for an update of the *Healthy People* report—this time setting goals for 2000.

Novello's designated topics included vaccination promotion, childhood nutrition, and initiatives aimed specifically at the Hispanic community. She hosted a series of regional workshops in Chicago, New

York, Miami, Los Angeles, and San Antonio to get a sense of Hispanic health issues on the local level in preparation of a national report. She endorsed medical screening for signs of domestic violence. And she spoke out against drunken driving and underage drinking, including a speech to members of Mothers Against Drunk Driving ("a group that didn't need much convincing," one reporter observed).[30]

Hers was a dissatisfying performance, many felt, especially in the wake of Koop. "She never focused on stuff with any kind of depth on the subject matter and, to me, she lacked substance in what she did," said Jeff Koplan, who ran the CDC in the late 1990s and early 2000s.[31] Meeker than Koop, Novello seemed happy to perpetuate female stereotypes. She decorated her office with teddy bears. She joked during speeches about being disappointed that Gucci pumps did not go with the surgeon general's uniform. She liked to take female visitors shopping, even if the visitors were esteemed researchers coming to see her on business. And with men, she could be surprisingly flirtatious. "You got the feeling that if Toni could wear her uniform just a little bit tighter she would do it, because that's one of the weapons she thought was fair to use," said James Gavin, a former Public Health Service officer who has held a variety of corporate and academic leadership positions since then. Not that men in the health bureaucracy always acted appropriately; stories were told of men in earlier administrations who hit on female underlings in the Public Health Service. But fairly or unfairly, Novello's personal manner was more widely noted.[32]

Yet many liked her, including Gavin, who said she was refreshing and "was probably the most gregarious of all of the surgeon generals I knew." Some fondly recall Novello visiting major league baseball clubhouses during spring training, poking players in the bicep, and telling them to stop chewing tobacco because it was a negative influence on boys. Another admirer was Walter Orenstein, who in the early 1990s was a CDC infectious disease specialist involved in the agency's response to a terrible resurgence of measles. "I got this call from the Surgeon General, and she wanted to know how she could help! I almost dropped dead," he said. "I was always thankful to her for that. I wasn't in a position [to plan or influence public education efforts]. . . . I think she was a big, big help early on in the initial efforts to promote immunization."[33] Indeed, some argue that she was a very good speaker and capable health official whose main failing was simply that she wasn't Koop. "Koop was a very hard act to follow," said Jeff Levi, executive director of the

Trust for America's Health, a Washington, D.C.–based public health advocacy organization.[34]

Years later, in a doctoral dissertation in which she evaluated seven of the eight surgeons general who served from 1961 to 2000, Novello discussed her views of negotiating the job of surgeon general. (She did not evaluate herself, saying she wouldn't be able to muster the required degree of intellectual detachment for that task.) She repeatedly focused on each doctor's ability to work within the surrounding political framework. She praised Luther Terry for his public relations acumen and ability to adapt to political realities. She complimented William Stewart as a realist who never let what he wanted cloud his judgment as to what was feasible within HEW. And she lauded Koop—not, as many others did, for his outspoken independence, but rather for his political savvy. "As he became more secure in his position, he thought carefully about the players and their power, then mapped the political terrain. He built linkages with other stakeholders. He recognized the value of personal contact and face-to-face conversations. Above all, he understood and masterfully used moral persuasion to achieve goals. At the end of his tenure he was as much a politician as medical expert," she wrote. Her harshest assessments were for Jesse Steinfeld and Joycelyn Elders (her successor), two of the surgeons general most aggressive in using the bully pulpit. Novello wrote that Steinfeld was unnecessarily confrontational, didn't know his place, and failed "to understand the boundaries of his job and that of the three ASHs under whom he served."[35]

Novello's departure from office came with Bill Clinton's election as president in November 1992. On Tuesday morning, December 15, 1992, Novello was getting ready for work when she heard on the radio that the president-elect was going to name someone else surgeon general. A few weeks earlier, Novello had said she planned to stay in office for the remaining fifteen months of her term. But Clinton wanted Elders, who had run the Arkansas Health Department while he was the state's governor. Phil Lee, who had agreed to come back to government service as Clinton's assistant secretary for health, was charged with negotiating Novello's departure.

"It was my job as the Assistant Secretary to give Toni a job but also to convince her to leave gracefully and not raise a stink," Lee recalled, adding "they wanted to give her [Novello] a job in a hurry." Lee talked to the head of UNICEF and secured Novello a job as special assistant to the director. Novello was interested in international health and agreed. "She was very decent about it," Lee said.[36]

Novello left office in June 1993 and became a special representative for the UN on health and nutrition issues. In 1999, she was named commissioner of health for the State of New York, serving under Governor George Pataki. She held the position for seven years, but her tenure was marked by scandalous behavior.

In early 2009, the New York inspector general's office issued a report finding that Novello had abused her position by having staff members act as personal chauffeurs. She was provided a state car and staff to drive her on official business, but she kept two security guards "on call" to drive her on weekend shopping sprees and transport her mother and friends to and from the Albany and Newark airports. The guards also picked up her dry cleaning, got her mail, and moved furniture for her. When Novello was in New York City, a state health department investigator there was used to drive her to Macy's and Saks Fifth Avenue. State officials had told her to stop using staff for personal business in 2003, but she continued. From 2004 through 2006, she inappropriately had staff work overtime on at least 260 occasions. She tried to cover it up, telling on employee to falsify his time sheet. She also understated the taxable benefit she received from the personal use of a state vehicle.[37] Reportedly, she was also something of a tyrant with the employees who did all this scut work for her: Security guard Charles Williams told investigators she "always yelled" if she bought expensive items and he didn't carry or handle them correctly. Novello "would embarrass you anywhere," he said.[38]

Investigators estimated that over the full seven years of her time in office, taxpayers footed the bill for nearly $50,000 in unwarranted overtime related to the shenanigans. Inspector General Joseph Fisch said Novello "shamelessly and blatantly exploited and abused her staff, adding new dimension to the definition of 'arrogance' and 'chutzpah.'"[39] He turned his findings over to the Albany County district attorney, who pursued felony charges. In May 2009, Novello was arraigned on an indictment whose twenty counts included defrauding the government and theft of services. She faced a jail term of four to twelve years, but avoided the slammer through a plea bargain in which she admitted guilt to one count of offering a false document for filing, a minor felony related to paperwork. She agreed to pay $22,500 in restitution and a $5,000 fine and to do 250 hours of community service at an Albany health clinic.[40] She kept her medical license and returned to a job she had previously landed, as a vice president at the Florida Hospital for Children in Orlando.

JOYCELYN ELDERS

The selection of Joycelyn Elders as the next surgeon general hit conservatives like a stomach punch. An outspoken liberal who had endorsed providing condoms in schools, Elders once said abortion opponents needed to "get over their love affair with the fetus," during a January 1992 appearance at a pro-choice rally. "It's ominous to see her in a position of so much authority," said Wanda Franz, president of the National Right to Life Committee, in an interview with the *Washington Post* the day after Elders's name surfaced as Novello's proposed replacement.[41]

More than any other person who has worn the surgeon general's uniform, Elders was a polarizing figure. People either prized her for voicing what no other health official would dare say about controversial issues . . . or they detested her for it. She continually generated controversy and media attention, and forces on the right end of the political spectrum vilified her. Conservative radio host Rush Limbaugh ridiculed her on an almost weekly basis.

Elders endured a stormy confirmation process, and ended up serving less than fifteen months—the shortest term of any surgeon general. But in that limited time she became one of the most famous, and nearly two decades later ranks second only to Koop in name recognition, according to many of the Public Health Service veterans and advocates interviewed for this book.

What made her memorable was also her undoing. She directly, frankly, and impolitically answered questions about the legalization of drugs and about masturbation that gave her enemies artillery-grade ammunition. Elders had her science right, but she did not sound like a white-coated medical expert simply stating the facts; she was more like an advocate begging for a fight.

Babies from Watermelon Seeds

No surgeon general before her faced as many social and economic disadvantages as Elders. She was born Minnie Lee Jones on August 13, 1933, named for a grandmother who taught her to always tell the truth. Her birth and childhood were in the tiny town of Schaal, Arkansas, in a rural area west of Little Rock. The oldest of eight children, she grew up poor in a sharecropper family, picking cotton as a child and helping her father stretch raccoon hides to sell. For a time, the family lived in a three-room cabin with no plumbing or electricity, and the only reading material was a copy of the Bible and a weekly farming newspaper her father got, called *Grit*.[42]

As a child, she had little exposure to doctors, who were too distant from Schaal and too expensive. The first time she could remember anyone going to a doctor was when she was nine. Her brother Bernard's stomach swelled and his fever wouldn't break. Her father placed Bernard on a mule and took him to see a doctor, who treated him for a burst appendix and then sent him right home, as there were no hospitals in the area taking black children.

Health information was scarce. No one used—or had ever heard of—aspirin. Her first menstrual period was a terrifying experience; she recalled practically hyperventilating in school, shocked that she was bleeding and trying to cover her lap so no one noticed. When she did learn about menstruation, it was from a home economics teacher who handed out Kotex package inserts as educational material.[43] "Sex was a secretive thing, not to be mentioned," Elders later wrote in her autobiography, *Joycelyn Elders, M.D.* "Children were told that babies were brought by storks, or that they came from swallowing watermelon seeds. As youngsters we spent a lot of time trying not to swallow a watermelon seed."[44]

She was valedictorian of her high school class, an achievement that opened two doors. First, she gave the valedictory speech at the diploma ceremony—a nervous address about doing your best that was her first big brush with public speaking. Second, she was awarded a full-tuition scholarship to Philander Smith College, a well-regarded Methodist institution in Little Rock. It was there that she changed her name from Minnie Lee to Minnie Joycelyn, then just Joycelyn. The name came from a peppermint candy she liked, and was part of her attempt to distinguish herself from the other Minnie Joneses in her family. It was also at Philander Smith that she grew interested in medicine. Edith Irby, the first black medical student at the University of Arkansas, gave a speech at the college that inspired Joycelyn.

Joycelyn earned her bachelor's degree in 1952 and married a fellow Philander Smith student, Cornelius Reynolds. She followed him to Milwaukee, where he got a job with the IRS and she took her first job in health care as a nurse's aide in a Veteran's Administration hospital. But the couple quickly realized the marriage was a mistake. Seeking a new direction for her life, she enlisted in the army in 1953, enticed by the promise of GI Bill tuition benefits that could help her extend her education.[45]

During her three years in the army, she trained as a physical therapist and was assigned to a military hospital in Denver, where she treated President Dwight D. Eisenhower after his heart attack. (Pleasant and grateful when the physical therapy was over, he said little during the sessions, she later recalled.) At the time, she was taking several classes, including one on public speaking taught by a Catholic priest at a Denver Jesuit school. The priest taught her how to speak with rhythm, and to never read from paper while giving a speech. His lessons were later supplemented with advice from her brother Chester Jones, a Methodist minister, but her undisputed skill for rousing a room was born in that Denver class. "Probably the most valuable course I've ever taken," Elders said.[46]

After the army, she went to the University of Arkansas Medical School, just like her hero Edith Irby. She graduated in 1960 and married a Little Rock basketball coach, Oliver Elders. Joycelyn Elders doggedly pursued her training through an internship and a pediatrics residency and by earning a master's degree in biochemistry. In 1967, she became an assistant professor of pediatrics at the University of Arkansas Medical Center, then moved up the academic ranks there to become a full professor in 1976. She focused on pediatric endocrinology and became an expert on childhood sexual development, and one of the state's leading medical authorities on hermaphrodites and children with a condition known as ambiguous genitalia.

It was about the time she became full professor that she first encountered Bill Clinton, then the state's young attorney general. They met at a political function, and he later attended the funeral of Elders's brother, Bernard, who had been abducted and slain by a jealous acquaintance of Bernard's wife. When Clinton became governor, he decided to reinvigorate the state health department and discussed it with his friend Bob Fiser, a top official at the University of Arkansas Medical Center. Joycelyn Elders's name came up, and in 1987 he appointed Elders director of the Arkansas Department of Health.[47]

Initially, Elders was hesitant to take the job; she saw herself as from the world of medicine, not public health. But Clinton cajoled her and she finally agreed.

Almost immediately, she became something of a legend. In her first press conference with Governor Clinton, a reporter asked how she would attack the state's teenage pregnancy rate, which was the second highest in the country. Elders responded that school-based clinics were in the works. Another question: would she hand out condoms in schools? "We're not going to put them on their lunch trays, but, yes," she replied. Her response was candid, frank, and—in a socially conservative state—incredibly politically incorrect. Clinton, a liberal, turned crimson as reporters immediately asked almost in unison if he agreed with that. "I support Dr. Elders," he said.

Clinton was true to his word, supporting Elders as she embarked on a controversial tenure as the state's health officer. She leaned on Tom Butler, the deputy director, and the two formed a good working partnership that resulted in improved immunization rates and childhood health screenings. She visited more than one hundred public health clinics, studied the health care needs of the state, and helped drive up rates of breast cancer screenings and HIV testing. She also pushed local school boards to support her school-based clinics, and parried with state legislators who tried to prohibit distribution of condoms in schools. ("I will not turn those children over to their vile affections," one state representative said.) Elders was the powerful voice of the campaign, and made her case at legislative hearings and during visits to schools and health facilities around the state. "When we see a 10-year-old or a 13-year-old girl pregnant, she hasn't been promiscuous, she's been abused," she told one gathering. To another audience, a group of black clergymen, she said: "You've been preaching abstinence for a hundred years. I've still got a problem. I've still got thousands of teenagers having babies every year."[48]

Her passion for addressing the teenage pregnancy problem led to an incident that was repeatedly raised later: In 1991, after the Arkansas health department learned that condoms being distributed in the state's public health clinics had an unusually high rate of breaking—50 per 1,000 condoms, much more than the FDA's safety-standard maximum of 4 per 1,000. Elders quietly ordered the recall of undistributed condoms, but declined to disclose the problem to the public, fearing it would scare people away from that form of birth control. "We made a decision for the greater public good," she later said, in a U.S. Senate hearing.[49]

Elders was certainly controversial, but was deemed successful. In 1992, she was elected president of the Association of State and Territorial Health Officers, her peer group in public health. And later that year, President Clinton—acting only a month after his election as president—told Elders he wanted her to be his surgeon general.

She wasn't interested. "I felt the job I had as Director of Health for the State of Arkansas was, frankly, a better job. I was . . . responsible in a direct way for more people," she said. But Clinton convinced her that she could do something about teenage pregnancy on a national level. Elders's elderly mother was also persuasive: "She told me she saw the president on TV today and he just looked pitiful, and she said, 'You need to go on up there and help him,'" Elders recalled.[50]

She agreed, and controversy followed. Within a couple of weeks, news reports told of Elders's plan to advocate the use of medical marijuana and to support condom advertising on television. She also supported giving the contraceptive implant Norplant to drug-addicted prostitutes, gratis. (Her race—she stood to be the first African American to hold the office of surgeon general—received little public comment.) The *New York Times* lauded her as "an unflinching realist," but opponents called her the "Condom Queen." Social conservatives opposed her nomination, alarmed by Elders's Arkansas crusades and her pugilistic pro-choice statements, including her reported characterizations of pro-lifers as "religious non-Christians with slave-master mentalities." "A Surgeon General of the United States must hold the respect of the entire country, and these are not the remarks of someone who is able to unite and work with different groups," wrote Beverly LaHaye, president of Concerned Women for America.[51]

The confirmation process dragged on, as Republicans probed Elders on a number of issues, including shoddy lending practices that occurred at the National Bank of Arkansas while Elders was serving on its governing board. One senator accused of her being anti-Catholic for saying in 1992 that the Church's hierarchy had long been vocal in opposing abortion but had been silent about the Holocaust and during years of slavery in which blacks "had their freedom aborted." (Clinton asked to her apologize to Catholic leaders while her confirmation was in limbo, which she did.)

Clinton was pressured to drop Elders, but he knew that doing so could cost him dearly in the black community. He had already dumped Lani Guinier, his candidate for civil rights chief at the Department of Justice, after her nomination exploded in June 1993 when Republicans and some Democrats assailed her academic writings as evidence of radical views on minority rights. The NAACP and other groups sharply protested Clinton's handling of Guinier; backing away from Elders would have further alienated many of his supporters.[52]

Elders helped her own cause in a July 1993 Senate hearing, calmly parrying most of the attacks against her. Two months later, she was confirmed by the Senate by a vote of 65 to 34.[53] Characteristically, she was not cowed by the political battles she had just weathered and immediately took to the road, giving speeches and press interviews at a pace unmatched by any of her predecessors.

Elders and the Bully Pulpit

From the very beginning of her term, Elders was in high demand as a speaker. She traveled across the country, speaking at colleges, medical conferences, schools, churches, and many other forums. In fifteen months, she gave more than three hundred speeches—sometimes three a day.

She had an agenda, topped by issues like violence prevention, minority health, smoking, and of course comprehensive sex education. But it wasn't simply a matter of Elders pushing her message on different groups, said Phil Lee, who as assistant secretary for health was Elders's boss. "It was more a pull. People wanted her to speak because they knew she would speak out on issues that were controversial," Lee said.[54]

Not only was she controversial; she was also very good—arguably, the best orator among all the surgeons general. She held up well in comparison even to Koop, the beau ideal when it came to using the bully pulpit. Elders was nearly as polished as Koop in presenting scientific evidence; indeed, none of her many critics ever really succeeded in making a case that she had her facts wrong, though they hated the conclusions she drew from them. Koop had also had the ability to stir emotions, at times thundering away like an Old Testament prophet. But Elders was better at eliciting a lump in the throat or a clench of the fist, in the style of a New Testament gospel preacher. Largely writing her speeches herself, she used alliteration, powerful imagery, and frank assessments to grab attention, and organized many speeches in a problem-then-solution format meant to help listeners journey with her to a rightful conclusion. She spoke from the gut about the poor and disenfranchised and children at risk, at times with so much conviction that she shook, as if God's words were coursing through her. "We have buried our heads in the sand for too long," she said in one 1993 speech. "While we have been sitting on the beach sipping lemonade saying 'Just Say No,' our children have been drowning in an ocean of sharks—alcohol, drugs, violence, teen pregnancy, STDs and AIDS. We have got to get in the lifeboats known as 'common sense' and throw out the lifeline or we are going to lose an entire generation of young people."[55]

Many public health veterans were deeply impressed. "Listen to her, and you'd be sitting on the edge of your chair, practically. She was that good," Lee said.[56] Some remember one of her first trips to visit the CDC in Atlanta, speaking to a science-oriented crowd not known for being a passionate audience. "She got three standing ovations. Three," one former CDC official recalled.[57] The reaction was even stronger in a speech she gave to a large crowd of Georgia state health department employees, many of them African American. "It was so thrilling to see so many of my staff, who never would respond to me that way, get that excited about being in public health and see a leader they could relate to," recalled Kathleen Toomey, a Public Health Service veteran who at the time was Georgia's state epidemiologist. "People were crying. When she finished, they had their hands up, trying to touch her. I had to whisk her off so she wouldn't get trampled. It was like dealing with Mick Jagger."[58]

Elders had free rein in her pulpit. Lee, as assistant secretary for health, handled most administrative matters pertaining to the traditional Public Health Service agencies and had no desire to upstage her. And Donna Shalala, the secretary of health and human services, rarely meddled. "I always spoke to anybody I wanted to. . . . Nobody told me what I was going to say, either," Elders said. That was true of her dealings with the press as well, she said. She enjoyed talking to reporters, and HHS press secretaries didn't funnel calls away from her.[59]

Notably, however, the Clinton administration did not make the controversial Elders a point person for its national health reform initiative. The night Clinton unveiled his health plan to Congress in late September 1993, Elders was seated next to Hillary Rodham Clinton in the House gallery—guaranteeing the new surgeon general would be repeatedly on television when the cameras panned to the First Lady. It was not surprising: Elders had known the Clintons for years, was eloquent on the need for health reform, and had even served on a health care reform committee appointed by President Bush. But sitting on the other side of Mrs. Clinton that night was the revered Koop, and it was Koop that the Clintons used as a leading spokesman as they attempted to sell their proposal to Congress, the public, and special interest groups. Indeed, in her memoir, *Living History,* Hillary Clinton makes no mention of Elders at all but praises Koop repeatedly. "He could deliver the hard truth and get away with it," she wrote. "He could say, 'We have too many specialists in medicine and not enough generalists,' and an audience filled with specialists would nod in agreement."[60] Elders had a penchant for irritating people, and on this most sensitive matter, she was allowed only minimal input and was ignored when she critiqued the completed task force report.[61]

Elders got into trouble in early December 1993 when—in response to a question at a National Press Club luncheon—she said legalizing drugs could reduce crime and the idea deserved further study. She was not the first health official to voice the idea: during the Nixon administration, Assistant Secretary for Health Merlin DuVal had quietly suggested to HEW officials that they hold a public dialogue on the legalization of heroin.[62] And Elders, with years of training in medical science, was simply saying what most scientists would have said—more study is needed. But Elders aired her thoughts in public, at a time when battles between the Clinton administration and Republican lawmakers were escalating.

The fallout was intense. Clinton's press officers immediately distanced the president from Elders's remark, saying he was firmly against legalizing drugs and had no desire to study the issue. Nevertheless, Republican governor Pete Wilson of California called on Clinton to fire Elders. Mischaracterizing her comment as an outright call for the legalization of drugs, Wilson called her words an insult to the narcotics officers who bravely fought drug trafficking. Senate majority leader Bob Dole was more temperate, but knew political ammunition when he saw it. "Americans must be wondering if the Surgeon General is hazardous to our health," Dole said to the *New York Times*. "I am relieved that the president has disassociated himself from Dr. Elders' remarks but remain concerned with this administration's commitment to fighting drugs."[63]

Things got worse less than two weeks later when an arrest warrant was issued for Elders's twenty-eight-year-old son, Kevin, to face a charge that he had sold cocaine to undercover agents. Elders said she supported her son. Shalala told the press she supported Elders, but privately she expressed her displeasure, and made a point of telling others that Elders had never been her personal choice for surgeon general.[64]

The arrest hung over the Elders family the rest of the year, but she was undaunted in her public speaking. In January, she said she remained convinced that the legalization of drugs merited further study. In February, she said the Medicaid program must have been developed "by a white male slave owner" because "it fails to provide services to poor women to prevent unwanted pregnancies, and this failure contributes to poverty, ignorance and enslavement." In March, *The Advocate* magazine published an interview with Elders in which she said an irrational fear of sexuality was behind conservatives' anti-gay behavior.[65]

She put out one report on smoking (this one on kids and tobacco use), but went beyond reporting on the problem by calling for the government regulation of tobacco products. She thanked abortion providers for helping women. She told Congress that sitting in a smoke-free section does not adequately protect nonsmokers' health. She pushed to get school-based clinics in all underserved schools.

Conservatives got angrier and angrier.

In June 1994, eighty-seven Republican House members called for Elders to resign, and former secretary of housing and urban development Jack Kemp—who was considering a run for president in the 1996 election—said he felt Elders "should have been bounced or fired for her views," which, he said, were "far, far, far to the left on social policy of the American people."[66]

In October, the *Washington Post* reported it had obtained a memo to a group of lobbyists prepared by Representative Newt Gingrich, the House Republican who was leading political attacks on Clinton. The memo discussed the upcoming midterm election and outlined Republicans' efforts to portray Clinton Democrats as "the enemy of normal Americans." Elders was one of his prime examples. Her advocacy of abortion rights and of making contraception available in schools put her way out of step with Americans of many religious faiths, Gingrich argued.[67]

Whether Elders was on the minds of many voters during the November election is hard to say. There were many heated issues that fall, including the Clinton's controversial health reform proposal and the Brady bill and assault weapons ban, which the National Rifle Association had focused on in attacking at least a dozen Democratic incumbents in the House of Representatives. But Elders's tongue certainly didn't help matters. The Democrats were decimated. More than a half-dozen seats in the U.S. Senate swung Republican, giving the GOP majority rule in the Senate for the first time since 1986. In a much bigger surprise, more than fifty seats in the House of Representatives swung to the Republicans, who became the ruling party in the House for the first time since 1954. Gingrich became Speaker.

Conservatives, emboldened by the election, put out a new call for Elders to resign. Some leading House Republicans said they would renew their call for Elders's resignation when Congress reconvened in January, and promised to hold rancorous hearings. The Traditional Values Coalition, a group claiming to represent the members of 31,000 churches, mailed letters supporting Elders's ouster to several hundred thousand supporters. Even some Democrats had had enough. Representative Dave McCurdy, a Democrat who lost a bid for Senate in the

November election and was perhaps looking for a scapegoat, thought the infamous surgeon general had been a factor in the Republicans' success and asked the president to get rid of her.[68]

How Elders Lost Her Job

At times through gritted teeth, Clinton had supported his surgeon general. But his breaking point came in December, following an offhand comment she made about masturbation.

On December 1, Elders gave a speech at the United Nations for World AIDS Day. Afterward, during a panel discussion, a middle-aged psychologist named Rob Clark asked her a question. He wanted to know if she thought the campaign against AIDS should include discussion about—and promotion of—masturbation. Elders said she advocated comprehensive health education starting at an early age, and that masturbation is a part of human sexuality and perhaps should be taught.[69]

For several days, her comments went unmentioned in the press. But a reporter for *U.S. News & World Report*—a national newsmagazine that had been focusing on complaints about Elders—learned what the surgeon general had said and planned to include it in an article in an upcoming issue.[70] White House chief of staff Leon Panetta had warned Elders about her off-the-cuff remarks before, and was wearied by yet another Elders-spawned headache. The decision was made that she had to go. "There have been a number of statements where the president has indicated he disagreed with her views, and this is just one too many," Panetta said at a December 9 news conference announcing her departure.[71]

But when Panetta asked for her resignation, Elders said no. She said she had to hear it from the president. Clinton called her and, in a brief conversation, told her he wanted her to resign immediately. "At any other time, we probably could have faced the heat," Clinton later wrote, in his autobiography *My Life*. "But I had already loaded the Democrats down" with a controversial budget, the health care proposal, and a variety of other politically sensitive initiatives. "I decided I had to ask for her resignation. I hated to, because she was honest, able and brave, but we had already shown enough political tone-deafness to last through several presidential terms," he wrote.[72]

Elders briefly weighed staying in office anyway, but only briefly. While she had a four-year term and could not technically be terminated by the president, she realized she could not stump without a travel budget or other support from the administration. Asked about her accomplishments during her fifteen months in office, Elders acknowledged that her push to get school-based clinics in all underserved schools ultimately failed, as did health care reform and some of the other calls to action she was involved in. "I think my proudest accomplishment is that I really increased the awareness of the American people about the sexual health of our people, the problem of teenage pregnancy," and other issues, she said.[73]

Immediately after her dismissal, the *New York Times*—which had praised her only a year earlier as "an unflinching realist"—now tsk-tsked her and deemed her a failure:

> The articulate former health director of Arkansas looked like just the person to talk sense to the nation's adolescents. But she was never able to win widespread support or become the conscience of the nation on health issues. Instead her blunt comments on drugs and sex served as red flags to conservative opponents who bashed her unmercifully. . . . Dr. Elders had been warned repeatedly by the White House to mind her tongue. She proved unwilling to listen. The result was a regrettable but inevitable loss. This is not a White House that can be passing out ammunition to its critics.[74]

While the *Times* chastised, others found the whole thing amusing. On December 10, just one day after Panetta announced Elders was out, the TV show *Saturday Night Live* led its broadcast with a skit with cast member Ellen Cleghorne playing Elders speaking at a news conference. Regretfully announcing she would be stepping down, she lamented that many high school graduates were still only masturbating at the fifth-grade level.[75] Not long after that, a comic folk group called The Foremen won attention and laughter around Washington with a ditty that used Elders's ouster as a euphemism for masturbation. The song's title: "Firing the Surgeon General."[76]

After her dismissal, Elders returned to her old job at the University of Arkansas, and there was one final flurry of opinion pieces commenting on her departure. Among the bitter was a letter to the editor of the *Seattle Times* by a reader named Alison Slow Loris, which said in part:

> Over and over she (Elders) has spoken out for common sense and honesty and the value of knowledge. It's not surprising that the Republican commitment to upholding ignorance, and Clinton's commitment to apparently nothing at all, have succeeded in driving her out of office. . . . I suppose we can count on the next surgeon general being afraid to speak up about anything at all. Since public speaking is virtually the only power or duty attached to the office, the post might as well be abolished. It would save some money.[77]

Loris was not the only one to voice such thoughts. Elders's departure was followed by years of nasty political fighting over who should replace her, and whether the Office of the Surgeon General should simply be shuttered. Not until 1998 would a distinguished physician named David Satcher agree, after repeated entreaties, to take the job.

CHAPTER 10

"You're on Your Own"

Less than three weeks after David Satcher was sworn in as the sixteenth surgeon general, a U.S. senator tried to shutter his office.

It was nothing personal, according to Conrad Burns, the Montana Republican who introduced the bill. "This legislation is not about Dr. Satcher, or about any previous Surgeon General," Burns said when he submitted the bill on March 6, 1998.[1] Rather, he said, the office had become too politicized and distracting in recent years, under both Republican and Democratic presidents. Other government officials spoke out on health issues, making the surgeon general redundant. "This legislation will sunset an office that has become a political football and has long since outlived its usefulness."

Burns and some other Republicans had been trying to abolish the position for years, but they were hardly neutral about David Satcher—a distinguished black physician whom they saw as an embodiment of a liberal public health agenda. In his earlier job as director of the CDC, Satcher had endorsed the distribution of condoms in schools, championed research targeting guns as a cause of death and injury, and supported programs providing clean needles to drug addicts. Senator John Ashcroft of Missouri, who joined with Burns and twenty-one others in voting against Satcher's confirmation, sniffed, "I believe an individual who supports needle exchange programs . . . is not the type of person who ought to be leading our culture as it relates to drug policy or health policy."[2]

In fact, Satcher was exactly the type of person needed to take over the Office of the Surgeon General. He rebuilt the position's prestige and temporarily rescued it from political cannibals. An effective, professorial public speaker with a distinctive look—his trim white beard and mustache a sharp contrast against his deep-brown skin—he was careful with his words and selective about which controversies he plunged into. Yet he contradicted the Clinton administration by endorsing needle-exchange programs and angered the Bush administration by issuing a report on sex that called for schools and communities to teach kids about birth control and support clinics that provide contraception.

The public has grown to expect the surgeon general to be more candid and forthright than the political animals that dwell in the surrounding branches of the federal health bureaucracy. Satcher was in huge demand from the get-go. "Oh gosh, when he came in, there had been a reservoir of demand," said Damon Thompson, the U.S. Department of Health and Human Services press officer assigned to Satcher during his four-year term. "People were just relieved to start talking to the surgeon general again, and the phone started ringing off the hook—even before he got sworn in."[3]

"JUST LIKE DR. JACKSON"

David Satcher was born March 2, 1941, on a farm outside Anniston, Alabama—a town known at the time as the "soil pipe capital of the world" for its production of sewer pipes. It was also a segregated place where white doctors did not treat black patients.

Satcher's first memories were of coughing and straining to breathe at age two, from a case of whooping cough and accompanying pneumonia. Satcher's parents had lost a child to whooping cough the previous year. David's father, a foundry worker, went to town and found Fred Jackson, the only black physician serving Anniston at the time. The next day, on his day off, Jackson came to the Satchers' forty-four-acre farm. Jackson doubted the boy would survive but told his mother what she could do to try to keep his fever under control and his lungs clear. The boy did recover, and his mother told him almost daily about how the noble physician had saved his young life.[4]

At age five, David said he wanted to see the doctor who saved him, and his parents agreed to take him to the hero physician for the boy's sixth birthday. Jackson died of a massive stroke at age fifty-four, before the meeting took place. But the doctor's influence had already taken root: "By the time I turned six years old, I was telling anyone who would listen that I was going to be a doctor—just like Dr. Jackson," Satcher said.[5]

Satcher came from a family of ten. Although they had little formal education, his parents—Wilmer and Anna Satcher—loved and respected learning. Having taught himself to read, Wilmer became known as one of the community's leading Bible scholars. Their children took to reading, too. While doing chores, David and his older brother called out words to each other from the *Reader's Digest* in a vocabulary-building game.[6]

David attended the only black high school in the county, and was so good at math formulas and other lessons that teachers would ask him to teach class when they were ill.[7] He excelled even though he had to do most of his studying on the bus, because after school and on weekends he worked at the foundry where his father was employed.

In 1959, Satcher got a full scholarship to Morehouse College, a private, all-male, historically black institution in Atlanta. Part of what is known as the Black Ivy League, Morehouse was led by Benjamin Elijah Mays, a minister, scholar, and social activist who would become a mentor to Martin Luther King, Jr., a 1948 graduate of Morehouse. Satcher arrived on campus as civil rights activism was coming into full swing thanks to student leaders like Julian Bond, a Morehouse student two years older than Satcher who led student protests against segregation in Georgia movie theaters, lunch counters, and parks.

Satcher was immediately drawn in. His father had been barred from better foundry jobs because of his race; Wilmer Satcher had to train and say "Yes, sir" to younger white men who knew less about the foundry and were not as good at their jobs. At Morehouse, David joined the local chapter of the Student Nonviolent Coordinating Committee (working with Bond). He was arrested five times when he and others went to restaurants and peacefully declined to leave after they were refused service. After one arrest, he and his fellow protesters refused bail and went on a one-week hunger strike.[8]

But he remained conscientious about his studies, carrying books with him to each protest to read in jail in case he got arrested. Fellow demonstrators teased him about it, but while some of his protesting peers drifted in and out of school, Satcher shined academically. Satcher also fell in love with a woman from Anniston, Callie Frances Herndon, who was attending Atlanta's Spelman College. They later married, in Anniston, in December 1967.

Satcher graduated Morehouse in 1963 with honors, then attended Case Western Reserve University in Cleveland, graduating with an M.D. and Ph.D. in cell genetics in 1970. Next came residency training at the University of Rochester, where he focused on pediatrics. Then came a turning point: he was on track for a successful career in academic medicine, though not necessarily one that would have given him many leadership opportunities, when he decided to veer from that path. Satcher and his wife moved to Los Angeles, where he joined the brand-new Martin Luther King Jr. General Hospital in Watts, a public hospital opened after the deadly riots of 1965 to fulfill a promise to L.A. to address inadequate health care services. Satcher became director of the hospital's sickle-cell disease center and was interim director of the King-affiliated Charles R. Drew Postgraduate Medical School.

The Satchers had four children, and the family was doing well until Callie was diagnosed with breast cancer in 1976. She died two years later. In an interview more than thirty years later, tears welled as Satcher recalled her last days. "When she was in the hospital, we talked a lot, and I told her I was never going to remarry. At first she was happy to hear that. And then one night she said she wanted me to promise that I would try to find somebody who loved me and loved the kids," he said.[9]

He remarried nearly two years later, to Nola Richardson, a California divorcée and mother of five. They had worked together at King Medical Center and had become friends after she presented him with a poem about sickle-cell disease that he encouraged her to get published, and she had cared for Satchers' children when Callie's health deteriorated.[10] Nola raised his four kids; the two youngest called her Mom.

The new family moved to Atlanta when Satcher took a job at Morehouse as head of community and family medicine. The next move was to Nashville, in 1982, where he became president of Meharry Medical College—the nation's largest private, historically black academic health center dedicated to educating minorities in the health professions. While there he founded the *Journal of Health Care for the Poor and Underserved,* which became known as the premier journal concerning the health of medically needy people in North America.

Satcher's successes had placed him on the radar of people in Washington. In the late 1980s, he was appointed to the Council on Graduate Medical Education (COGME). The panel advises the HHS secretary, who at the time was Otis Bowen. "Dr. Bowen is the person who really got me involved in government," Satcher later said.[11] Satcher became chair of COGME and issued a series of reports that bolstered his stature as a national authority on medically underserved people and on related issues such as the future of the health care workforce. In 1993, Satcher was appointed to the task force working on the Clinton national health reform proposal. The same year, the Clinton administration tapped him to be director of the CDC.

THE CDC YEARS

Traditionally, CDC directors were veterans of the federal Public Health Service, many of them having gained years of experience at the agency in important administrative positions before they were selected. The one exception was Bush appointee Bill Roper, but he at least had worked in public health in Alabama. Satcher had zero experience in public health. But Satcher spent about five years as CDC director, and gained a reputation as a forceful voice on controversial topics, including three—the Tuskegee Study, gun violence, and needle exchange—that would carry over into his service as surgeon general.

The infamous Tuskegee Study had been placed under the CDC's oversight from 1959 until it was stopped in 1972. The study became a deep stain on the Public Health Service, and a reason for the black community's enduring mistrust of government health officials. Those connected to the study admitted no wrongdoing, and the government was slow to compensate the families of the men who suffered during the experiment.[12] Satcher felt penance was long overdue, and appointed a committee to study how to prevent such a thing from happening again. HHS Secretary Donna Shalala, with Satcher, called President Clinton with the committee's findings, and Clinton instantly agreed to make a formal apology to the families of the experiment subjects. The ceremony was held in May 1997. Satcher was there, receiving credit for making it happen.[13]

Gun violence was more controversial. In the 1980s, the CDC began focusing research dollars on the role guns played in U.S. deaths and injuries. The work rose in prominence while Satcher was at the helm of the CDC with the 1993 publication of a controversial, CDC-funded study in the *New England Journal of Medicine* that concluded having a gun in the home made it three times more likely that someone who lives there will be murdered. The National Rifle Association and its allies in Congress increasingly objected to the CDC fostering this kind of work. In 1996, federal legislators tried to take away the $2.6 million in firearm research funding from the CDC. Satcher battled in Washington to restore the money, and it was put back, but it wasn't much of a victory.

While the CDC retained the money, it was directed to brain trauma research, and CDC appropriations bills from 1996 forward stipulated that research money for injury prevention and control could not be used to advocate or promote gun control, even if such policy was the logical conclusion of CDC research. Satcher saw it as a defeat, but others applauded him. Phil Lee, the assistant secretary for health under Clinton, praised Satcher for "his willingness to take that on, his willingness to deal with people on the Hill who were confronting him about that, his willingness to work very hard to prevent the kind of clobbering of the program that would have occurred had he not been there."[14]

Needle exchange had landed on the CDC's agenda in the early 1990s when Roper saw a need for objective study of some of the needle-exchange programs such as those that had started in San Francisco and Tacoma, Washington, in the late 1980s.[15] Study results came back shortly after Satcher succeeded Roper, and they indicated the programs helped reduce the spread of HIV. Satcher endorsed further research and said that it appeared to be wise public policy. (His position on such programs would cause him problems later.)

The Clinton administration had considered Satcher as a replacement for Joycelyn Elders after her resignation in 1994. But Satcher—with a good job at the CDC—demurred. "I said I would rather not, for two reasons," Satcher said. "I was excited about being the director of the CDC, and so I didn't like the idea of going in and spending a few months and then leaving to become surgeon general. That was one thing. But there was another issue: I just didn't like the environment around the office with Joycelyn's firing. Now, I understood the logic of her firing. But I didn't want to walk into that situation as I saw it in 1994."[16]

So in February 1995, the Clinton administration instead nominated one of Satcher's Meharry colleagues, Henry Foster Jr. He seemed like a good, safe choice: a respected, consensus-building obstetrician who had been lauded for a program he'd founded at two public housing developments that taught kids to believe in themselves and make choices that steered them away from teen pregnancy. Indeed, President George Bush had cited the program as one of his "thousand points of light" recognition of significant volunteer service. Satcher told the media he couldn't think of anyone more successful than Foster at helping disadvantaged communities. "I just have to believe that America will listen to someone like that," Satcher said.[17]

But within only about one week, the nomination had turned into a debacle. Foster, it turns out, had performed abortions—a firestorm revelation at a time when the Clinton administration was battling conservative Republicans on a number of fronts. What's more, no one could get a straight answer about how many he had performed, indicating that the White House had done a poor job vetting Foster and that Foster was not being completely open about his past work in family planning.

By the time of Foster's Senate confirmation hearing, Republicans had found other stones to throw. Foster was from Macon County, home of the Tuskegee Experiment, and he had been vice president of the county's medical society in 1969 when CDC officials met with the medical society and briefed the physicians on the experiment. Foster said he had never attended a meeting where he was told that local syphilitic men were being denied treatment, and didn't become aware of the nature of the experiment until the Associated Press broke the story in 1972. Several senators intimated that Foster was lying, just as he had apparently lied about how many abortions he had done.

There was no clear proof that Foster in 1969 had known about, or fully understood, the implications of the Tuskegee Experiment. But the abortion question led key HHS officials to lose faith in Foster, and even Satcher wasn't sure if his friend was lying about that or not.[18] President Clinton liked Foster and refused to withdraw the nomination. But in late June, the Senate ended the matter when, by a vote of 57 to 43, it failed to bring the nomination to a vote.

The Foster mess sparked Conrad Burns and others to begin introducing bills to do away with the surgeon general. Those bills failed, Clinton delayed naming a replacement, and the net effect was a two-year limbo. In the spring of 1997, Clinton officials again looked at Satcher, this time not only for surgeon general but also for assistant secretary for health. The structure and personnel at HHS had been changing. Phil Lee had served as the ASH in the mid-1990s as a favor to the Clinton administration. But in 1997, Lee was getting ready to retire, he advised Satcher to also ask for the ASH job.[19] The position commanded a larger budget and staff than what was available to the surgeon general, and it would guarantee that Satcher would be the top public health advisor to the secretary.

SATCHER'S TURN

The White House formally announced Satcher's nomination in September 1997, with Satcher pledging to demystify science and preach good health.[20] His advocates noted that the carefully vetted Satcher had a talent for choosing his words carefully and was respected on Capitol Hill.

The nomination process began smoothly. In an appearance before the Senate Labor and Human Resources Committee in October, Satcher efficiently fielded charges that the CDC had lobbied for gun control; he replied that the agency hadn't financed a lobbyist or done any lobbying, and that CDC researchers didn't go into their work with an anti-gun bias. At the end, the committee's chair—Senator James Jeffords, a Vermont Republican—predicted the Senate would act quickly on Satcher's nomination.[21]

But one month later, a group of Republicans ground things to a halt. They had been poring over Satcher's responses to questions about late-term abortion, a rare and gruesome procedure in which a doctor compresses the skull of a fetus before extracting it from the womb. Satcher said he would support a ban on such abortions only if exceptions were made for situations in which a pregnant woman's life or health was in jeopardy. Senator John Ashcroft—the Missouri Republican who would emerge as Satcher's most vocal critic—said Satcher's words amounted to support of partial-birth abortion. Ashcroft contended that Satcher's position was at odds with the rest of the medical profession—even though the American Medical Association, the American Academy of Family Physicians, and other doctors' groups had been enthusiastically supporting Satcher.[22]

Ashcroft found more to throw at Satcher in two editorials that had been published in the *New England Journal of Medicine* in September, just a week after Clinton formally announced the surgeon general nomination. The editorials questioned U.S.-funded clinical trials of AIDS drugs in developing countries, including a study funded by the CDC and the National Institutes of Health that looked at preventing transmission of the AIDS virus from infected pregnant women to their newborns. In the study, some women were given the drug AZT and others were given a placebo. But AZT had already been shown to be an effective treatment, and critics said it was wrong to withhold it from any of the participants. In one of the editorials, Marcia Angell (who later would become the journal's editor) likened the research to the Tuskegee Study.[23]

Satcher and NIH director Harold Varmus defended themselves in a coauthored response editorial published the following month. AZT was an extremely expensive and complicated treatment, and the study would answer questions about both the safety and feasibility of doing it in those settings, they argued. Also, they wrote, the experiment was done with the blessings of the host countries.[24]

Ashcroft used the controversy for his opening salvo at Satcher's confirmation hearing in February 1998. "It is pretty clear that when there is a known therapy, medical ethics say you are not allowed to give people just sugar pills and send them on their way, watching them die," he said. He also blasted Satcher's position on needle exchange: "I believe an individual who supports needle exchange programs, who would accommodate drug use instead of seeking to curtail drug use, . . . is not the type of person who ought to be leading our culture as it relates to drug policy or health policy."[25] Satcher believed Ashcroft was grandstanding to establish himself as a leader among conservative Republicans.[26] Ultimately it mattered little: Ashcroft and the other Satcher critics were clearly in the minority. "You had to put up with the noise, but we had the votes," Shalala said.[27] The new surgeon general was confirmed by a vote of 63 to 35.

Satcher was sworn in three days later. Initially, he said, he planned "to listen for a while" before determining a list of priority issues.[28] But he soon made headlines for speaking out—on needle exchange.

In 1989, Congress said no federal money could be spent on needle-exchange programs until the government could show that they both reduced transmission of HIV and did not increase drug use. In early 1998, health officials believed they had that evidence, thanks largely to CDC-backed research. A press conference was scheduled for Monday, April 20, at which Shalala—flanked by Satcher and Varmus—would declare the administration's intention to lift the ban.

Late the night before the Monday press conference, Clinton got cold feet. The White House called Shalala just before 9 A.M. to tell her the ban would stay in place, and HHS scurried to replace the full news conference it had scheduled with a smaller, no-cameras-allowed briefing.[29] It was a political decision. "The science was there," Satcher later said. "But they had counted votes, they knew that it was not going to pass Congress and they knew that it was going to be used against him [Clinton]."[30]

It was a crucible moment for Satcher. As the assistant secretary for health, he was a political employee expected to fall in line with the president's wishes, just as Shalala—a strong supporter of needle exchange—was about to. But as surgeon general, he had a duty to take positions based on the best science and public health practice, even if it put him in conflict with Clinton.

At that press conference, he wore the ASH hat. He and other government scientists looked uncomfortable as Shalala announced the administration would not try to lift the ban, but none of them voiced disagreement. Later that week, Satcher was more forthcoming about his feelings. He talked to the media again and said he was disappointed with the decision.[31] His statements provided fodder to editorialists who called Clinton spineless, but Satcher didn't get in trouble. Shalala had told him and other administration health leaders they could publicly disagree with Clinton's funding decision, without repercussions. "We never backed off from our position that needle exchange was a good thing. We just didn't have permission from the president to use CDC money for it," Shalala said.[32]

But Satcher's stance had little practical effect, as the funding ban stayed in place. "He wasn't listened to," said Anthony Fauci, the longtime director of the National Institute for Allergy and Infectious Diseases and a health official known as a master communicator.[33]

THE REPORTS

Surgeons general have tended to have their most lasting impact through their reports. Satcher's first, released in late April 1998, was a 332-page tome on smoking. It was the twenty-fourth surgeon general report on that topic, but this one offered a new wrinkle: it was the first to focus on the dangers of smoking to specific minority groups, noting, for example, that American Indians smoked at much higher rates than most other groups and that smoking was rising faster among black teenagers than either white or Hispanic kids. Satcher presented the report to Clinton in a ceremony on the South Lawn of the White House, an unusually high-caliber launch for a surgeon general's report.[34] But it fit well with Clinton's desire to see Satcher play a starring role in efforts to address racial disparities.

On a Saturday in February, only about a week after Satcher took office, Clinton announced that he was putting Satcher in charge of outreach for a new initiative to eliminate racial and ethnic health disparities by 2010. Health disparities would become something of leitmotif for Satcher over the next four years and beyond.

Satcher pursued the issue as both advocate and measured academic. In so doing, he balanced roles a bit like he had in his Morehouse days. He was now a national leader on issues of race, regularly meeting with the Congressional Black Caucus, speaking to the Southern Christian

Leadership Conference, and discussing racial health disparities with the ethnic and mainstream media.[35] But he was also the nation's doctor, at times disagreeing with black church and civil rights leaders, and pushing them to move beyond an abstinence message and embrace condom use and other strategies to prevent the spread of sexually transmitted diseases.

He was speaking on the issue at a time when a growing body of studies indicated shameful differences in the health and medical care received by minorities. The surgeon general reports issued by Satcher spotlighted the disparities, and were followed by important reports on the same topic by the Institute of Medicine and others. Years later, Satcher would coauthor one of the first medical textbooks on the subject. "He opened up a whole field of scholarship and research," said David Kessler, the former FDA commissioner.[36]

During Satcher's first summer as surgeon general, a second theme of his administration also began to emerge—mental health. Some surgeons general had previously tried to bring mental health to the fore. Most notably, Thomas Parran in the 1940s stumped about the need to recognize mental illness as a public health issue, and pushed successfully for congressional funding for clinical research focused on psychiatric disorders. Some presidents had addressed mental health, as well, most notably Jimmy Carter, who created a commission on mental health in 1977 that proposed ambitious changes for improving mental health treatment. Nevertheless, mental illness remained stigmatized and poorly understood by much of the American public, and advocates lamented the government's inaction concerning inequities in insurance coverage for mental illness compared to maladies involving other parts of the body.

Tipper Gore, the vice president's wife, had long been an advocate for the mentally ill and had sensitized Satcher to the problems of mentally ill children when they met at a conference in the late 1980s. He agreed to work with the Clinton-Gore White House to do something about it, and announced a series of recommendations designed to make Americans more aware of mental illness, to increase depression screenings, and to remove barriers to psychiatric and psychological treatment.

In October 1998, Satcher unveiled an anti-suicide initiative. Suicide was the nation's eighth leading cause of death at the time, with an estimated daily average of 85 suicides and about 2,000 attempts. Satcher made preventing suicide one of his priorities—the first time a surgeon general had given that kind of prominence to the issue.[37] In July 1999, he issued a report on suicide, at a press conference with Tipper Gore.

Except it wasn't a surgeon general's report, technically speaking. Only twenty pages long, it seemed a mere pamphlet compared to some of the doorstops put out by earlier surgeons general. Those kinds of reports took years to produce, and were long and dry "state of the science" documents more often talked about than actually read. Satcher wanted a leaner document that might be quicker to produce, one that mixed some advocacy in with a summary of research—something with less heft but as much policy-swaying punch. He named the resulting document a Call to Action.

"It was just a very brief articulation of the situation as it existed and some kind of an—I won't say agenda—but kind of a blueprint for people who wanted to take action," said Damon Thompson, Satcher' press secretary.[38] There was pressure to get it out quickly, in part because youth violence and suicide dominated the news following the shocking April 1999 massacre at Columbine High School in Colorado, in which two teenagers killed twelve students, a teacher, and then themselves. (The massacre triggered work on a separate surgeon general's report, on youth violence, released in 2001.) Satcher reasoned that public interest in the issue might fade in a year or two. He also worried suicide could become an overlooked issue in the context of another pending report, a more encompassing one on mental health.

The Gores had asked for the larger mental health report, one of only two of the Satcher surgeon general's reports born of an outside request. (Shalala initiated the other, a 2000 report on oral health. She got the idea for it from her dentist, John Drumm, who asked her why there had never been a surgeon general's report on dentistry.[39]) Work on the mental health report started in 1997, before Satcher was in office, but he unveiled it in December 1999 with Shalala and Tipper Gore. It drew front-page coverage in newspapers across the country with findings that one in five Americans experience a mental disorder each year and half of all Americans suffer a disorder during their lives. It also said most people never seek treatment for their depression or other problems, perhaps because they fear being stigmatized or are unable to pay for effective treatment. And it strongly argued for expanding mental health services and ensuring parity in health insurance so that mental illnesses were given coverage equal to that for other conditions.

Advocates celebrated Satcher's report as a potential game-changer. "This is a historic day. It's wonderful that we have a surgeon general talking about mental health and mental illness, in a voice that has not been used in Washington before," said Michael Faenza, president of the

National Mental Health Association, in an interview with the *New York Times*. He added, however, that much depended on whether politicians would have the enduring interest and willpower to act on the recommendations.[40]

The White House, the true propelling force behind mental health reform, took additional steps. A half-year before Satcher's report came out, Clinton had directed the U.S. Office of Personnel Management to institute parity in the health insurance of federal employees. When George W. Bush was elected in 2000, he too pledged an interest in mental health, and in April 2002, he created a commission on mental health that used Satcher's 1999 report as its scientific foundation and repeated Satcher's goals.[41] But efforts to get Congress to close the loopholes in mental health parity dragged on for years. It was not until 2008 that Congress finally passed the kind of full-parity law that advocates had long been awaiting.

OBESITY AND SEX

Meanwhile, Satcher also began to work on two other issues that were, ultimately, much more controversial—obesity and sex.

The importance of being physically fit had been instilled in Satcher as a child when he worked on the family farm and struggled to keep up with his fast-walking grandmother, but also saw his mother struggle with her weight. He thought of his mother later in life as he grew to understand obesity's relationship to heart disease, diabetes, and other illnesses that disproportionately struck African Americans, and he did his best to avoid the same problems. He ran track at Morehouse and remained a jogger for much of his life (he was the first surgeon general, incidentally, to run a marathon).[42] He was a strong proponent of exercise, and his staff at the CDC had put together a 1996 surgeon general's report on the importance of physical activity, issued by acting surgeon general Audrey Manley.

Indeed it was Satcher's CDC that first shoved the nation's weight problem onto the public health policy agenda. Obesity had long been perceived as a relatively unusual condition, but when Satcher was CDC director, the agency's chronic disease scientists developed a striking time-lapse series of maps that showed increasing obesity rates across the United States. No state reported obesity rates greater than 15 percent in 1985, but more than half had achieved that fatty status by 1995—and a sizable number hit rates of 20 percent and more a few years later. "Rather than simply showing a trend, the maps conveyed something far more urgent—a spreading infection," writes the political scientist J. Eric Oliver in his book *Fat Politics*.[43]

By the late 1990s, the concept of an obesity epidemic had begun to take hold in the media. Satcher, now surgeon general, carried the issue forward. He solicited comments from researchers, doctors, advocates, and others to put together a summary of the problem and offer proposals to address it. His work would not be completed until late in his term when as surgeon general he produced a thirty-nine-page Call to Action document in December 2001.

Oliver calls it "the first shot in the federal government's current war on obesity," and it certainly turned some heads.[44] It estimated that 300,000 deaths a year were attributable to people being overweight and obese, putting the problem in the same ballpark as cigarette smoking, which was blamed for 400,000 deaths. Satcher recommended that the restaurant and food industry promote more reasonable portion sizes, that communities create safer playgrounds and places to walk, and that schools provide daily physical education at every grade and healthier food options. The report also led to continuing medical education programs for doctors who cared for obese children. "I think Dr. Satcher's report really helped put childhood obesity on the radar screen," said Joe Thompson, the surgeon general for the state of Arkansas, who has led efforts to fight childhood obesity in that state.[45]

Nevertheless, the childhood obesity problem continued to worsen.[46] Even some scholars who believe the Call to Action was important question how much impact it actually had. "It certainly was timely. But it's hard to know, was this leading the charge or just parts of the zeitgeist of the time?" said John Parascandola, a former historian for the U.S. Public Health Service.[47]

Sexual health represented an even more sensitive set of issues. Teenage pregnancy, sexually transmitted diseases, and other fornication-related public health problems had caused officials to wring their hands for decades. But sex, of course, is what had sunk Satcher's predecessor Joycelyn Elders; her December 1994 comment that perhaps we should be teaching children how to masturbate had been the final straw that caused Clinton to call for her resignation.

Satcher had long ago learned of the life-changing impact of STDs and teen pregnancy, especially on minority communities. One of his sisters (Olivia) was adopted by his parents from Satcher's cousin, a teenager who had gotten pregnant and was in no position to keep and care for the child. "I didn't come at the sex thing from a very liberal perspective.

I came at it out of concern we needed to do something to improve the lives of people," he said.[48] In June 1999, he formed a work group to focus on promoting healthy sexual practices, and held conferences on the topic in Newport, Rhode Island, and Warrenton, Virginia. As Clinton's second term drew to a close in 2000, Satcher pushed to synthesize the information he'd gathered and proposed putting it out as a report or Call to Action. Donna Shalala said no.

Shalala had been a steadfast ally of Satcher's, using him as a trusted advisor and a high-profile spokesman, encouraging him to speak his conscience on controversial issues like needle exchange, and signing off on virtually all of his formal reports and Calls to Action. But not this time. President Clinton had been famously disgraced for having sexual liaisons with White House intern Monica Lewinsky and then, in 1998, lying about it on national television. It was still a source of shame for the administration in 2000, and a shadow over Al Gore's presidential campaign. Shalala told Satcher she would not sign off on a report or Call to Action on sexual health. In an interview years later, she said there was no political motivation or White House directive behind that decision. "It wasn't finished. Organizationally, it needed a lot of work," she said.[49]

Satcher, and others, had a different understanding of what happened. Satcher said the work was substantially finished. Shalala had talked to the White House about it and then told him he could submit something to a medical journal on the subject—fine. But no report. "She made it very clear that they felt the press would take that and embarrass the White House," he said.[50]

He assembled an article and approached the *American Journal of Preventive Medicine,* which agreed to publish it. But Satcher then changed his mind, feeling strongly that it should be a meatier, official release. It seemed possible, or even likely, that Gore would get elected and that Satcher would continue on as surgeon general. There was even speculation that he might be chosen as Gore's HHS secretary. With patience, Satcher might get an opportunity to release the report in the next administration.

He did get that chance, though under dramatically different circumstances than he'd imagined.

A NEW ADMINISTRATION

After George W. Bush won the closely contested election of 2000, Satcher told officials in the new administration that he was willing to forfeit the last year of his term and resign. He expected they would want to appoint their own surgeon general. But the new administration told him they wanted him to finish his term. In fact, Bush's new HHS secretary, Tommy Thompson, had a little time left in his term as Wisconsin's governor and asked Satcher to serve as acting secretary during the two-week interim following Shalala's departure. Satcher attended Bush's first Cabinet meeting on January 31, 2001, and was greeted warmly. "When he [Bush] saw me there," Satcher recalled, "he immediately came over and shook my hand and said how pleased he was to have me there. Then, when it was over, he came back over and said; 'Well, what did you think? How'd you like it?'"[51]

Thompson started work on February 2 and gave hearty thanks and praise to Satcher, and the two developed a good rapport. But Thompson was different from his predecessor. Donna Shalala had come to the Clinton White House from a career in higher education, including a stint as chancellor of the University of Wisconsin at Madison. She was an effective public speaker and shrewd politician, but had hired a roster of stars as agency heads—people like NIH director Harold Varmus, a Nobel Prize–winning scientist—and gave them wide latitude to rule and speak as they saw fit. Thompson, in contrast, was a career politician who held much tighter reigns and preferred to be the one with the microphone. *New York Times* columnist Frank Rich once wrote that Thompson "comes across as a Chamber of Commerce glad hander."[52] The new HHS secretary certainly meant business, and quickly instituted a "One Department, One Voice" policy for the department. "It was sold as an attempt to make sure that the administration speaks with one voice on matters and people aren't flying around willy-nilly," said Damon Thompson, Satcher's press secretary. "They put in tough rules about when you could comment, what you had to do before you could comment."[53]

Satcher told Thompson about the sexual health report and sent him a copy. Not long after, Thompson came to the HHS's Parklawn office building in Rockville, Md., where Satcher's office was located. It was a spring day, and Thompson was there to handle starting-gun duties for a five-mile footrace in which Satcher was participating. They were standing together before the start, and Thompson said he'd read the report and felt the American people needed to read it, too.[54] The surgeon general took that as a blessing to release it. "So I called him one day and told him that I had scheduled a press conference to release the report," Satcher recalled. "I think he almost fainted on the other end of the line. But when he recovered, he asked me if I would wait, and I said, 'Tommy, you know, we've already paid the money for the hotel and everything to release this report, so we've got a lot of people coming and so we'd rather not wait.' He said 'I'll get back to you.'"[55]

Other political appointees were brought in to review the report, which had been through many drafts. CDC director Jeffrey Koplan was with Satcher when administration officials picked over it, wanting to change dozens of parts of the latest iteration. "You know, 'We don't like this, we don't like that.' David said, . . . 'I'm not changing that stuff,'" Koplan recalled.[56]

Ultimately, Thompson said he could not sign off on the report, but he would not stop Satcher's press conference. "He said, 'David, go ahead, but you're on your own. I'm not going to be able to protect you on this one," Satcher said.[57] Satcher released his thirty-three-page Call to Action on sexual health at a Thursday press conference in late June 2001. Thompson, the ever-present emcee at HHS announcements, was not there. Nor were any other HHS staff aside from Satcher's own people. They didn't want to be near the ensuing firestorm.

Citing a range of studies, the report concluded there was no good evidence that teaching abstinence prevents teens from having sex or that a gay person could become straight. It also said that although sex was best and safest if done in monogamous relationships, the relationship didn't have to be a marriage.

It was not something the family values crowd wanted to hear—a slap to those who believed discussion of condoms had no place in schools and who classified homosexuality as aberrant behavior. (And to some, it may not have helped that it was a black man lecturing the nation on sexual behavior. Carol Moseley Braun, the only black U.S. senator when Satcher was confirmed, told him at the time: "Promise that you will stay away from sex. The worst thing that could happen would be for a black man in Washington to be talking about sex. Don't give them an excuse to lynch you.")[58] The media lapped up the sexual health report; the Bush administration grimaced. "The president understands the report was issued by a surgeon general that he did not appoint, a surgeon general who was appointed by the previous administration," Bush spokesman Ari Fleischer told reporters. "The president continues to believe that abstinence and abstinence education is the most effective way to prevent AIDS, to prevent unwanted pregnancy."[59]

That report ended any hope Satcher might have had of Bush appointing him to a second term, political observers said. But more than that,

Satcher found himself sidelined in the following months, even in a situation where the surgeon general's silence hurt the administration.

9/11 AND ANTHRAX

On the morning of September 11, 2001, Satcher was being driven to the train station to take a trip to Princeton, New Jersey, for a speaking engagement that afternoon. When he heard the news that hijacked airliners had hit New York's World Trade Center and the Pentagon, and that Washington, D.C., was being shut down, his driver took him home to the NIH campus, which that day was rapidly being turned into an armed camp. He understood the government's reaction; NIH was the center of federal medical research, and a potential target for the kind of terrorism that seemed to be unfolding. But as permanent fences and car-search stations went up, he liked the place less and less. He had enjoyed jogging around the campus and walking through it with his wife, Nola. "But after that, none of us enjoyed being there much," he said.[60]

Traveling again by early October, he was in Boston on October 4 at an awards ceremony when he learned of a new terror beginning to unfold. Robert Stevens, a Florida-based photo editor for a tabloid newspaper called *The Sun,* had been diagnosed with an inhaled form of anthrax. It was the first case of inhalation anthrax reported in the United States in twenty-five years.

Satcher was also informed that Tommy Thompson was the official speaking to the media about it. No one told the surgeon general to be silent on the subject. "They just said, 'You're in Boston, here's what you need to know, and the secretary is going to be making a statement,'" said Damon Thompson, the press secretary, who was with Satcher on the trip.[61] The secretary spoke at a White House briefing, accompanied by Scott Lillibridge, his special advisor on bioterrorism. Thompson did nearly all the talking. He said the CDC had just confirmed the diagnosis of anthrax in a sixty-three-year-old man in a Florida hospital, and it appeared to be an isolated case. With 9/11 fresh in their minds, the first question from reporters was whether the man's illness was the result of terrorism. Thompson said there was no evidence of that. He added that the patient had recently traveled to North Carolina. A reporter asked about possible sources of anthrax infection. Thompson replied; "That's why the doctor is here," and briefly ceded the floor to Lillibridge, who said contact with wool and animal hides were possibilities.[62]

But then Thompson took back the microphone, and made a series of statements that would later be remembered as a blunder in crisis communication. He volunteered that investigators knew the man was an outdoorsman who, during his North Carolina trip the previous week, drank water from a stream. Thompson said the case was still under investigation, and the stream water was only one possible explanation for the man's illness. But he was very reassuring—sounding more certain as the press conference went on—that there was no need for the public to worry. "This is an isolated case and it's not contagious," he concluded.[63]

Here is what the media heard: the government thought Stevens got anthrax from drinking stream water, and was investigating to substantiate that theory. But though that's what the HHS secretary conveyed, that was not what the government actually thought. "Everybody suspected this was terrorists, but we had no idea how he got it," Damon Thompson said later.[64]

It turned out not to be an isolated case or to have anything to do with drinking water from a backwoods stream. The next week, NBC News anchor Tom Brokaw developed skin anthrax after opening a letter. Two days later, Senate majority leader Tom Daschle's office was quarantined after a staffer there opened a letter containing anthrax. More reports followed about anthrax letters received at ABC News, the *New York Post,* and other media companies. And on October 17, thirty-one congressional staffers tested positive for anthrax and the House of Representatives was shut down.

Tommy Thompson continued to be the HHS spokesman in those initial weeks, consistent with the "One Voice" philosophy practiced within the department. HHS public affairs officers funneled all questions about anthrax to Thompson for two weeks after the October 4 press conference.

But public panic escalated as more poisoned letters turned up and more buildings were evacuated. Hospital emergency rooms and health departments were deluged with calls from the worried well. HHS experts quietly cringed at Thompson's lack of specialized knowledge, on full display as increasingly anxious reporters peppered him with questions. Some wags within the department joked that the HHS media relations motto should be changed to "One Department, One Voice—Not His." Outside the department, some politicians and others began demanding to hear from the experts. "If the people with expertise are not allowed to speak, then I get a little bit worried about what is being hidden from me," said U.S. Representative Christopher Shays, a Connecticut Republican who chaired a House subcommittee on national security. "The experts have to be able to answer the questions."[65]

From the beginning, reporters sought out CDC director Jeffrey Koplan because of his agency's leadership in the investigation, and HHS officials finally approved Koplan to begin appearing on television. But Koplan was a reluctant spokesman and flatly rejected an on-camera interview request from 60 Minutes (in part because he didn't feel an investigative news program was the appropriate venue to disclose information on what was still a very uncertain situation). His resistance stiffened when HHS officials scripted answers that said anthrax was not a big problem. "I thought, 'We don't know if this is a big problem or not!'" recalled Koplan, a Clinton appointee who would leave the CDC director job early the following year.[66] Koplan also was beginning to come under fire, as the CDC at times seemed off-balance, changing its guidance to local health officials as it struggled to learn exactly what it was dealing with.

As the situation spiraled, HHS began calling on Satcher, NIH scientist Anthony Fauci, and others to answer questions. "An explosion of spokespersons" ensued, recalled Georges Benjamin, executive director of the American Public Health Association. But that too, was problematic. "The national public health voice had gotten confused," Benjamin observed.[67]

The surgeon general should have been the government's health authority, Benjamin and other experts believe. Satcher was the natural point person for anthrax. He had been steeped in bioterrorism and disaster planning experience from his years at CDC and as assistant secretary for health. He was also a calm and careful presence, in marked contrast to the shoot-from-the-hip HHS secretary. Besides, there was a long tradition of surgeons general being the main communicators at a time of public health crisis. Rupert Blue had spoken as the nation's doctor during the terrible Spanish flu pandemic in 1918 and 1919. Leonard Scheele had delivered the news about illnesses caused by the Cutter polio vaccine in 1955. C. Everett Koop had been the government's sage voice during the AIDS crisis in the 1980s. The public respected the surgeon general, and so did the public health workforce. "Our people consider him our leader," said Mohammad Akhter, at the time the American Public Health Association's executive director.[68]

But Satcher had been benched during the crucial early weeks of the crisis. Many believed the administration's lingering distaste with the surgeon general over the June sexual health document was a main reason. Others said that's a misinterpretation. Bill Pierce, then HHS deputy assistant secretary for public affairs, said Tommy Thompson was simply accustomed to speaking for the organization, and the department did its best to deal with a complicated and worsening situation that was not only a public health emergency but also the subject of a criminal investigation. But Pierce also acknowledged that Satcher should have at least had a place at the dais from the very beginning. "Had we had the surgeon general at the secretary's side at the initial announcement, we probably could have avoided a lot of criticism," he said.[69]

Results from a Harvard University telephone survey, released in early November 2001, showed that Satcher and Koplan were the two government health officials the public trusted most. Later that month at a House subcommittee hearing on national security, experts voiced a similar conclusion, arguing that Satcher should have been the one informing the public about anthrax.[70] Satcher, however, was already winding down his term. That month he told reporters he would not seek reappointment when his term expired the following February.

During his last week in office, he shared with reporters his worries about what would happen to the Office of the Surgeon General after his departure. The office's $1 million budget could barely cover the cost of generating even one surgeon general's report, and the lack of a "meaningful budget" would damage the office, he said. He also opined that it was essential that his successor be "independent enough to report directly to the American people on the basis of public health and science."[71]

Satcher left office in February 2002. He moved back to Atlanta to take a position with the Morehouse School of Medicine, leading a new health care program focused on addressing medical disparities.

In an era in which the primary power of surgeons general is their bully pulpit, the officeholders are judged largely on their communication skills. Satcher was good but not great. He was a skillful speaker, schooled from his youth in the cadence and rhythm of Baptist sermons and using a populist style—without raising his voice—to discuss science and dispense public health wisdom. "I always liked David's style," said Koplan. "It's low-key without being soporific."[72]

Satcher never became an outsized national presence like the charismatic Elders or the commanding Koop. But that wasn't really his goal. He was more interested in following the example of Julius Richmond, the thoughtful Carter-era health official who was the only other physician to simultaneously serve as surgeon general and assistant secretary for health. With the ASH position came control over more people and resources within HHS, meaning that the two lowest-key people to serve as surgeon general in the past forty years were also the most powerful. They had greater ability to assemble and release the reports that are a surgeon general's most influential and enduring form of communication.

Satcher was a consensus builder, and there were battles he chose not to fight. For example, as surgeon general he said relatively little about the public health menace posed by guns, despite the CDC research that convinced him of the dangerous role they played in suicide and violence. But on other topics, Satcher was unswervingly willing to say what he thought needed to be said. As Elders once said, "Only do-nothing surgeon generals are not controversial," and Satcher was.[73] Repeatedly discouraged from putting out the sexual health report, he joined Koop in the tiny ranks of surgeons general who issued a report against the wishes of White House officials. "He said, 'I'm willing to be fired for it, if need be,'" said Damon Thompson.[74]

He probably would have gone that far, others opined. "Satcher was the kind of guy that if they had tweaked him too much, he would have walked out," Fauci said.[75]

His successor was different. Richard Carmona, an emergency room physician and hard-charging former Green Beret from Arizona, was a popular choice who seemed destined to be a star in the office. But he never took the kind of stands the soft-spoken Satcher did, and virtually disappeared into the government bureaucracy.

PART FOUR

Plummet, 2002–Present

CHAPTER II

MIA

If ever there was a candidate who seemed likely to restore the Office of the Surgeon General to Koop-like prominence, it was Richard Carmona. Here was an outspoken trauma surgeon who had grown up in Harlem, shined as a Green Beret in Vietnam, and won media attention for a heroic cliffside rescue. A combination SWAT team member and university professor, he had the respect of both Republicans and Democrats. He sounded like a hero from a dime novel.

But once he was in office, Carmona proved to be the lowest-profile surgeon general the nation had seen. He was a "do-nothing surgeon general. He faded into the woodwork," said Kim Elliott, former deputy director of Trust for America's Health, a Washington, D.C.–based public health research organization. "He was MIA."[1]

Indeed, Carmona's biggest moment as surgeon general didn't occur until nearly a year after he completed his single, four-year term in office. He began making pointed comments about the Bush administration, saying he was continually muzzled by political overseers who believed theology and ideology should guide public health messages to the public, and landed squarely in the headlines following a July 2007 congressional hearing at which he laid it all out. "I was often instructed what to say or what not to say," Carmona testified."[2]

Although some praised Carmona for speaking out like that, others judged it as too little, too late. They argued that Carmona could have quietly told members of Congress while such interference was going on, or made a more public stand. "When these things are happening to you, at a certain point you give voice to that," said Jeffrey Levi, executive director of Trust for America's Health. "He's wanting us to see him as a hero in retrospect."[3]

GUNS AND AMMO

Richard Henry Carmona was born on November 22, 1949, and grew up in Harlem. His parents had both come to New York from Puerto Rico. His childhood was harrowing. "Richie," as he was known, was the oldest of the four children born to Raoul Carmona and Lucy Martinez. His father was an alcoholic who was frequently absent and unemployed. His mother, also a hard drinker, was an uneducated chainsmoker. When Carmona was six, the entire family was temporarily homeless and living in the streets until they were taken in by Maria Anglade Carmona, his paternal grandmother—or *abuelita* to little Richie. The family later lived in a roach-infested tenement, subsisting on food brought to them by his abuelita. At age twelve, Richie Carmona's mother hit him with a broom when he confronted her about buying a bottle of rum instead of groceries needed to feed the family.[4]

Not surprisingly, schoolwork was not his focus growing up. Whereas other surgeons general were hardworking academic prodigies as children, Carmona was frequently truant and ultimately dropped out of high school. But his life changed when he met Sal Hasson, an Army Special Forces officer who was visiting a neighborhood soda shop. Carmona was so impressed by Hasson's stories of military life and world travel that he decided to talk to an army recruiter and, at age seventeen, enlisted. "In retrospect, it was the best thing I ever did," Carmona would say years later in speeches as he recounted his life story. "It gave me a platform to be successful the rest of my life."[5]

In the army, Carmona earned a general equivalency diploma, a necessary step for him to emulate Hasson and qualify for the Green Berets. After his training, Carmona was sent to Vietnam and became a sergeant with a Green Beret unit, working as both a weapons specialist and a battlefield medic. He was part of a twelve-member team but often was sent on stealth missions that involved just two or three soldiers, often working with Montagnards or other Vietnamese friendly to U.S. forces. He was tasked to do such things as surveillance and finding downed pilots. One of his most harrowing missions—one for which he was later awarded a Bronze Star—involved locating an underground hospital assumed to exist (a plausible explanation for what happened to Viet Cong soldiers who were wounded on the battlefield but quickly disappeared). The mission started on New Year's Day 1970, and went awry after Carmona and his comrades were discovered about the same time they found the hospital. They survived an ambush and multiple firefights, however, and escaped without a casualty.[6]

Carmona earned a variety of service awards and decorations, including two Purple Hearts. (He was wounded in the shoulder, back, and legs, leaving him with bullet fragments that would pain him for decades afterward.)[7] Leaving the army after three years' active duty, he married his childhood sweetheart, Diane Sanchez. Two of his uncles arranged a position for him as an apprenticed electrician, but Carmona decided to go to college instead.

He started at Bronx Community College, where he made the dean's list and in 1973 graduated with an associate degree in liberal arts—and a 3.73 grade point average. Then he headed west. In 1974, Carmona took California's state nursing exam, which was based on the Special Forces curriculum. He passed and worked as an emergency department nurse while taking a premed college course load at the University of California, San Francisco. That's right: Carmona was the first nurse to become a surgeon general.

He graduated with a bachelor's degree in biology and chemistry in 1976, then rolled right into medical school at UCSF, graduating in 1979. "I had average intelligence, but I had a great deal of tenacity. . . . It's something Special Forces instills in you," Carmona said. As he completed medical school, he won an award he would frequently mention the rest of his life, a gold-headed cane, awarded to the senior medical student who—in the assessment of his classmates and the medical faculty—best exemplifies the qualities of a "true physician." Carmona completed his residency training in San Francisco, but it would take him another eight years to get his board certification as a surgeon, as he failed the board examination twice before passing it.[8]

Next came another move, this time to Arizona. In 1985, Carmona was recruited by Tucson Medical Center—the city's largest hospital—to lead the region's first trauma care program. In 1986, he became a doctor for the Pima County Sheriff's Department and a leader of its SWAT team. Just as when he was Green Beret, Carmona had responsibilities not only in the world of medicine but also in the world of violence.

He became a celebrated action hero in the 1990s because of two incidents. In 1992, he was part of a helicopter rescue team that responded when another helicopter crashed during a snowstorm on a mountainside in the Coronado National Forest, roughly one hundred miles from Tucson. The pilot and a flight nurse on the downed medical evacuation helicopter died, but a flight medic—though critically injured—remained alive. Carmona carried the medic to safety. (Some producers planned to make a television movie about the incident, but the film was never made.) The rescue story was told and retold, and years later it inspired a joke from President George W. Bush: "When I first learned that Dr. Carmona once dangled out of a moving helicopter, I worried that maybe he wasn't the best guy to educate our Americans about reducing health risks."[9]

In 1999, while driving to work, Carmona stopped at the scene of a traffic accident where a man driving a pickup had hit another vehicle and was threatening the other driver with a gun. Carmona repeatedly ordered the truck driver to put down the gun. The man—Jean Pierre Lafitte—fired at Carmona, grazing his scalp. Carmona (who'd earned a sharpshooter badge in the army) fired back seven times. Three shots hit Lafitte, killing him. A few hours later, Lafitte's father was found stabbed to death, and investigators concluded Lafitte had murdered him earlier that day. Lafitte's mother was nevertheless bitter about her son's death and the publicity Carmona got from it. "This man keeps putting himself in the media. This is not professionalism," she said to a *Tucson Citizen* reporter.[10] The discomforting idea of a doctor blowing someone away was mitigated by initial media reports that suggested that after Carmona shot the man, he rushed over to give him medical attention. But those reports were wrong. Carmona stayed at his car, reloading and then training his gun on the unmoving man.[11]

Carmona was involved in many conflicts. He was fired from Tucson Medical Center in 1993 after TMC officials said he had alienated doctors and administrators with his "street-fighter" attitude. Carmona filed a wrongful termination suit, claiming he was fired for protesting illegal and unethical practices at the hospital, including what he said was substandard care by one doctor and unnecessary consultations by other physicians. The suit was settled, with Carmona reportedly receiving $3.9 million and a full-page newspaper advertisement in which the hospital apologized and praised his skills.[12]

In 1994, he was hired to run Tucson's small, financially troubled Kino Community Hospital. Carmona eliminated the operating deficit in two years, and was promoted in 1997 to run the county hospital's parent organization. But financial reports later showed that mounting uncollectible accounts made Kino appear to have more money than it actually did. He also butted heads with various physicians, hospital workers, and county politicians over his handling of a range of issues. After years of tumult, Carmona agreed to resign in 1999.[13]

He was teaching surgery, public health, and family and community medicine at the University of Arizona when George W. Bush was elected in November 2000. When it came time to replace Satcher, Bush wanted a surgeon general who could be a good point person on emergency preparedness issues. Carmona, a trauma specialist with a favorable résumé, wanted a health post in the new administration. He most likely received a boost from a prominent southern Arizona businessman named Jose Canchola, a former mayor of Nogales, restaurateur, Bush supporter, and part owner of the Arizona Diamondbacks baseball team. Canchola was a good friend to have, and his support helped land Carmona the nomination.[14] In March 2002, Bush announced Carmona was his pick for surgeon general.

Reporters were impressed; one newspaper called him a real-life Indiana Jones. He was a hit in Congress, too. Republicans liked him because he was a law-and-order type committed to working on bioterrorism and emergency preparedness. And Democrats thought he seemed enough of a maverick to be a strong and independent voice within the Bush administration. In July 2002, the Senate confirmed him without debate—the first time in decades that a surgeon general nominee sailed through the process so smoothly. Carmona was sworn in to office on August 5.

The fifty-two-year-old Carmona was as giddy as a child about the opportunity. "It is as if the fairy godmother reached out and touched me and cast me in the best Disney movie ever made," Carmona said at the time of his confirmation hearing.[15] But his four-year term would prove to be more like a depressing political film that nobody went to see.

CARMONA AND THE BULLY PULPIT

Carmona's first full month on the job—September 2002—included meetings at the White House and Pentagon, an event at the National Press Club, and speaking engagements in California, Arizona, and Illinois. His prospects in the bully pulpit seemed promising. HHS Secretary Tommy Thompson had become more gun-shy on public health matters following the anthrax debacle, theoretically allowing Carmona a fair amount of opportunity to be a lead communicator. Eve Slater, the assistant secretary for health when Carmona took office, was not considered a competitor. A quiet and reasonable administrator, she had allowed Satcher speaking freedom even after he was on the outs with the Bush White House, and was not interested in restricting Carmona, either.

And Carmona proved to be a very good speaker. Not a Koop or Elders, perhaps, but animated and interesting enough to hold an audience. In his standard talk, he narrated his life story with humor, humility, and passion (almost always paying homage to his abuelita), and then finished with a discussion of health disparities or whatever other health topic was being spotlighted. Some HHS staffers, including his speechwriters, had prodded Carmona to tell stories about himself.[16] Audiences seemed to respond well; it made him more human and easier to connect with.

Unfortunately, the script rarely changed much. "It's a nice story—up from a tough neighborhood, poor background, rose through this and did all these things, and now look where he is," said Jeffrey Koplan, the CDC director. "But after a few times, you got it, and you gotta move on to something else."[17] Cristina Beato, who for a time would be Carmona's boss, once said she frequently heard the same complaint. "I cannot tell you how many times—and I don't mean to be flippant about this—that people would tell me, 'I am sick and tired of hearing about his abuelita.'"[18]

Another problem was that his topics were not appetizing to the press. Health disparities proved a particularly hard sell. It was, after all, old news; Satcher had addressed it extensively. It also was too complicated a topic for a short, punchy news story. "It's not a thirty-second sound bite," observed Georges Benjamin of the American Public Health Association.[19]

Meanwhile, Carmona undermined his own credibility from the start by dodging reporters' questions about controversial topics. In August 2002, at one of his first public speeches, Carmona was asked about his position on abortion at a San Antonio summit on Hispanic health care. It was not a surprising question for a surgeon general, and Koop and Elders had been clear about their thoughts on the topic. But Carmona responded that abortion was something that he would "deal with when it comes up as an issue." Another example occurred the following month. Carmona appeared at a bioterrorism conference in Tucson, where he was billed as one of the nation's experts on bioterror response readiness. But when a reporter asked him whether all Americans should be vaccinated against smallpox, Carmona replied, "All I can say is, the best scientific minds in the world are working on it."[20]

So, for various reasons, Carmona quickly lost visibility. "Where is he?" asked U.S. Representative John Peterson, a Pennsylvania Republican, during a hearing in March 2003 (less than eight months after Carmona had taken office). "There's been a big drop-off in that office."[21]

Carmona resurfaced in early June, during his appearance at a congressional hearing on smokeless tobacco and "reduced risk" tobacco products. After Carmona spoke about the dangers of tobacco, U.S. Representative Ed Whitfield—a Republican from the tobacco-growing state of Kentucky—asked Carmona if he would support the abolition of all tobacco products. "I would at this point, yes," the surgeon general replied. Carmona's answer got little reaction at the moment he said it, but Whitfield later said he was disappointed and shocked. "I've never heard anything like that from any public official" or even from anti-tobacco advocates, Whitfield said. The exchange got front-page coverage in the *Washington Post,* with the White House distancing itself from Carmona's comments. "That is not the policy of the administration," White House spokesman Scott McClellan told reporters later that day. "The president supports efforts to crack down on youth smoking, and we can do more as a society to keep tobacco away from kids. That's our focus."[22] Of course, Whitfield was the one at fault for pushing a public health official to say such a thing. "Why would you, a legislator [from a tobacco state], ask the surgeon general of the United States that question?" asked Georges Benjamin. Nevertheless, Carmona was the one who seemed to pay for the statement, and he was placed on a noticeably tighter leash following the hearing.[23]

But in fact, Carmona was getting static from his bosses before that incident. As early as August 2002, internal HHS e-mails show Carmona was questioned about making travel plans without completely following an approval and scheduling process demanded by politically appointed higher-ups. Hundreds of e-mails on that topic—some of them nasty—circulated over the next three years. One issue was the high number of trips he made to Arizona and to San Diego, where his homes were. (Twelve of the nineteen trips he took in his first six months in office were to those two locations, one HHS officials complained.)[24]

Ground transportation was another recurring theme. One string of e-mails discussed Carmona's requests for reimbursement for taxi fare on days when records indicated he had used a government car and driver. (Carmona later characterized the problem as one of clerical error, noting it was resolved when he paid back $3,580 he had received in excess travel expense reimbursements.) Another series spoke of

Carmona's preference for a chauffeured sedan over taxis, and a recurring clash between him and Assistant Secretary for Health Eve Slater over use of a government car.[25]

Another dustup occurred when HHS officials learned through a newspaper article that Carmona was planning a spring 2004 trip to a neglected military cemetery in New York—a trip they hadn't approved. One more involved what was seen as a surprise change of plan by Carmona regarding a weekend trip. He tried to bring with him, without what was seen as proper prior clearance, an attractive speechwriter named Jennifer Cabe (whom one peeved official referred to as "Jennifer Babe").[26] "Apparently, the SG forgets that he reports through an organization!" wrote William Turenne, a former Eli Lilly executive working as a high-level consultant to the HHS secretary.[27]

The surgeon general clearly sparked some of his own problems, but he was dealing with one of the most dysfunctional Public Health Service front offices of all time. The cast included HHS Director of Intergovernmental Affairs Regina Schofield, a den mother for political appointees, who had previously worked eight years as a sales representative for the tobacco company Philip Morris; and Turenne, a consultant who had no real line authority but was a friend of HHS Secretary Thompson and acted like the political officer in a Soviet battalion.[28]

And then there was Cristina Beato, a toxic presence who succeeded Eve Slater as assistant secretary for health. Known for her conservative ideology, Beato was ultimately ousted following allegations she had lied on her résumé. (She ascribed the résumé fabrications mostly to clerical error.)[29] Carmona said she pushed him to give more credit to the White House in his speeches. She alleged that Carmona assigned a driver to pick up his laundry. Amid the smoke of accusations and denials, it was clear that she helped implement a level of bureaucratic control greater that Carmona could stomach. "He and Cristina Beato could not get along if they were the last two people on the face of the earth," said one person who worked with both. "They would kill each other rather than cooperate. It was as ugly as anything I've ever seen."[30]

Beato wasn't alone in her contempt for Carmona. Turenne, especially, had little use for the surgeon general. In a September 2002 e-mail, he worried that Carmona was not focused on strengthening the public health infrastructure, defending President Bush's position on stem cell research, defending Bush's position on smallpox vaccine, or doing and saying other things that the administration wanted him to. Turenne saw Carmona as a political surrogate to be used to argue the Bush administration's perspective on health matters, as a show dog to occasionally be displayed at Republican fund-raising events, and as an understudy spokesman who could fill in when the secretary was too busy. He kept up his criticism of Carmona for years, sometimes in the context of the discussions about Carmona's travel. He found ceremonies in which Carmona was being given awards particularly galling. In one e-mail, he wrote: "How many trips to Arizona? How many trips to Mexico? How many self-congratulation celebrations?"[31]

(Turenne and Beato did not respond to interview requests from the author.)

In 2005, Bush administration officials tried to undercut Carmona's involvement in a landmark government lawsuit against tobacco companies. The case, which had been filed by federal prosecutors in 1999, during the Clinton administration, contended that cigarette makers had violated civil racketeering laws by conspiring for decades to withhold from the public information about the dangers of their products. Prosecutors decided to use Carmona as a witness, thinking the surgeon general would put a persuasive face on the government's case. But Bush administration officials were unhappy about Carmona's involvement, believing it would suggest the White House supported the lawsuit.[32]

After the Department of Justice put Carmona on its witness list, prosecutors were told Carmona's participation had not been approved by the political bosses at HHS. When it came time for the surgeon general to testify, a top-level, Bush-appointed DOJ attorney—Daniel Meron—tried to warn the lawyers away from Carmona, said prosecutor Sharon Eubanks. "Everyone says he's a buffoon. You don't want him testifying because he'll ruin our case," Meron said, according to Eubanks's 2012 book about the case. When Eubanks responded that she had worked with Carmona and found him to be sharp, Meron reportedly replied: "He had better do well. If he doesn't, you'll be blamed. This is on you."[33]

Carmona did testify and "was magical," Eubanks said. He appeared in dress uniform, striding confidently down the center of the courtroom to take his place. His voice was clear and authoritative. The judge was deferential to him and made sure the defense attorneys remained respectful too. And he was persuasive, Eubanks said. "It wasn't just what he said; it was how he said it. You could tell he believed in what he said."[34] In 2006, a federal judge ruled in favor of the government and ordered the tobacco companies to stop using descriptions like "mild," "natural," "light," "ultra light," "low tar," and other words that could make a consumer believe one brand was less hazardous than others.

Carmona was well aware of the gravitas he possessed. "The fact of the matter is, when it comes to health and science, there is no more credible source of information than the surgeon general of the United States," he said.[35] He was wrong on that point, however. On most public health topics, there was another leader in the department who had come to be regarded as more credible than Carmona—CDC director Julie Gerberding.

Through the years, CDC directors had gradually acquired the components of the platform on which the surgeon general's pulpit was originally based. The surgeon general had once overseen the epidemic-investigation and disease-prevention efforts of the Public Health Service. Now the CDC handled those jobs, and the daily boss of public health was the agency's chief, not the surgeon general. CDC staffers often did the bulk of the work behind the renowned surgeon general reports, and the forewords to surgeon general smoking reports had been authored or coauthored by CDC directors since 1989. Nevertheless, CDC directors had kept a fairly low profile over the years. The job's traditional focus was running the agency, and CDC directors tended to be staid personalities accustomed to deferring—often happily—to HHS higher-ups when it came to media appearances and public messaging. (It helped that the CDC is located in Atlanta, away from the horde of national media in Washington, D.C.)

Gerberding, however, was very comfortable taking the lead in health communications. In 2001, when she was a lower-level CDC official, she had impressed Tommy Thompson with her handling of media questions about the anthrax scare. He elevated her to CDC director in 2002 (about the time Carmona became surgeon general), making her the first woman to head the CDC. Thompson was comfortable with her speaking for the government on the range of scary, urgent public health matters that fell under the CDC's purview, including SARS (severe acute respiratory syndrome), food poisoning, and the threat of a deadly new type of influenza. She was a collected and clear orator who strengthened the agency's communications staff to make the CDC more responsive and pro-active in addressing the public. She spent roughly 25 percent of her time in Washington, often to speak to Congress in public hearings or to appear at press conferences, though she also spoke directly to the White House more often than her predecessors had. Indeed, some at HHS considered her a bit of a rogue; a powerful voice with a remote base (in Atlanta) who was a bit harder to control than the crew in Washington.[36] Gerberding certainly could play to the spotlight: for a profile in *Vogue* magazine, she posed for a full-page color photograph in a gray Chanel suit and white Marc Jacobs high-heeled shoes.[37]

How good was she? It's nearly impossible to gauge the influence and effectiveness of one federal health official compared to another, but Gerberding was far more visible than her predecessors. One analysis found that from 1998 to 2002, Surgeon General David Satcher was mentioned in newspaper and wire reports more than 5,500 times—or roughly 3.5 times more often than CDC director Jeff Koplan. The tables turned when Carmona and Gerberding were in office together. Gerberding was mentioned or featured in news reports more than 4,000 times from 2002 to 2006, or nearly twice as often as Carmona. What's more, health reporters rated her as more newsworthy and credible than Carmona, the HHS secretary, or other top federal health officials, according to one survey of journalists.[38] The perception may have rubbed off on the general public, which through the decade continued to rank the CDC as one of the most trusted federal agencies.[39]

SUPPRESSION AND TRANSFORMATION

In early 2004, the Union of Concerned Scientists issued a report detailing twenty-one incidents of suppression or distortion of scientific findings by Bush administration officials. The group included twenty Nobel laureate scientists, and they presented examples of actions that represented stark contradictions with what surgeons general had been preaching for decades. Bush's Department of Health and Human Services pushed abstinence-only programs as a way to prevent unwanted teen pregnancies and the spread of venereal diseases, even though most studies showed that the approach didn't work. Not only was the Bush administration spending more than $1 billion on abstinence-only programs, but it also changed the guidelines on how such programs were assessed (for example, attendance and attitude were used as success measures, but not pregnancy rates in female participants).

There were more examples. A National Cancer Institute website was altered to suggest strong scientific evidence existed of a link between abortion and breast cancer, when there was no such link. A CDC website was changed to make it seem as if there was sharp scientific debate about the HIV-preventing effectiveness of condoms, when there wasn't. And after an advisory panel took steps to expand the definition of lead poisoning to include more children, HHS Secretary Tommy Thompson became unusually involved in the appointments of the panel's members, adding at least two people with financial ties to the lead industry. As a result, the definition change was tabled for years.[40]

Such shenanigans had a particularly forceful impact on the surgeon general's office. Carmona came into office with great ambitions for releasing reports on a variety of important topics. Work on some was already well under way, and in 2004 two came to fruition.[41] But several others never saw the light of day. For example, in 2003, Carmona told a crowd at a national conference for prison medical staffers that his office was working on a Call to Action on correctional health care, but it never came out. Administration officials were worried a report that pointed toward improved health measures in prisons would make them seem soft on crime, Carmona said in an interview years later.[42]

But the report-that-never-was that ultimately got the most attention was one on global health.

The document was to be a Call to Action, a shorter and more nimble document than the staid and voluminous surgeon general reports. Satcher had had some success tackling timely health topics through that format, and Carmona deemed it a good way to address the link between poverty and poor health in countries and to open discussions about what corporations and the U.S. government could do to improve health conditions in foreign nations.

The work started well. Carmona got the money and manpower to do the global health document from the HHS Office of Global Health Affairs. Most of the work was done by subject-matter experts, including people from the NIH, some universities, and the Catholic Medical Mission Board. An initial draft was ready by 2005, and the Commissioned Officers Association organized a global health summit in Philadelphia for that June, in expectation that Carmona would release the report there in a keynote address.[43]

But the Bush administration scotched those plans after finding some parts of the sixty-five-page report unpalatable. Carmona's draft discussed the importance of ratifying an international tobacco treaty, something the U.S. Senate had not done. It talked about the importance of health care systems providing access for all patients, and acknowledged that the U.S. system had failed to do that. It noted that pollution spread across international borders, and that gaps between the richest and poorest people were linked to gaps in health among different economic and social classes. It called on the federal government to spend more on global health improvement and to emphasize global health more in its foreign policy. And it broached the topic of global warming and extolled the benefits of condom distribution.

William R. Steiger, the man in charge of the HHS Office of Global Health Affairs, emerged as the most visible obstacle to the report's release. Steiger was the kind of political appointee who made scientists shake their heads until their necks hurt. A sandy-haired man in his mid-thirties who looked like a college fraternity president, he seemed a little young for such a position and appeared to lack the right expertise—his college degrees were in Latin American history, not public health. But his political connections were impeccable. His father was a former Republican congressman from Wisconsin who had once hired a young Dick Cheney as an intern; his mother had been appointed chair of the Federal Trade Commission by the first President Bush.[44] The capper? The elder Bush was Steiger's godfather, and HHS Secretary Thompson was a friend of the family.

Steiger carried out his job like someone who never forgot who put him there. Earlier, he had challenged a plan by the World Health Organization to fight the global obesity epidemic. Calling the science in the report questionable, he argued—as junk food manufacturers had—that combating obesity should be less about criticizing how foods are made and marketed and more about personal responsibility. Steiger stirred further outrage in public health circles by implementing a vetting policy for government scientists invited to attend WHO meetings, designed to give the Bush administration more control over who participated in international scientific deliberations.[45]

As for Carmona's report, Steiger argued that it lacked scientific rigor. Steiger commissioned an alternate version to be produced by others within HHS, but Carmona—whose name would have been on the final product—refused to go along with some parts of the new version. And so it died.[46]

Meanwhile, Carmona was shouldering broader responsibilities regarding the Commissioned Corps. The Corps's nature had changed as decades passed and the plagues of the nineteenth century were tamed. The elite cadre of physicians gradually became less regimented, as its officers stopped wearing their uniforms routinely and were more likely to be assigned to a laboratory or hospital than be dispatched to a diseased port or quarantine station. At the beginning of the twenty-first century, most Corps members worked in offices alongside the "civilians" of the Public Health Service, and the Corps was little more than a parallel personnel system within HHS that offered slightly different benefits. Koop had tried to revitalize the Corps in the 1980s, but his successors were less gung-ho. A reorganization in the 1990s moved the Corps out from under the surgeon general's oversight.

Some critics deemed it wasted effort and continued to view the Corps as an unnecessary anachronism. The 1990s iteration of that grousing had focused on James Felsen, a Corps officer working at the Health Resources and Services Administration who was the subject of a lengthy *Washington Post* article in 1996. Felsen made $117,000 annually in a do-nothing job where he'd been parked after running afoul of his bosses. To pass the hours each day, he constructed a large arch out of Styrofoam coffee cups in his office.[47] Conservative commentator Jessica Gavora wrote that Felsen was emblematic of what was wrong with the Corps. "Originally designed to provide the nation with a mobile, readily deployable cadre of medical personnel, over the years the [Corps] has drifted far from its mission. Today no one is sure what it's supposed to do, but there is growing agreement on this: What it does, it does too expensively, and probably shouldn't be doing at all," Gavora wrote, in an essay that advocated dismantling the Corps to save taxpayers $130 million a year. Gavora reminded everyone who was at the top of this problematic organization: "The Surgeon General is the highest-ranking and most prominent of the Corps."[48]

Early in the Bush administration, criticism of the special status of the Corps persisted. But the terrorist attacks of September 11, 2001, seemed to change some minds—most notably, that of Tommy Thompson. On that Tuesday morning, Thompson was meeting with a group of high-level government health experts for a briefing on the specter of pandemic flu. As the horrors of the attacks unfolded, Thompson became preoccupied with responding to the unfolding tragedy and wanted to know if HHS doctors were prepared to go wherever they needed to be sent. "September 11 really gave the Commissioned Corps a raison d'être," said Walter Orenstein, a CDC vaccination expert who was one of the scientists in the 9/11 briefing.[49]

In July 2003, Thompson announced what was to be the Corps's "most sweeping transformation since its creation." The stated goal was to put in place a new system so that by the end of 2005 every single member of the Commissioned Corps was trained and ready to go to whatever situation HHS officials deemed in need of response.[50] Carmona was designated a leader in the transformation, and that role made sense. The military had turned his life around when he was a young man, and he seemed at ease in the vestments and culture of uniformed service. This surgeon general was happy to preside over the many ceremonies and traditions that went with being a Corps member. He also spoke frequently with officials in the Department of Defense to improve relations between the Commissioned Corps and other uniformed services. He emphasized the uniform service identity heavily and pushed to recentralize his authority over his uniformed officers. Corps members recognized his passion, and Carmona strengthened the esprit de corps in the organization. "I don't think Corps morale was ever higher than when he was surgeon general," said Gerard Farrell, executive director of the Commissioned Officers Association of the U.S. Public Health Service.[51]

But Carmona encountered interference. Under Beato's authority, the responsibilities for compensation and other Corps personnel issues were split up and distributed to different HHS officials. "Nobody was quite sure anymore who was in charge," Farrell said.[52]

This scattered management of the Corps persisted in the days after Hurricane Katrina hit the Gulf Coast in August 2005. It was one of the deadliest hurricanes in U.S. history, killing more than eighteen hundred people during the storm and its subsequent floods. The government decided to mobilize Corps members. But, while Carmona was the titular head of the Corps, he did not simply call up people and send them out. The HHS assistant secretary for public health emergency preparedness coordinated the personnel response, telling Carmona how many people were needed in which location for what purpose, and he put together the groups of individuals who made the trip. But individual public health agencies, like the Indian Health Service, sometimes had different plans for their employees who were Corps members. There was at least one instance in which some deployed to the hurricane zone were called back by the IHS two days later.[53]

About two thousand officers—a whopping one-third of the Commissioned Corps—were deployed. They were sent to Louisiana, Mississippi, and elsewhere to treat patients, monitor for disease outbreaks, and perform a variety of other services. Not only did they provide crucial aid, but their uniforms lent an air of stabilizing authority that was sometimes useful. But if the uniforms helped the Corps officers in some situations, they were a source of anxiety in others. During the Katrina response, it became clear that many Corps physicians and scientists had not quite mastered uniformed services behavior. Some were so worried about flubbing salutes, they crossed the street to avoid directly passing army or navy personnel.[54]

To remedy such a problem, the three-day Corps introductory class was expanded in 2007 to two weeks of more intensive indoctrination at a campus in Lansdowne, Virginia. The program included important training about what kind of challenges an officer might face upon deployment. But significant time was also spent on things foreign and silly to many of the M.D.'s and Ph.D.'s who attended—things like standing in formation, participating in a flag squad, or learning rules about the size of earrings, the length of fingernails, and whether men could have beards and mustaches. Women were coached on how to fix their hair in a perfect bun. Established federal scientists found themselves having to wear uniforms on a daily basis and began to worry about the nuances of the dress code. (Indeed, online PHS chat forums sometimes carried as much chatter about clothes as the pages of *Glamour,* only with more of an anxious twist.) Some veterans found it all very irritating, including the salutes thrown their way by younger, newly indoctrinated Corps members. "They said 'Why are you doing that?' or 'Don't do that,'" said Robin Toblin, who was a young CDC Epidemic Intelligence Service officer during the transformation.[55]

CARMONA'S DEPARTURE

As Carmona approached his four-year anniversary in office—and the end of his term—it was clear that his accomplishments had been modest. He'd put out only two full reports, both of them released in 2004, and neither had gotten quite the degree of media attention that accompanied the higher-profile reports of his predecessors. He wanted to get at least one more major document out, and he succeeded.

In late June, Carmona released a 727-page report focused on the hazards of secondhand smoke. He had been involved in it from its early stages, frequently asking questions and pushing for a consequential conclusion. That was a bit unusual: surgeons general tended to be largely hands-off on reports as they were being drafted, often becoming significantly involved only when the report was in its final stages. In the process, Carmona said, he did his best to fend off meddling from some administration officials who were trying to "water down language so as not to offend the tobacco industry."[56] The resulting report looked back on two decades of studies and concluded that even trace amounts of cigarette smoke is dangerous to nonsmokers. "The debate is over as far as I'm concerned," Carmona told the media. "Based on the science, I wouldn't allow anyone in my family to stand in a room with someone smoking."[57]

Items checked out to:
LANGER MARTHA JANE

*Remember to renew your materials before
the due date at http://library.arlingtonva.us*

Title: Death money / Henry Chang.
Barcode: 202065388953
Due Date: 05-05-15

Title: The devil's chair / Priscilla Masters.
Barcode: 202065410237
Due Date: 05-05-15

Title: Sorrow bound : [a Detective
Barcode: 202070118719
Due Date: 05-05-15

Title: Surgeon General's warning : how
Barcode: 202065403539
Due Date: 05-05-15

Title: Spineless : portraits of marine
Barcode: 202070153840
Due Date: 05-05-15

*Free Wi-Fi available at every Library
location plus public PCs for accessing the
web, word-processing and more.*

It gave Carmona his biggest media splash since his "ban all tobacco products" comment in 2003. Anchorman Charles Gibson led the *ABC World News Tonight* broadcast that evening with news of Carmona's report, emphasizing the finding that even a brief exposure to smoke could cause harmful cellular changes. Carmona was on CBS's *The Early Show* the next morning, advising cohost Hannah Storm not to go into any room where someone was smoking.[58]

Some celebrated the report as providing crucial fuel for advocates in assorted localities who were working to enact smoking bans in settings like bars and restaurants. But that movement was already well under way, with no-smoking laws already on the books in seventeen states and more than 460 U.S. towns, cities, and counties. Generally speaking, local lawmakers seemed less influenced by what the surgeon general had to say than by the experience of other, bolder governments that had already taken such action (including New York City, which had enacted its ban in 2003). Still, Carmona's report was cited by state legislators and city council members across the country as they tried to create their own smoking bans. "It helped move things along," said Stanton Glantz, director of the Center for Tobacco Control Research and Education at the University of California, San Francisco.[59]

But the report's splash caused few lasting ripples. Surgeons general had been warning of the dangers of secondhand smoke since the 1970s, and a common view was that Carmona was not breaking ground but rather just piling on in a fight health officials were already winning. (One study has indicated that the proportion of nonsmokers with signs of nicotine in their blood had dropped to 46 percent in the early 2000s, down from 84 percent a decade earlier.[60]) Carmona's document didn't lead to congressional briefings or hearings, as was seen following past surgeon general reports. It did not help along any federal tobacco-control legislation. "There was nothing" in terms of the report's impact on Capitol Hill, said Sherry Kaiman, who at the time was a staffer for U.S. Senator Christopher Dodd of Connecticut and who later became director of policy development at Trust for America's Health.[61]

Apparently, there also was little impact on the general public's opinion about secondhand smoke, either. A Gallup poll conducted in early July, less than two weeks after the release of Carmona's report, found attitudes were basically unchanged on the subject, with about 56 percent considering secondhand smoke to be very harmful. That was about the same finding of a similar poll the previous summer.[62]

What's more, the report didn't even end the debate over the dangers of secondhand smoke, despite Carmona's assertion that it did.

Some critics believed that like some surgeons general before him, Carmona had ventured beyond the evidence when it came to secondhand smoke. Scientists had established that people who smoked regularly were in much greater danger of lung cancer and other illnesses, but Carmona was going further than that, saying a nonsmoker with even a brief exposure was putting themselves in danger. That claim seemed to contradict a five-hundred-year-old scientific precept that "the dose makes the poison'—that is, that chemicals are toxic when consumed, inhaled, or absorbed in certain concentrations, and not deadly below those concentrations.[63] One critic was Michael Siegel, a professor at the Boston University School of Public Health. "One can say that there is no safe level of exposure to any carcinogen," Siegel blogged after the report came out. "There is no safe level of exposure to car exhaust. There is no safe level of exposure to the sun's rays. . . . For that matter, there is no safe speed at which you can drive without risk of injury or death."[64]

In fact, federal officials had already negated that precept in some instances (the Environmental Protection Agency, for example, had said there is no safe level of exposure to asbestos). And many scientists had come to agree with Carmona that even small amounts of exposure to cigarette smoke can trigger harmful changes in the heart and blood vessels (though some remained skeptical that those changes were necessarily permanent or led to cancer).[65] Overall, the public health establishment strongly agreed with the new report's findings and considered the issue indeed settled. "I think we're at a point, with the 2006 report, where you could say the next person who's funded to look at whether secondhand smoke causes cancer or heart disease ought to get arrested," said Thomas Glynn, a Cancer Society official who has been involved with surgeon general smoking reports since Koop was in office.[66]

But some skepticism endured, and the surgeon general didn't help his cause when he declined to call for dramatic federal measures to snuff out smoking, despite the report's dire warnings. He maintained it was his role simply to provide information to Congress and the public, not to advocate policy, but that rationalization struck some as disingenuous. "How can you, as Surgeon General, truly believe that a brief exposure to secondhand smoke causes heart disease and lung cancer and fail to recommend that this devastating health hazard be eliminated?" Michael Siegel wrote.[67]

Carmona had only a limited opportunity to defend himself. About six weeks after the report's release, his term expired. He had hoped to be reappointed to a second term, and had reason to believe he would be. Several months earlier, some Republican pols approached him about running for political office. (Karl Rove was among the party leaders Carmona spoke with about it, Carmona said.) Carmona met with President Bush to talk about the prospect, and Bush gave Carmona mentoring advice about pursuing political office only when the time felt right. "He said 'I'm happy with your work, and if you want to stay as surgeon general, that's ok,'" Carmona recalled.[68] But as his term neared its completion date, he heard nothing from the Bush administration about a reappointment. "They were moving boxes out of his office, and he still hadn't been told officially from the president that he was not to be renewed," said Karen Near, who served as Carmona's senior science advisor.[69]

Finally, days before his term expired, he was called into HHS Secretary Mike Leavitt's office. Leavitt was not present, but roughly a dozen others were, including some lawyers. Carmona was told he would not be reappointed and had only a few days to clean out his office and vacate the surgeon general residence on the NIH campus. There would be no going away ceremony. "Not even a thank-you," Carmona said.[70] Some outraged commissioned officers did organize a retirement ceremony for Carmona, but it was held at a Marriott hotel in Bethesda since there was no approval for one to be held on government property.

Officially, news of the end of Carmona's service came when the surgeon general announced his resignation in late July 2006. HHS officials made no statement themselves, and referred questions to the White House, which declined to comment. In public health circles, some speculated that Carmona's discharge must have had something to do with the final smoking report having perturbed the Bush administration.[71] Asked about it in an interview three months later, Carmona said he had no idea why the administration had declined to renew him. In an interview six years later, he said he believed neither the president nor the vice president drove the decision; rather, it was the work of political appointees—he declined to name names—who had become his antagonists.[72]

Karen Near and some of her colleagues said they were sorry to see him go. Carmona had carried out his job with honor, they said. But others said the relative silence over his departure was apropos of his entire term. "It's hard to remember another Surgeon General who was so largely invisible as he has been, and that's a tragedy," said Sidney Wolfe, of Public Citizen's Health Research Group, in an interview with the *Arizona Daily Star*. Michael Murphy, an Arizona state health department spokesman, was even harsher: "Went out with a whimper, didn't he?"[73]

Carmona's detractors called him a good soldier within the Bush administration who followed orders, when what the public needed was a self-governing surgeon general. Good riddance, these critics said. However, less than a year later, Carmona would write himself a second act.

CARMONA SPEAKS OUT

After Carmona, the Bush administration endeavored to name a new surgeon general who would hold the office for years after Bush left the White House. The candidate list seemed lamentable. One physician reportedly considered was Zachariah P. Zachariah, a Fort Lauderdale cardiologist and successful Republican fund-raiser. But the White House decided not to forward his name after learning he was under investigation by the Securities and Exchange Commission for allegedly using nonpublic information to make more than $500,000 in illegal profits.[74] In 2010, he was exonerated of all charges. The White House interviewed at least four other prospects, but found each of them flawed.

Bush officials were pleased, however, when they settled on James Holsinger Jr., a sixty-eight-year-old University of Kentucky preventive cardiologist with an impressive résumé. Holsinger had been Kentucky's secretary for health and family services, had taught at several medical schools, and was a retired major general with the U.S. Army Reserve. Beyond those attributes, he shared the Bush administration's interest in addressing childhood obesity. A *National Public Radio* report, aired shortly after his nomination was announced, called Holsinger "one of the nicest guys around."[75]

But within two weeks of the announcement, the nomination began to founder because of a revelation about Holsinger's longtime involvement in the United Methodist Church. *ABC News* unearthed a 1991 paper that Holsinger had written that attempted to make a medical argument that homosexuality is unnatural and unhealthy.[76] Holsinger suddenly became fodder for late-night talk show hosts and a bit of an embarrassment to the Bush administration.

Koop, former HHS Secretary Louis Sullivan, and conservative groups endorsed Holsinger's nomination. Elders, the American Public Health Association, and an array of AIDS and gay and lesbian organizations stood against it. The Republican legislators tasked with moving his nomination through the Senate began sounding ambivalent. "Dr. Holsinger has not had the opportunity to speak publicly about the allegations and concerns raised against him," said U.S. Senator Mike Enzi of Wyoming, the ranking Republican on the Senate Committee on Health, Education, Labor, and Pensions, in his opening statement during Holsinger's July 12, 2007, nomination hearing. "I look forward to his testimony today so that he can finally address them. I hope that the Committee gives him a fair hearing and will listen to his responses so that we can determine his qualifications to be the next Surgeon General."[77]

In the hearing, Holsinger said his views had evolved since 1991, and that he believed strongly in standing against discrimination of any kind. But his performance wasn't enough. The controversy had become a headache the Bush administration didn't want. Within a few months, the White House stopped responding to the HELP Committee's requests for more information, and the nomination was quietly dropped. (Asked about it years afterward, Holsinger said he never withdrew his nomination, but he declined to comment further.[78])

Meanwhile, Carmona had been making some noise.

In January 2007, while speaking at the annual dinner of the Public Health Service Commissioned Officers Foundation, he complained about his experience in the Bush administration. "I increasingly witnessed a government that was more and more using theology and ideology to drive its policies and its people: stem cells, abortion, Plan B, the war and many more," he said.[79] Sitting in the audience was Arthur Kellermann, a noted emergency medicine physician on a health policy fellowship working for the U.S. House Committee on Oversight and Government Reform. Kellermann relayed Carmona's comments to the committee chairman, Henry Waxman. Waxman recognized a potent new example of the degradation of federal public health practices under the Bush administration's ideological rule.

On July 10, just two days before the Holsinger nomination hearing, Waxman convened a hearing on the politicization of the Office of the Surgeon General. At Carmona's urging, Koop and Satcher appeared with him.[80] Each talked about moments when the presidential administrations under which they served hindered their attempts to use the bully pulpit. But Carmona was clearly the star of the show. He said he was instructed not to address controversial issues like emergency contraception and abstinence-only education, and was denied permission to issue reports on a wide range of topics, including mental health, prison health, global health, and even emergency preparedness. "I was given lots of different reasons," Carmona testified when asked why he wasn't allowed to do an emergency preparedness report. "'This might scare the people; you should think about it.' 'The new Department of Homeland Security will be responsible, and why should the Surgeon General do this?' I was given lots of reasons, from the cost to everything else, not to move this forward."[81]

Carmona also said he was directed to attend what were essentially political pep rallies for the Republican Party. In subsequent media interviews, Carmona said he was discouraged from attending events that might benefit prominent Democrats, including a speech at the Special Olympics (an organization strongly supported by the Kennedys). He also said he was ordered to mention President Bush in speeches at a rate of at least three times per page.

The hearing made headlines for several days, and both Waxman and Senator Edward Kennedy introduced bills to protect the Office of the Surgeon General from political interference. Both bills died quickly and quietly, to virtually no one's surprise. The Bush administration showed little appetite for this kind of legislation: it vehemently opposed a bill to strengthen the Office of the Inspector General. And there was little confidence that it would get enough votes to clear the Senate. "These were symbolic bills," said a former staff member on Waxman's oversight committee.[82]

Carmona was cheered by prominent health leaders for raising the issue, but some also faulted him for waiting too long. Koop and others had urged him to take a stand—and walk away from the job, if need be—while Carmona still held the job, believing his words would have had even more impact then. "I said two things will happen," Koop once said, recalling a conversation with Carmona while the latter was still in office. "'Either you'll get the freedom [necessary to do the job right] and everyone will shut up, or they'll fire you. But you're ahead either way.' But he wouldn't take the chance on the firing."[83]

Sharon Eubanks, the prosecutor, strongly disagrees. She believes that if Carmona had spoken up, he would have quickly been shown the door, à la Joycelyn Elders, and wouldn't have been able to accomplish anything else. Carmona deserves credit for speaking out in 2007, a year after his term ended but while the Bush administration was still firmly entrenched, she added. "That takes courage. There were some powerful people he was going up against when he said that," she said.[84]

Interestingly, Carmona later decided to go into politics. Registered as an independent voter since 1989, he remained that way even after joining the Bush administration, and some Republicans in 2006 had urged him to run for Congress to fill the House seat for the district near Tucson.[85] In 2011, he was approached again, this time by the Democratic Party. They wanted him to run for a U.S. Senate seat in Arizona—a state where the majority of voters were Republican. President Barack Obama himself called Carmona as part of the effort to recruit the former surgeon general.[86]

Carmona announced his candidacy in November 2011, and essentially decided to run for Senate as surgeon general. His campaign page on Facebook was dominated by photos of Carmona in his white PHS uniform with gold shoulder bars—in one he's kneeling and a little girl is touching the three white stars on the shoulder bars. Likewise in his speeches and media appearances, he routinely referred to his time as the nation's doctor. ("As I look at this through the eyes of the Surgeon General, it doesn't make any sense," Carmona told Rachel Maddow during a March 2012 appearance on her television show, after she asked him about an Arizona bill to defund women's health services.[87]) Invoking the past cut both ways, however, his Republican opponent, U.S. Representative Jeff Flake, ran a TV campaign spot featuring Cristina Beato. "Carmona is not who he seems," Beato said in the ad. "He has issues with anger, with ethics, and with women."[88]

Campaigning as surgeon general didn't work. Although the race was closer than many expected, Flake defeated Carmona in the November 2012 election. Some had hoped that had Carmona become senator, he might have tried to resuscitate and champion legislation to protect the Office of the Surgeon General from political meddling. But that was not to be.

Carmona failed to be the hero many had expected when he was first chosen as the nation's doctor, but at least he had a few moments of prominence, fighting the good fight. His ultimate replacement would barely register in the public's consciousness at all.

CHAPTER 12

"America's Doctor"

In April 2010, Anne Schuchat glimpsed something in the *New York Times* that made her excited about Regina Benjamin's potential impact as surgeon general. It was a short promotional blurb for an article in the newspaper's coming Sunday edition, about "America's doctor." "I thought 'Finally,'" said Schuchat, a high-ranking CDC flu expert who is also an assistant surgeon general.[1] Finally, she meant, a major media spotlight on Benjamin. The blurb's phrasing seemed a sure giveaway; "America's doctor" had long been the unofficial title for the surgeon general, and that was how Benjamin referred to herself in speeches.

But when the Sunday paper came out, Schuchat was disappointed to learn the article was actually about Mehmet Oz, a sort of surgeon populist who was a near-constant presence on television and in other media. The *Times* feature included a full-page photo of a trim Dr. Oz jogging in full stride on a treadmill, and discussed his varied pushes to make Americans healthier. It made no mention of Benjamin or her office.[2]

The omission was understandable. Benjamin proved to be the lowest-profile surgeon general—less visible, even, than the sat-upon Richard Carmona. Even people working in public health struggled to conjure her name.

One was Stanton Glantz, a University of California, San Francisco, researcher who has been a longtime critic of tobacco companies and a contributor to surgeon general reports. Glantz can easily list relatively obscure CDC scientists who work on smoking issues. But when a surgeon general report on smoking was released during Benjamin's term, "I had to go look up her name."[3] Many others would be equally stymied, said William Schaffner, a Vanderbilt University infectious diseases expert often quoted in the national media. Standing in a hallway outside an Atlanta meeting of national vaccine experts in June 2013—nearly four years into Benjamin's term—Schaffner nodded toward the closed doors and said; "Among the people in that room, I think many would not be able to give you her name spontaneously. And this is a highly educated group. If you go out to the average doctor, let alone the public, they could not name the surgeon general. That's not the office being used to its best."[4]

Benjamin's personality was no doubt a reason for her obscurity. Self-effacing and possessing a low-key charm, she had an inspiring past that caused some to liken her to a living saint. But not all saints are good preachers. When it came time to step into the surgeon general's pulpit, Benjamin frequently came off as uneasy and unprepared, interrupting her speeches with pauses and shuffling papers as she grasped for the next scripted words. She was unwilling to badger or criticize anyone—not tobacco companies, not gun manufacturers, not alcohol distillers, not marketers of unhealthy foods, and not ordinary citizens who were stuffing or poisoning themselves to death.

Also working against her, surprisingly, was the Obama administration. The George W. Bush administration was infamous for discouraging scientific discourse that conflicted with certain political messages, and it was widely assumed the next administration would be an improvement. But the Obama people—intently focused on getting health reform legislation passed and implemented, and intent on minimizing distractions—seemed no more interested in having a freewheeling surgeon general than the Bush people had been.

"She's controlled," said Benjamin's mentor, former surgeon general David Satcher.[5]

TOO GOOD TO BE TRUE

Regina Marcia Benjamin was born October 26, 1956, in Mobile, Alabama. She grew up in nearby Daphne, known as "the jubilee city" for an occasional phenomenon in which a bounty of shrimp, crab, flounder, and other marine life washes ashore from Mobile Bay. Young Regina spent a lot of time on the bay's eastern shore, fishing and crabbing.[6] That seafood was important, because the family was poor and broken. Her parents separated when she was two (they never actually divorced), and her mother—Millie—supported Regina and her brother, Charles, by waiting tables and fixing women's hair.[7]

She attended an African American Catholic Church that her mother and grandmother had helped establish after segregation policies had forced them to sit in the back of their old church. "I was a good Catholic girl growing up," who never smoked marijuana or got into other kinds of trouble, she once told the *New York Times*.[8] Her tenth-grade biology teacher at Fairhope High School remembered her as a bright, well-spoken and hardworking student who was always prepared for class. Others remembered her as a popular cheerleader who wore pretty dresses instead of the jeans and T-shirts others kids favored.[9]

Benjamin graduated from Fairhope High in 1975 and then traveled about 140 miles west to attend Xavier University, a small, historically black Catholic school in New Orleans. She initially considered becoming a lawyer or pharmacist and, while exploring possible career choices, got a summer internship with the Central Intelligence Agency—her introduction to working for the federal government. But ultimately she decided to go into medicine, partly because it was popular with other students. ("Premed was the big thing to do," she recalled.) Xavier has a good track record of placing students into medical schools, and faculty believed Benjamin had a lot of promise. "She was always very, very concerned with people and I always thought that she would be the kind of doctor I would want to go to," said J.W. Carmichael, her premed advisor at Xavier, in a 2009 interview with the *Times-Picayune*.[10]

For medical school, she went to Atlanta to be part of the new Morehouse School of Medicine, which had just been established in 1978 (the year before Benjamin graduated from Xavier). The dean was Louis Sullivan, who years later would become secretary of health and human services. The head of the department of community medicine and family practice was David Satcher, the future surgeon general, who would become something of a role model for Benjamin. But in the school's first years it was an abbreviated and unaccredited program: students started at Morehouse but finished their medical school training at other, accredited institutions. Benjamin transferred to the University of Alabama, Birmingham, where she got her degree in 1984.[11]

She paid for medical school by signing up for the National Health Service Corps. The program—which Jesse Steinfeld had helped create—provided scholarships, and repaid medical school loans, in exchange for a young doctor's commitment to work in a medically underserved area.

Benjamin was assigned to a clinic just outside of Bayou La Batre, a somewhat isolated fishing village southwest of Mobile with only about 2,000 residents. After two and a half years, she decided to open her own practice in the town. She rented a storefront near a pool hall, which her boyfriend at the time—a carpenter—helped fix up.[12]

Benjamin opened her office in 1990, and struggled. Many of her new patients couldn't pay their bills. She worked late-night shifts at various hospital emergency rooms to keep afloat, and decided to go back to school to develop the business savvy necessary to run the practice. (She got an MBA at Tulane, commuting to New Orleans to take classes.)[13]

She began serving on state and national medical association panels, and started to draw attention in the medical community. Doctors from other backwoods communities called and wrote asking for advice. In 1995, she gained national attention when a colorful reporter for the *New York Times* wrote a news feature about her entitled "Poor Town Finds an Angel in a White Coat." In the article, Rick Bragg painted her as a living saint, saying she eschewed conventional success, made house calls in her Ford pickup, and cried when her patients died. Wrote Bragg, "Dr. Benjamin is a soft-spoken woman, quick to smile, slow to brag, too good to be true it seems."[14]

Benjamin's growing legend was boosted by a series of disasters. In 1998, flooding from Hurricane Georges destroyed her clinic. In 2005, Hurricane Katrina trashed it. In 2006, on New Year's Day, a fire gutted it. Each time the clinic was rebuilt, thanks to volunteers and Benjamin's determination. While C. Everett Koop had been likened to Moses, Regina Benjamin was more akin to Job—the innocent, nobly enduring loss after loss after loss. "Through floods and fires and severe want, Regina Benjamin has refused to give up," President Barack Obama would one day say of her.[15]

Benjamin never married, and didn't even own pets. ("I have trouble keeping silk plants," she once joked. "I'm gone a lot."[16]) But she became prominent in organized medicine, and in 1995—when she was still in her thirties—was elected to the American Medical Association's Board of Trustees, making her the first black woman elevated to the governing board of what had long been the nation's most powerful physicians' organization. In 2002, she became president of the Medical Association of the State of Alabama—the first woman and the first African American to win that post. In 2008, she was elected chair of the Board of Trustees of the Federation of State Medical Boards. Though never a household name, even in southern Alabama, she began to make money from speaking engagements and got a consulting gig with Burger King. Her reported personal income was $184,000 in 2007.[17]

In 2008, she won a MacArthur Foundation "genius grant," good for $500,000 over five years, and vowed to use it to build up her clinic.[18] Nearly a year later, when he nominated her for U.S. surgeon general, Obama celebrated her as a selfless example for the rest of the nation.[19]

She was not, however, his first choice for surgeon general.

Just a few weeks after he was elected president, Obama met for more than two hours in Chicago with Sanjay Gupta, an Atlanta neurosurgeon and high-profile medical reporter for CNN. Gupta was just thirty-nine years old and extremely telegenic—a few years earlier he'd been voted one of *People* magazine's "Sexiest People." He had also been a White House fellow in the late 1990s, writing speeches for First Lady Hillary Rodham Clinton and getting a sense of life in a Democratic presidential administration. Obama reportedly wanted Gupta not only to be surgeon general but also to have a job at the new White House Office on Health Reform; he would be a leading spokesman for the Obama administration's efforts to fix the nation's troubled health insurance system. The *Washington Post* broke the story in early January 2009, noting Gupta did not deny he planned to accept the positions. Indeed, he was thinking about it hard, and flew to New Hampshire to consult with C. Everett Koop.[20]

The news seemed to instantly resuscitate the moribund Office of the Surgeon General. Gupta, already a household name, stood to become the most influential surgeon general in decades. Joycelyn Elders—the last surgeon general to consistently excite audiences—enthusiastically endorsed him. Others did too, arguing that an effective surgeon general must not only be willing to boldly discuss what public health science dictates when political bosses disagree, but also have the confidence to walk away from the job to preserve that principle. Gupta certainly seemed to fill that bill. "The odds of being able to shut him down are pretty slim. The last thing I would want, as a politician, is someone of Sanjay Gupta's media savvy to be resigning in protest," said Jeff Levi, executive director of Trust for America's Health.[21]

But there were many critics. Some current and former Commissioned Corps officials grumbled that Gupta had no background or qualifications in public health. Some medical journalists faulted Gupta's TV work, noting instances when he seemed to shirk traditional journalistic values like objectivity and distance and go in for puffery and self-promotion (he reported on himself treating wounded soldiers in Iraq in

2003 and on a Haitian infant earthquake victim in 2010). The trend lines of his coverage "too often fail to scrutinize medicine [or] ask the tough questions about medicine, and [he] too often glamorizes medical advances," said Gary Schwitzer, a former CNN newsman who operates a website critiquing health care journalism.[22]

Meanwhile, problems arose for the man who was to be Gupta's boss. Tom Daschle, the former U.S. senator from South Dakota, was to be Obama's secretary of health and human services and the leader of the new administration's health reform push. But during his nomination process, Daschle admitted he owed the government at least $140,000 in back taxes and interest. He also acknowledged he had worked closely with health care businesses and health insurers in his years since leaving the Senate, an apparent conflict of interest. Amid controversy, in early February Daschle withdrew his name, saying he had become too much of a distraction to the new Obama administration.

Gupta was no doubt uneasy about the roster change. He reportedly had spoken at length with Daschle about defining the next surgeon general's role within the Obama administration. Nearly a month would go by before the Obama administration announced a new nominee for HHS secretary—a no-nonsense former Kansas governor named Kathleen Sebelius. During those many weeks of limbo, Gupta remained mum about his plans.

Finally, three days after Sebelius was formally announced, Gupta told the media he had withdrawn his name from consideration. He gave a variety of reasons, including that his wife was expecting their third daughter and a new, travel-intensive job based in Washington would be too much for the family. He was also uneasy about giving up his lucrative gigs as a TV medical correspondent and part-time physician. "I was in my 30s. . . . In order to be Surgeon General, I wouldn't have been able to practice. . . . So it just wasn't the right time," Gupta said in a 2012 interview with a Canadian newspaper.[23]

More than four months would pass before the Obama administration would propose another candidate for surgeon general. The delay was understandable: the Daschle debacle had caused a backlog, with more important appointments within HHS delayed until a new secretary was on board. The new FDA commissioner was not sworn in until May, the CDC director was not in place until June, and the NIH director was not confirmed until August.

Meanwhile, the government was dealing with a new strain of influenza—known as novel Type A H1N1, or swine flu—discovered in

California and Mexico in late April. It was the first flu pandemic since the late 1960s. Many of the early cases identified were severe, which gave the impression that this flu was especially dangerous, particularly for younger adults and children. As the public began to fret, a still-being-assembled health bureaucracy was doing its best to manage, with a number of different officials fielding reporters' questions. It was a golden opportunity for a strong and expert surgeon general to calm and inform the public. But it was not until July 13 that Obama announced Regina Benjamin's selection, and it would not be until late October that she was confirmed. The swine flu pandemic had already peaked, and public concerns about it had waned, by the time Benjamin settled in to her office.

"LOOK THE PART"

That Regina Benjamin was not a major spokesperson on swine flu is understandable, given the jumble of events in 2009. It was more surprising that she was little consulted on a topic many expected to be a main focus of the next surgeon general—obesity.

David Satcher sounded an early alarm that obesity was becoming epidemic in America. Richard Carmona called it "the terror within." Bush nominee James Holsinger had pledged to make the issue his main priority, and all indications were that Obama's appointee would do the same. Indeed, many expected that the next surgeon general would not just walk the talk but also run the 5K. Satcher, after all, was a former college athlete who led fitness races. Carmona worked out ninety minutes a day, looked fighting trim, and was praised for it by his bosses. "Not only does he believe in what he's doing, he practices it," gushed HHS Secretary Tommy Thompson at a press event in 2004. "I thank the Surgeon General for being an example of what healthy living is all about."[24]

But here was Regina Benjamin, shaped more like an apple than an athlete. (Once of average weight, she had put on pounds in her forties because of a thyroid problem, long work hours, and family stresses.[25]) Her appearance was noted—and denigrated—in weeks of criticism following the announcement of her nomination. Bloggers, TV commentators, and chat room denizens snickered at the selection of someone who looked so out of shape. "I wouldn't hire a poor person as my financial advisor. I wouldn't hire a couch potato as my personal fitness trainer. And I wouldn't hire a fat person as the nation's chief proponent for healthy behavior," commented a *Washington Post* reader on one of the newspaper's blogs.[26] Also among the Benjamin bashers was Michael Karolchyk, who ran a Denver fitness center notorious for its crass commercials. In an interview with Fox News anchor Neil Cavuto, Karolchyk called Benjamin "obese," "lazy," and someone who made "poor food choices." He continued, "If you're going to be the man who's going to be the Surgeon General, or the female, you should look the part."[27]

Benjamin found the uproar about her weight—and the idea that she needed to shape up—hard to listen to. "It was very hurtful. It was very hurtful," she said, in an interview shortly after she took office. She also said she didn't think her weight would work against her ability to preach health behaviors to the public, noting that two-thirds of adults were either overweight or obese. "I understand what Americans are going through. We're going through it together."[28] Benjamin—who refused to give her weight—exercised regularly and during her time as surgeon general hiked the Grand Canyon and led a series of one-mile walks in different cities. She frequently encouraged her audiences to think of exercise as a fun thing to do, and smiled and danced to demonstrate. But the preconfirmation brouhaha over her weight turned out to be her highest visibility on obesity, because someone else in the Obama administration took over that topic.

Michelle Obama—a trim, striking, Harvard-trained lawyer with glamorous style—had emerged as something of a role model to young women. As the new First Lady, she was ambitious to lead a substantive health initiative that would complement the White House's health reform efforts. In late October 2009, at about the time Benjamin was being confirmed by the Senate, she decided to consolidate and boost efforts to fight childhood obesity. Her "Let's Move!" campaign was officially launched in February 2010, with a White House pledge of as much as $1 billion over ten years and the stated goal of ending childhood obesity in a generation. Benjamin was at the campaign kickoff ceremony, but as just one of more than a dozen dignitaries sitting in the audience. The football player Tiki Barber was the only adult on stage with the president's wife.[29]

Mrs. Obama believed previous efforts to address the childhood obesity epidemic had been small, scattered, and ineffectual—an assessment that included the work of previous surgeons general. She was an outsider to public health, but leaders within the field did not disagree. "Thanks to Mrs. Obama, the country is beginning to tackle the epidemic. We hope that this is just the first step," said Jeff Levi of Trust for America's Health.[30] It seemed more like a rocket-boosted leap than a step, with the "Let's Move!" campaign featuring the kind of supporting cast that a surgeon general's initiative could never hope to attract. The singing superstar Beyoncé Knowles contributed a song and appeared in a video, dancing with children. The National Football League made prominent players available. And a variety of other celebrities appeared at campaign functions, including the celebrity chef Rachael Ray.

But the biggest star was Michelle Obama, who continually promoted the campaign, often by impressively exercising herself. A media tour in early 2012 to mark the second anniversary of "Let's Move!" included a stop on the *Ellen* show at which the First Lady did more pushups than host Ellen DeGeneres; a visit to *Late Night with Jimmy Fallon* where she outmuscled Fallon in a comedic tug-of-war; and an appearance on prime-time TV's *The Biggest Loser* where the dieting reality show contestants came to the White House to work out with—and be inspired by—the First Lady.

The effort was largely about pushing children and their parents to take personal responsibility for eating right and exercising. But as it was originally conceived, it also involved pushing food and soft-drink companies and other organizations to decrease the amount of fatty and sugary items placed in front of children at schools, restaurants, and supermarkets. It borrowed from the anti-smoking campaign, which not only advocated that people stop smoking but also pointed fingers at cigarette manufacturers for Joe Camel–style marketing that helped hook kids. As Koop and other surgeons general had scolded tobacco manufacturers, the First Lady started her campaign by chiding—gently—the companies that made processed foods. "We need you all to step it up," she said, in a speech to the Grocery Manufacturers Association in March 2010. "We need you not to just tweak around the edges, but to entirely rethink the products that you're offering, the information that you provide about these products, and how you market those products to our children."[31]

But Michelle Obama was no C. Everett Koop. By the spring of 2012, critical analyses were beginning to appear that faulted the White House for letting the powerful food industry off the hook. Fodder for their grousing came when the administration dropped an attempt to discourage marketing of foods to kids that didn't meet certain nutritional guidelines. Indeed, Michelle Obama had gradually clammed up about new food standards or other substantive changes, and many noticed. "I'd focus more on exercise, too, if my husband was up for re-election," said Margo Wootan, director of nutrition policy at the Center for Science in the Public Interest, in an interview with Reuters.[32]

In the summer of 2013, signs emerged of a national decline in child-hood obesity, for which the White House tried to take partial credit. But the evidence was specific to low-income preschoolers fed through the federal WIC program (the Special Supplemental Nutrition Program for Women, Infants, and Children), and experts said the major reason was not the First Lady's boosterism but rather a 2009 policy change that limited or eliminated less healthy options from what WIC provided.[33]

Significantly, few suggested that Regina Benjamin had anything to do with it.

BENJAMIN'S ISSUES

With childhood obesity—one of the most pressing public health issues of the day—removed from her plate by the White House, what was the surgeon general to focus on?

When Benjamin took office, her agenda was unclear. (There had been no confirmation hearing at which senators might have publicly asked about that. In an unusual maneuver, the Senate approved her nomination on the night of October 29 through a voice vote on a con-sent agreement.[34]) But it seemed likely she might be eager to address several health issues that had personally pained her.

One of them stemmed from the death of her only sibling, her brother, Charles, from an HIV-related illness at age forty-four in 1996. The nation continued to struggle with AIDS, with HIV infection an escalat-ing problem in young gay men and in heterosexual African Americans of both genders. Perhaps Benjamin would focus on finding new ways to persuade the people most at risk to use condoms and get tested. Or perhaps she would address the fact that although sex education was common in U.S. schools, only two-thirds of teens were actually being taught about birth control methods.

Her mother, Millie, a smoker, had died of lung cancer in 1997 at age seventy-five. Millie's brother—Regina Benjamin's Uncle Buddy—also died of smoking-related causes. The surgeon general was the historical leader of the nation's public health battle against tobacco, and smoking remained the leading preventable cause of death in the United States. Indeed, the decline in adult and teen smoking rates had essentially stalled, and the time was ripe for a federal health official to try to pump up the fight.

Benjamin had spent nearly two decades serving an impoverished community where people had traditionally lacked the money, health insurance, or other means to get needed medical care. She seemed the ideal person to speak passionately on the need for health reform (more ideal, at least on paper, than the affluent neurosurgeon and TV personality Sanjay Gupta).

Beyond the issues that had personally touched her, there were other pressing public health needs that could be addressed by a forceful education campaign pursued by a strong surgeon general.

Melanoma incidence rates had been increasing for decades, and the World Health Organization in 2009 determined that tanning beds were a carcinogenic contributor to that problem—meaning that someone needed to persuade indoor tanners (the majority of them young women) to drop the stupid and dangerous habit. Simple sunburns were also part of the problem. A CDC survey would later show that the percentage of Americans who'd had a recent burn rose from 45 percent in 2005 to 50 percent in 2010, prompting some experts to comment that health officials were failing to make headway with their warnings.[35]

The nation was facing an alarming rise in antibiotic resistance, dangerously weakening the medical arsenal against bacterial infections. By one CDC estimate, as much as half of all antibiotic use was inappropriate, partly due to pervasive public ignorance of the fact that antibiotics are not useful against viral illnesses. The issue was ripe for a forceful education campaign led by the nation's doctor.

When Benjamin took office, only one in three teenage girls had rolled up their sleeves for an expensive vaccine against cervical cancer that had come on the market in 2006. It was controversial: because it protects against a sexually transmitted virus, some parents felt taking their daughters to the doctor for the shots was a tacit endorsement of sexual activity. But health experts worried the low vaccination rate meant many young girls were at needless risk for future cancer.

Misguided parent groups had for years been raising alarms that vaccines caused autism. Studies had failed to back up that belief, but celebrities like Jenny McCarthy had continued to espouse the theory on *Oprah* and in other forums, often unrebutted by federal health officials. McCarthy and vaccine opponents apparently were persuasive: a Harris Poll in 2011 found 18 percent of Americans believed vaccines cause autism and another 30 percent weren't sure.[36] And the number of parents seeking exemptions for school attendance vaccination rules kept climbing.

Nevertheless, the day after her swearing-in ceremony, when asked what topics she wanted to tackle, Benjamin said, "I'm a family doctor. I like everything. I like all of health care. . . . I didn't have any specific issue. My only issue is caring for the patient." She added that she'd be happy to work as part of a team on whatever the administration assigned her.[37]

The Obama administration assigned her little of substance. It was focused on a historic push to create and implement health reform, sell it to the American public, and protect it from assaults by political enemies. Benjamin's close ties with the AMA seemingly qualified her as a key salesman of health reform not only to the general public but also to the nation's physician community. But within HHS, responsibility for the effort rested with the secretary, Kathleen Sebelius.

Sebelius was an inherently political person: the daughter of a Democratic Ohio governor, the wife of the son of a former U.S. congressman, and a former lobbyist and governor of Kansas before she joined the Obama administration. Trim, white-haired, and with a no-nonsense midwestern manner, she picked her battles. In 2011, she would become known as the first HHS secretary to ever publicly overrule the Food and Drug Administration. The issue was whether the agency should allow emergency contraceptives to be sold over the counter to girls younger than seventeen. The FDA had deemed the prescription medication safe for teenage girls. But Sebelius, pulling rank, said she was not satisfied that enough research had been done. Her decision was widely perceived as one based on politics, not science: By taking that action, one year before the 2012 presidential election, she spared the Obama administration a social controversy over parental control of their daughters' contraception.[38]

Clearly, the HHS brass did not want any distractions, and that concern extended to the surgeon general. A committee was appointed to vet all the speaking invitations Benjamin received. Among the members with significant veto power was Dori Salcido, the communications director for Assistant Secretary for Health Howard Koh. (It was a process far removed from the days of Joycelyn Elders, who used to make the speaking decisions herself.) Benjamin initially shared a speechwriter with Koh, but after a year lost that person. She became her own speechwriter, though most of her talks relied heavily on notes and data supplied by HHS staffers. Her speeches were not formally vetted, but she stayed within the guidelines that senior HHS officials set out regarding which topics were assigned to others.[39]

She was in over her head. Having defined herself for years in terms of her jobs and professional memberships, Benjamin was confident she could succeed in the HHS milieu as well. But Washington was a much tougher, more unforgiving environment. She lacked experience in the federal government and had to lean on staff members who held allegiances to other political appointees. "She was put in a role she was ill-prepared for. But I don't think she believes she was ill-prepared," said David Rutstein, who served as her deputy before retiring in 2010.[40]

Benjamin was also a disappointing public speaker. She lacked not only the look-you-in-the-eye intensity that Koop and Elders exhibited as they thundered about a particular public health issue, but also the subtler aura of authority that Satcher, Carmona, and other surgeons general had routinely exuded from the podium. Like an unprepared novice, Benjamin sometimes seemed less a public health authority than a hostage being forced by her abductors to read a statement before a television camera. "Sad to report, she read a very low-key, uncomfortable, scripted talk, stretched out to fit the allotted time, that was the opposite of charismatic," said Alan Blum, director of the University of Alabama's Center for the Study of Tobacco and Society, summarizing a speech she gave in April 2012 before the Medical Association of the State of Alabama.[41]

As one government scientist put it: "She doesn't absorb the facts and have a full command of the issue so she can speak from the heart and say, 'Here are the five reasons we need to do this!' She's more like; 'OK, where are those five reasons? There was this one and this one . . .' Things get a little mixed up."[42] Several health officials interviewed for this book declined to speak on the record about her performance as a public speaker, but her weaknesses were commonly acknowledged. When asked about it, Carmona replied, "That is a criticism I've heard repeatedly."[43]

In her unscripted remarks, Benjamin sometimes stumbled. An unfortunate gaffe occurred in the spring of 2011, after a devastating earthquake and tsunami in Japan caused meltdowns at three nuclear reactors and the evacuation of hundreds of thousands of residents. The catastrophe led to a wave of concern on the U.S. West Coast that a nuclear cloud could drift to the shores of California, causing a run on potassium iodide tablets by panicked people wanting to protect themselves from radiation. As luck would have it, Benjamin was in California's San Mateo County at the time, touring hospitals to learn about their work with minority communities and with medical records. A television reporter there asked the surgeon general about the run on the pills. She replied she wasn't aware of people stocking up, but didn't think such a step would be an overreaction. "It's definitely appropriate," and good to be prepared, she added.

The problem? Other health and emergency officials had been saying there was no significant risk to Californians from the Japanese reactor meltdowns, that detection devices had not seen increased radiation, and that buying up or taking the pills was a waste of valuable medicine and could even cause severe allergic reactions in some people. A California Emergency Management Agency spokesperson noted that if a nuclear power plant in the state did release radiation, pills would be issued only to people living within ten miles of the plant. For people to buy and take pills because of the Japan incident was ridiculous. "There is no reason for doing it," said Martin Fenstersheib, Santa Clara County's public health officer, to the *San Jose Mercury News*.[44] Two days later, President Obama emphasized at a press conference that people in the United States need not take any precautionary measures, and an HHS spokesperson e-mailed the media that Benjamin wanted to clarify that there was no need for Californians to get potassium iodide.[45]

Benjamin also took some heat for comments she made in 2011 about the role of hairstyles in women's willingness to exercise. She posited that a significant number of women—especially black women—were shunning exercise because they'd invested time and money in hair-straightening chemical treatments that can be undone by sweat and motion. Indeed, some small studies had suggested a significant proportion of black women who didn't exercise said they were worried about messing up their hair. So she made a valid point, and appeared repeatedly at an Atlanta trade show for hair dressers to encourage them to explore offering exercise-friendlier styles.

The *New York Times* reported on her effort in August 2011, giving it national attention. But for a surgeon general who had been operating off the public sonar, it was an odd way to resurface. Critics were skeptical that hairstyle maintenance was a major reason for the nation's ample waistlines, and wondered aloud if this was the kind of issue a surgeon general should be prioritizing. "The role of the surgeon general is traditionally, and appropriately, to take on big issues," Jeff Stier, a senior fellow at the National Center for Public Policy Research, a conservative think tank, told the *Times*. "I don't know whether the Surgeon General's role is to engage in smaller issues like this. It strikes me as bizarre."[46]

One high-level federal health official, speaking on condition of anonymity, said Benjamin has been a disappointment to the administration, and suggested that her weaknesses in the pulpit drove decisions not to assign her big topics. But the feeling was that though her performance was lamentable, it wasn't a major problem. "The fact that we don't have an effective person in that role right now is not harming the health of the U.S.," the official said. "It's a lost opportunity, but it's not harm done."

Lost opportunities steadily came and went during Benjamin's term.

One came in July 2012 when the American Cancer Society Cancer Action Network wrote Sebelius asking for a surgeon general's report on how sodas and sugar-sweetened beverages were affecting the public health. New York City mayor Michael Bloomberg had thrust the issue into the national conversation by pushing for serving-size limits on sugary drinks and provoking a backlash by beverage makers and soda lovers. The Cancer Society's advocacy affiliate believed the time was ripe for a dust-settling report akin to the smoking report commissioned by Luther Terry. Two months later, U.S. Senators Richard Blumenthal of Connecticut, Frank Lautenberg of New Jersey, and Ron Wyden of Oregon (all Democrats) also called on Benjamin to investigate the possible link between sugary beverages and obesity. Benjamin said nothing, but in fact everyone was looking to Sebelius to green-light the report. Many months passed, and by the fall of 2013 HHS officials still had not announced a decision.[47]

Another lost opportunity came in the wake of a young man's horrific murder of twenty first-graders and six adults at an elementary school in Newtown, Connecticut, in December 2012. The tragedy prompted a number of physicians and public health leaders to renew calls for stricter measures against gun violence, calls that had been sounded in years past by surgeons general like Koop and Elders. (Koop had advocated restrictions on gun ownership, and Elders once told *Mother Jones* magazine that she was in favor of a total ban on the sale of automatic weapons and would prohibit handgun ownership for anyone under eighteen.[48]) Even Antonia Novello, who had been so careful not to upset her Republican political bosses, had written a stirring editorial in the *Journal of the American Medical Association* in which she called violence a public health emergency that demanded serious action.[49] But in the aftermath of Newtown, Benjamin said nothing.[50]

Benjamin did have some visibility in a role assigned to her through the Affordable Care Act—the sweeping health reform legislation signed into law in March 2010. It was nearly impossible for the surgeon general to be silent about the law, which touched on many aspects of public health, including not only health insurance but also topics like FDA authorization of generic medications and rules requiring restaurants to display the caloric count of menu items. The ACA also created a National Prevention, Health Promotion, and Public Health Council, tasked with developing a plan to increase the number of Americans who are healthy.

Benjamin was made the chair of that panel, but her role was not publicly prominent. It was nearly miraculous that the law got passed in the first place, given the staunch political opposition, and various provisions were under constant threat of repeal afterward. By all accounts, Obama administration officials did not want anyone—especially a fumbling surgeon general—saying anything that would help political enemies hack at the act. (One Republican lawmaker later opined to the *New York Times* that Sebelius had "a fortress mentality" about the ACA.[51]) The council had no dedicated funding of its own, and no control over the $15 billion Prevention and Public Health Fund. Seventeen federal agencies were represented on the council, but deputies and assistant deputies represented agencies at most of the meetings.

In June 2011, the National Prevention Council produced a strategy document that mainly cataloged current health-related initiatives. A year later, Benjamin released a follow-up "action plan" that listed scores of activities the government was undertaking to address obesity and other public health issues—but again, many already existed or were in the works, anyway.[52] Some believed Benjamin's work on the council could prove important in years to come, that her strategy document will influence future federal health grants. American Public Health Association executive director Georges Benjamin (no relation to the surgeon general) called it a "naive assessment" to expect any more than what she delivered.[53] Still, at the end of her time in office, the impact was at best uncertain and the work was not widely known.

So it was that Benjamin was barely visible, as primary communication for the great public health issues of the day were assigned to others. Michelle Obama handled childhood obesity. Kathleen Sebelius had health reform. And CDC director Tom Frieden and his staff did the bulk of the messaging regarding smoking, breastfeeding, the swine flu pandemic of 2009, and most other public health matters. (And they were effective, judging from a 2013 survey of 1,800 Americans, in which 75 percent said the CDC did a good or excellent job.[54])

In speeches, Benjamin continued to refer to herself as "America's doctor," employing a variation of a label for the surgeon general used for decades. But not many others used that phrase to describe her. Most of the nation was seeing another physician.

DR. OZ

The May 21, 2012, issue of *The New Yorker* featured a cartoon depicting a man waiting in a doctor's office. On the wall, next to the physician's diplomas, was a large sign that read: "THANK YOU FOR NOT MENTIONING DR. OZ."[55] The joke was easy to get. Mehmet Oz was seemingly everywhere.

Oz, the Harvard-educated son of Turkish immigrants, was a successful cardiothoracic surgeon in New York City. He ascended to celebrity status through repeat appearances on *The Oprah Winfrey Show*, the culture- and ratings-dominating daytime talk show. On the air, Oz proved to be a gifted communicator, able to deliver simple and audience-riveting explanations of a variety of bodily functions and health problems. It didn't hurt that he was athletic, capable of punctuating a point about the importance of exercise by dropping on the floor to do a set of seemingly effortless push-ups. He first appeared on *Oprah* in 2004, and Winfrey had him back on the show more than fifty times over the next five years. Her company, Harpo Productions, championed him: in 2007, it filed a trademark application to make sure the phrase "America's Doctor" was used to promote Oz. In 2009, the trademark went through and Oz officially became "America's Doctor."[56]

His media presence extended beyond *Oprah*. He also became a fixture on the radio and in bookstores, as co-author of a popular series of "You" books, including *You: The Owner's Manual*. Eventually it became nearly impossible to pass through a grocery store check-out line without seeing his face on the cover of some health or diet publication. When *Prevention* magazine put Oz on its cover in October 2011, newsstand sales shot up 45 percent. When *Shape* did the same thing a month later, sales jumped 10 percent.[57] He was huge on Twitter, with more than 1.7 million followers in May 2012. (Regina Benjamin's supporters have touted her efforts to communicate to the public through Twitter, but at the same point in time she had only 3,000 followers.[58])

As Oz soared, some failed to notice that his trajectory through popular culture had started from a scientifically shaky launching pad. Popular as it was, *Oprah* was considered something of a menace by public health and medical experts. The show had often been quick to hype certain medical treatments like a new wrinkle-smoothing procedure involving radio waves, while quickly skating past unknowns and downsides (like the fact that the procedure was very painful and could cause burns and scars).[59] On occasion, Oprah accorded expert status to celebrities as they voiced wayward opinions about medical issues, like Suzanne Somers extolling the virtues of unregulated hormone creams to preserve her youth, or the actress and former *Playboy* centerfold Jenny McCarthy asserting that a measles-mumps-rubella vaccination caused her son's autism and that a special diet and other unproven therapies cured him.

Oz was perhaps the most scientifically solid of the "authorities" in the *Oprah* stable, but he was a little out there, too. He had long been open to exploring and praising alternative therapies that had not weathered rigorous scientific testing. That bent came from his wife's family: Lisa Lemole Oz's mother had been a strong believer in homeopathy and meditation, and Lisa herself was a Reiki master who promoted such treatments. Back in the 1990s, Oz had helped establish an alternative-therapies center at New York–Presbyterian/Columbia University Medical Center that offered a hands-on energy healer who could "assist" in the operating room.[60]

Oprah went off the air in 2009, and *The Dr. Oz Show* debuted later that year. He was a ratings star, but proved an underachiever when it came to conveying conventional scientific wisdom. Supplements and alternative medicines were regularly highlighted, despite enduring questions within the medical community about a lack of good evidence that they work. (Among the barrage of tips from Oz to his fan base: banana leaf tea to boost the metabolism, butterbur capsules for sinus inflammation, raspberry ketone to burn fat, and eggplant to ward off cancer.) Meanwhile, he was sometimes too quick to raise alarms about conventional treatments and products.[61]

And then there were Oz's occasional forays into the afterlife. He featured the controversial clairvoyant Char Margolis in a show that suggested medical tests could be used to show a different form of consciousness in mediums, but neglected to explore the possibility that she was a fraud. He was agape at another self-described psychic medium, John Edward. Oz later enthused to *TV Guide*: "We had John on the show because I'm all about learning. I've always liked the guy. He seems authentic, not at all like a charlatan. I've learned in my career that there are times when science hasn't caught up with things, and I think this may be one of them."[62]

Oz had a point about science sometimes being behind. Surgeon General Jesse Steinfeld started warning about the dangers of secondhand smoke well before there was, arguably, enough scientific evidence in hand to warrant such a caution. But Steinfeld, a cancer expert, made his leap based largely on his medically trained understanding of biologic plausibility. Oz jumped to the other side based on the performance of a guy who "seems authentic."

Interestingly, neither Carmona nor Benjamin said they had a problem with Oz. Both have appeared on his show, and said the kind of health education he does is complementary to the surgeon general's work. "I don't see him as competition," Carmona said.[63] Others have been less benign about the TV doctor. "Oz scares me," said Paul Offit, an infectious diseases expert at the Children's Hospital of Philadelphia who has written books criticizing the antivaccine movement. It's a small tragedy, he added, that Oz has become "America's Doctor." "It certainly would be important for the surgeon general to have that role. You'd like to think the surgeon general would give advice that is science-backed, that is evidence-backed. Because Dr. Oz certainly doesn't."[64]

BENJAMIN'S DEPARTURE

"America's doctor" was not the only title Benjamin struggled to lay claim to. As Twitter emerged as a leading social medium, the identifier @SurgeonGeneral was taken by a rap artist, meaning that Benjamin went by the handle @SGRegina instead.[65]

Maybe that was fitting. The surgeons general remembered as difference makers were activists on controversial issues. Thomas Parran was a relentless campaigner against venereal disease, in an era when polite people didn't speak of such things. Luther Terry, best remembered for the report on cigarette smoking, also advocated for seat belt use when the culture frowned on wearing one.[66] C. Everett Koop browbeat Americans into changing attitudes on a variety of topics, most notably AIDS. Jesse Steinfeld, Joycelyn Elders, and even the mild-mannered David Satcher were activists as well, rankling their political bosses when they addressed important and unsettled public health concerns. In contrast, what was arguably Benjamin's single most concentrated public outreach effort was a campaign to encourage people to walk more.[67]

In early June 2013, Benjamin announced that she had decided to resign effective the middle of the following month—or five months short of the official end of her term. Obama administration officials were tight-lipped about her departure, aside from issuing short statements thanking Benjamin for her service. Benjamin did not say why she was leaving early, commenting only that her personal plans included a short break and a return to volunteering at her clinic in Alabama.[68] (In an interview a few months later, Benjamin said it was her decision to leave and that no one in the administration had suggested to her she wouldn't be reappointed. Indeed, she said President Obama expressed mild surprise when at a White house function she told him she would be leaving.)[69] She also said she would be replaced by Boris Lushniak, her deputy and a public health veteran whom department insiders described as a much more effective speaker than Benjamin, and who would be acting surgeon general until the White House decided to formally appoint someone else. In a statement released to the Commissioned Corps, Benjamin wrote: "I was called to serve, and I have truly enjoyed serving as America's Doctor, promoting prevention in everything we do. I will leave the Office of Surgeon General confident that we have paved the path for a healthier nation with a much stronger focus on wellness and prevention."[70]

Short news items about her stepping down appeared in newspapers and on media websites across the country. On a few sites, readers posted comments. Some were complimentary. Others—reacting to a photograph of Benjamin published with the article—made crude comments about her weight. And a few others revived the discussion about whether a surgeon general was necessary. "The post of surgeon general is nothing but a sinecure so that some political crony of the president's can wear a military-looking uniform and act important," posted one reader of the *Washington Times*. "Congress should abolish it."[71]

In November 2013, President Obama announced he planned to nominate a successor to Benjamin. His selection was Vivek Hallegere Murthy, a respected physician at Harvard-affiliated Brigham and Women's Hospital. Only thirty-six, he stood, if confirmed, to become the youngest surgeon general since John B. Hamilton in the nineteenth century. But he came to the Obama administration's attention not so much because of his age or Boston medical pedigree as for his experience as a wunderkind health and political advocate. In 1995, he had created VISIONS Worldwide, a nonprofit focused on HIV education in India. More important, in 2008, he had founded a national grassroots organization named Doctors for Obama to help the president get elected, and then morphed it into Doctors for America to support the Affordable Care Act.

Described by friends and colleagues as soft-spoken but idealistic, Murthy was widely expected to play the health reform salesman role once envisioned for Sanjay Gupta.[72] But few were forecasting he would develop into the kind of Koop-like maverick many have hoped for.

CHAPTER 13

The Surgeon General's Demise

In his novel *2030*, comedian Albert Brooks envisioned a future America incapacitated by debt, devastated by a giant California earthquake, and shaken by violent conflict between the elderly and the younger generations. Much of it sounded fairly plausible, actually, except for one detail: Brooks imagined that the government would still have a surgeon general and that the character would be an influential figure.[1]

Judging from how things stand now, that seems extremely unlikely. The Office of the Surgeon General has been sinking for more than half a century. In the 1960s, William Stewart was stripped of his oversight of 150 federal programs, 38,000 people, and a $2 billion budget, and reduced to a glorified health educator. Granted, the surgeon general is a health educator blessed with a unique bully pulpit, but as the years have passed, that pulpit has been used to diminishing effect.

Smoking—the surgeon general's bread-and-butter issue—illustrates the point. In the 1960s, Luther Terry issued a report that was the definitive turning point in the public's perception of smoking's dangers. In the 1980s, C. Everett Koop drove a national conversation about the dangers of tobacco that coincided with a substantial reduction in smoking rates. But in the past several years, with relatively little attention from the Office of the Surgeon General, the drop in teen smoking rates has stalled and adult rates have declined only slightly.[2]

Epidemic response is another example. The surgeon general was once the guiding hand who dispatched disease detectives to outbreaks, ordered quarantines, and told the public what was happening and how to protect themselves. Those responsibilities have passed to other health officials, and for good reason: It's been more than a decade since the nation's doctor has had infectious disease expertise comparable to the CDC director or other government health experts. Subject matter experts are not always the best communicators, of course. But the last two CDC directors have generally been considered at least as good—if not significantly better—than their surgeon general counterparts.

True, the office has been buoyed at times by rare and driven personalities aided by supportive administrations. (Koop was neither a smoking expert nor an infectious disease specialist when he took the job, but became a point man on both tobacco and AIDS.) But the necessary constellation of people and conditions for such success has become a rarity, and there's little reason to believe future administrations will be interested in employing the kind of quasi-independent, speaking-truth-to-power maverick the job really requires.

As of this writing, the office is at a nadir, and yet it still may not have hit bottom. With regret, it's my purpose to argue that it's probably time to do away with the surgeon general.

Many in the public health community may well recoil at the idea. Some—even in public health—believe (incorrectly) that the surgeon general is still a powerful federal health official, so the idea of abolishing the position might seem bewildering. Others, who have a better understanding of how bad things have gotten, may nevertheless object because they feel the potential for great things from the office still exists. Officially, anyway, "there is a freedom there that even the CDC director, or Tony Fauci, does not have," said William Schaffner, the prominent infectious diseases expert. He echoed a prevalent belief that the position could be brought back into prominence if filled by an individual "willing to give a bit of a stiff arm to the White House and perhaps to others in positions of power and leadership in the health arena."[3]

Undeniably, the title still has built-in prestige. Regina Benjamin, for all her weaknesses, was perceived by one national business magazine to be one of the "100 Most Influential People in Healthcare" for three years running. (Those rankings at times put her ahead of her boss Howard Koh, CDC director Tom Frieden, and U.S. Food and Drug Administration commissioner Margaret Hamburg.) Richard Carmona made the publication's list three times, too.[4] Heads do turn when a surgeon general enters the room, and the hefty reports issued by the office continue to be oft-cited references in the medical world. "We don't want to lose the brand," said Georges Benjamin of the American Public Health Association.[5]

Some voiced another concern, specific to the Commissioned Corps, which the surgeon general officially oversees. Corps members work in hard-to-fill positions in places ranging from prisons to mental health clinics to American Indian reservations, and are on call round-the-clock for disaster response. Yet the Corps's value and cost-effectiveness, too, have been repeatedly questioned over the decades. "If the Office of the Surgeon General is abolished, then it would logically follow that the Corps should be abolished," said Gerard Farrell, executive director of the Commissioned Officers Association of the U.S. Public Health Service. Regarding talk of doing away with the surgeon general or Commissioned Corps, Farrell said, "This is a really bad idea on many levels."[6]

Some also would resent such a move because it would be tantamount to "letting the bastards win." David Rutstein, Regina Benjamin's former deputy, likened the surgeon general to a proud animal that politicians had starved and crippled—and then wondered aloud if the right thing to do is put it out of its misery. "You start wounding something over and over and over, and when it gets to death's door, then you ask 'Is it viable?'" he said. "Well, probably not. But one answer is to stop wounding it."[7] The thing to do, optimists argue, is to enact legislative safeguards that would strengthen the Office of the Surgeon General. "I think it's an imperative public health issue that we corral this problem and fix it as soon as possible," said Howard Markel, a University of Michigan medical historian. "I think we have to come up with safeguards that are as ironclad as possible, . . . because our health depends on it."[8]

The call for safeguards includes a desire for measures that ensure strong nominees. The theoretical ideal is finding another Koop, but it's recognized that Koop succeeded through shrewd and intense effort, a formidable personality, and a hard-to-replicate set of circumstances. It's not sensible to expect a Koop to come along again. The more realistic models look to other influential surgeons general for examples of people who came from the world of public health, either by rising through the ranks of the U.S. Public Health Service or—as in the cases of David Satcher and Joycelyn Elders—by having experience leading other government health agencies.

Some believe all surgeons general should come from the Commissioned Corps, just as they did for the first century of the position's existence. (Richard Carmona, who did not come from the Corps, is among those who voiced this opinion.[9]) The argument is that such a career path would boost the Corps's psyche and perhaps end the snickering asides that occur when an outsider with only a dim understanding of federal public health is brought in and awarded the surgeon general's three-star uniform. But to work the bully pulpit, a history in the Corps is not strictly necessary. An accomplished history as a leader at the CDC, or of a major state, county, or city health department, or of a variety of other organizations might confer as much or more credibility with the public, and a sufficient amount of credibility with the Corps. These kinds of eligibility requirements can be written into legislation, as U.S. Representative Henry Waxman did in his 2007 bill when he proposed that six candidates had to be considered each time an HHS secretary selected a new surgeon general and that at least three of them had to come from the Commissioned Corps.

Who should draw up the list of nominees? Waxman proposed that the HHS secretary come up with the names, but that likely would mean a continuation of the current system in which nominees are selected for political reasons, such as trying to please political allies (as in the case of choosing Luther Terry and Koop); trying to satisfy campaign supporters (as was said to be the case with Carmona); or making a show of a commitment to racial or ethnic diversity (as with Antonia Novello).

Another option was suggested by the late U.S. Senator Edward Kennedy of Massachusetts. At about the time Waxman introduced his bill in 2007, Kennedy introduced his own bill for strengthening the Office of the Surgeon General. Kennedy proposed that each nominee be selected from a list of ten names drawn up by the Institute of Medicine (IOM), a nonprofit organization chartered in 1970 to serve as a national source for unbiased, research-based advice on matters of biomedical science and health. Its membership includes a lengthy and esteemed list of researchers and policy experts, most of them from universities. (Alternatively, perhaps organizations like the American Public Health Association or the Association of State and Territorial Health Officials could be asked to draw up initial lists of nominees.) Granted, entities like the IOM might not come up with an unexpected gem like Koop, but they likely would spare the nation from iron pyrite nuggets like Novello, Carmona, and Regina Benjamin.[10]

Ask some of the former surgeons general themselves, and they'll say that whoever selects future nominees should seek not only the proper credentials but also a bit of a swagger.[11] Indeed, self-confidence is crucial to success in the job, and a surgeon general must be accomplished—and determined—enough to be willing to walk away from the job if his or her ability to speak truth to power is significantly compromised. Koop and Elders, the best-remembered surgeons general of the past forty years, both emphasized that point to me in interviews for this book. "The first week I was in Washington, in an interview with the press, I said: 'If I am ever asked to say something that I do not believe, I will go home. And if ever I am asked not to say something that I do believe, I will go home,'" Koop said.[12] "I think it's an important attitude to have," Elders said of the confidence requirement. "I felt I was the people's surgeon general and I was there to serve and work in their best interest. I was not the president's surgeon general or the Congress's surgeon general."[13]

Of course, Elders was ousted from her job after little more than a year in what became an enduring lesson that such an attitude can get you fired. Optimists say her experience points to another needed safeguard for the Office of the Surgeon General—a greater guarantee of job security.

One idea is to borrow from the comptroller general, who is appointed to a fifteen-year term that allows the office to stand apart from the political scaffolding erected by any one president. The comptroller general, who heads the Government Accountability Office, is a maverick who watchdogs other federal agencies. He or she can be removed only for reasons of malfeasance or misfeasance, and such a dismissal requires a joint resolution of Congress. What's more, the GAO gets its annual budget through a congressional appropriation that cannot be restricted by the executive branch.

Another "general" model involves the inspectors general. IGs, as they are called for short, are positions established within federal agencies to investigate fraud and abuse. (There are more than seventy of them at the federal level.)[14] The Inspector General Act of 1978 gave IGs direct access to government records and information, authorized them to conduct whatever investigations they deemed appropriate, and allowed them to hire and control their own staff. A 2008 law took further steps to strengthen and improve the quality of IGs, including increasing their subpoena powers and requiring the Council of Inspectors General on Integrity and Efficiency draw up a list of qualified candidates for the president or agency heads to consider whenever there is an IG vacancy. Although each higher-level IG is under the general supervision of the secretary of his or her department, the IG has an independent relationship with Congress. The IGs over the postal service and the Capitol police have terms of seven and five years, respectively; the terms for other IGs are indefinite. They can be removed by a president or agency head, of course, but that's not easily done.[15] Per custom, IGs are not expected to step down when a new president is inaugurated.

In contrast to the comptroller general and the IGs, surgeons general never enjoyed such protections from meddling by others in the administration. But it once was common, at least, for surgeons general to hold office for a decade or longer. Although they have had four-year terms since early in the twentieth century, surgeons general routinely used to serve multiple terms through a variety of administrations. They were considered career professionals, expected to make the best decisions for the public's health regardless of who happened to be in the White House at the time. Back then, tradition ensured a degree of autonomy that set the office apart from the political appointees who swarmed in with each new administration and were swept out when it was over.

In the past fifty-five years or so, however, a pattern has developed in which each president has appointed his own surgeon general, and that surgeon general typically has left office no more than a year after his or her president vacates the White House. That pattern has made it clear that surgeons general have to dance with, and bow to, the chief executive who brought them.

Some think a longer term—at least six years—would buy resource-deprived surgeons general the time to make the connections and build the momentum needed to turn out significant reports or initiatives. Even the great Koop didn't hit full stride until his second term. Carmona, unable to stay in office more than four years, could not bring his global health report to fruition. Jesse Steinfeld, for all his ambition and aggressiveness, was thwarted by a term that ended too soon. "Jesse wasn't there long enough to have much of an impact," former HHS official Charles Edwards once said.[16]

Of course, a longer term won't protect the surgeon general from political interference. The greatest enemies of surgeons general have not been presidents or Cabinet secretaries but lower-level officials who see themselves as paladins of an administration's political agenda. (Recall that Carmona testified to Congress in 2007 that while he was surgeon general, underlings walled him off from media interviews, told him to read from scripted speeches, and suppressed his reports.) These second-tier officials are the men and women who restrict a surgeon general's budget, travel, and visibility. What to do about that?

Waxman and others proposed that the surgeon general should submit a proposal budget directly to the president and to Congress, rather than have the budget determined by HHS officials. They recommended that the surgeon general also have the ability to hire and fire staff, and be protected from HHS censorship. The surgeon general also should be granted more freedom to choose the topics for reports, Calls to Action, and other communications. It's been suggested also that the nation's doctor report annually to Congress on the state of the nation's health. Such a document might permit the surgeon general to frankly explore problems and issues that administration officials have chosen not to emphasize. It could also strengthen a surgeon general's connection to policymakers in Congress. But some experts doubt Congress could produce the kind of bulletproof legislation needed to truly protect a surgeon general. "I don't think laws like that do a lot of good in the real world. . . . There are all kinds of things in the federal government that are 'insulated.' It doesn't work," said former HEW Secretary Joseph Califano.[17]

Yes, lawmakers have gone to great lengths to install safeguards for IGs. But IGs are a far more popular cause. They are tasked with cracking down on waste, fraud, and abuse in the executive branch, often making them intriguing to whichever political party is not currently controlling the White House. Indeed, the Inspector General Reform Act of 2008 was most ardently championed by Democrats who were wary of the George W. Bush administration. And Bush signed it into law only after the White House took a great deal of heat for declining to turn over internal e-mails and documents to the Department of Justice's inspector general, who was investigating the removal of nine U.S. attorneys in 2006 for what appeared to be political reasons.[18]

Congress has shown very little interest in creating protections for the surgeon general, however. The last, best hope of making a change came in the summer of 2007, when congressional Democrats were briefly able to make political hay out of Carmona's disclosures about how he was muzzled by the George W. Bush administration. But the House and Senate bills introduced in the wake of that brouhaha never came close to a floor vote. And the architect of one of the bills acknowledged that because of political disinterest, there was never any real expectation that the legislation would be enacted.[19]

Expecting little help from the Hill, some surgeons general—namely, Julius Richmond and David Satcher—moved to gain additional power by simultaneously taking the job of assistant secretary for health. Satcher, especially, was able to parlay his dual appointment into an unusually productive term. Some strongly believe that standardizing that arrangement is the most practical approach for restoring luster to the Office of the Surgeon General. Yet Satcher himself expressed doubts about such a step. He said the dual appointment was advantageous to him at that point in history, given the hands-off management of HHS Secretary Donna Shalala and his need to reestablish the visibility and productivity of the Office of the Surgeon General after it had been vacant for four years. But he and others noted that the ASH is much more of a political line appointment, with greater pressure placed on the officeholder to parrot the messages of the HHS secretary and the White House. The surgeon general is supposed to be a less beholden voice, but that willingness to be independent is inevitably compromised by wearing both hats. Asked in an interview if a surgeon general today should also serve as ASH, Satcher replied, "That's not my preference."[20]

All that said, in an increasingly partisan and embattled Washington, we face the prospect of increasingly inconsequential surgeons general continuing to limp along. Pessimism about the ability to get the necessary legislation passed, and about whether it to be carried out properly, leads to the conclusion that the situation will only deteriorate.

There is some money to be saved by doing away with the nation's doctor. A surgeon general is a relatively small expense. (In 2012, Benjamin was paid about $192,000. She had only about ten staffers and didn't even have her own budget—all the money is funneled through the ASH.[21]) But modest as the sum is, it's not insignificant. At a time when federal, state, and local public health departments have had to slash funding and staffing for a wide range of disease-prevention and -investigation services, a few hundred thousand dollars can be well spent hiring epidemiologists or other necessary public health workers.[22]

There is an intangible, troops-rousing value to the position, given its status as ceremonial leader of the Commissioned Corps and unofficial monarch of the U.S. public health workforce. Elders was a master at such inspiration, and Carmona was pretty good at it as well, at least as far as the Corps was concerned. Someone with a similar talent in times like these may be well worth that expenditure, even if the surgeon general had a low profile with the general public. But even the surgeon general's ceremonial role is limited; for example, the highest award that the surgeon general can bestow at his or her own discretion is only the third most important award within the Public Health Service.[23] What's more, Benjamin showed little interest in bolstering the Corps, and her political bosses didn't penalize her for her apparent indifference. No doubt her successor will not be penalized for indifference, either.

In truth, the office has been wounded and weak for at least half a century now, and a crippled surgeon general has gradually become a given in the culture of presidential administrations. Washington logrollers prefer the position to be a paper tiger. And it's been more than a decade since a surgeon general has had the backbone to try to substantively change—in ways that might offend vested interests—the cultural norms and industrial practices that allow unhealthy behaviors and conditions to roost among the public. There may still be some degree of automatic prestige attached to the title, but even that mystique is fading. The problem is not just that most people no longer know *who* the surgeon general is; in my years of working on this book, when I talked to children or younger adults about the topic, I frequently found many had not even heard of the job title.

"I sort of suspect the surgeon general thing has had its time," said Hale Champion, the former HEW undersecretary during the Carter administration.[24]

"It's a useless office, the way it has been used lately," said the late David Sencer, the former CDC director, in an interview with me in 2007.[25]

As I was working on this book, I found myself thinking about Henrik Ibsen's classic play *An Enemy of the People*. First published in 1882, it centers on a physician named Thomas Stockmann, who runs tests on the water in his Norwegian town—water thought to have medicinal qualities. Indeed, the town's waters are the basis of a public baths project expected to bring tourism and new life to the struggling community. But Dr. Stockmann's tests show the waters are polluted and certain to cause illness.

Stockmann tries to publicize his scientific findings, and to push the mayor and local authorities to stop the project. But the mayor attempts to control him and threatens to fire him, and the people grow to resent his meddling in the town's gambit for prosperity. At the play's end, Stockmann is without a job, standing in the debris of his home after rock-throwing townspeople have shattered his windows. But he is resolute that he will tell the world of the health dangers lurking in his town, and will try to save the lives of those who attack him. "Remember now, everybody," he tells his frightened family, the only ones still at his side. "You are fighting for the truth, and that's why you're alone. And that makes you strong. We're the strongest people in the world."[26]

In the many interviews I did for this book, I was reminded of Stockmann's speech as I heard person after person express their enduring admiration for the job's potential. "Because of that bully pulpit, you have as much moral authority as you're willing to take on," said John

Santelli, a former CDC official who became a Columbia University professor of population and family health.[27] Old enough to remember when Koop and Elders were at the center of national health policy debates, I fully appreciated Santelli's words. Indeed, for a time I counted myself among the optimists who believe there must be some way to resurrect the nation's doctor.

But as seven years passed working on this book, and as I gradually absorbed the many ways in which the office has been declining, I came to conclude there will be no such change. Any recipe I could offer for resurrecting the nation's doctor would require the interest and involvement of an array of powerbrokers. Currently there are no powerful advocates for the surgeon general in Congress—certainly no one akin to the late U.S. Representative Paul Rogers, who rebuffed attempts by the Nixon administration to tamper with the Public Health Service. As the years pass, it's less and less likely that younger legislators will have heard of the surgeon general, let alone be interested in spending precious political capital fighting on the office's behalf. Public health advocates and lobbyists could try to put the issue on Congress's radar, but they have more pressing priorities like shoring up underfunded health services and disease-prevention programs. And they, too, are getting younger and less concerned with the status of a moribund health bureaucrat.

That's something of a tragedy. The surgeon general still is the nation's chief health educator and could play a pivotal role helping our society understand and accept medical evidence. A good surgeon general persuades people to stop smoking and drop other harmful habits. An effective surgeon general prods them to eat better and get disease-preventing vaccinations. A great surgeon general influences policymakers to act on behalf of the public health. Terry and Koop are perhaps the best-known success stories, but others in the post calmed fears, corrected misperceptions, and improved the public's health.

Such work is still needed. An important 2009 national survey found that fewer than 70 percent of U.S. adults thought parents should be required to vaccinate their children; only about half knew that antibiotics don't work against viruses; and only half believed people are causing global climate change.[28] The findings point to widespread misbeliefs that are not only wrong but dangerous, contributing to the resurgence and mistreatment of infectious illnesses and the further degradation of our environment.

More than ever, America needs a strong surgeon general. And who knows? Perhaps some unexpected occurrence—like a scandal gravely damaging the scientific credibility of the CDC director or HHS secretary—would prompt Congress or a president to rebuild the office.[29] Or maybe another Koop will come along to raise the position's profile. But that individual would be the kind of wild-card whom presidential administrations tend to avoid—a media-savvy maverick willing to defy political overseers and roil political waters as she or he preaches science to the public. Such scenarios seem far-fetched at best.

With faint expectation of a "Hail Mary" turn of events, it is perhaps time to shutter the Office of the Surgeon General, divert the money to a better purpose, and look to others for public health leadership. The surgeon general has become something of a farce: not the independent speaker of truth-to-power that many perceive, but rather a frequently muted mouthpiece for whatever administration is currently presiding. Indeed, it is arguably more harmful than helpful to allow the surgeon general to endure. The nation's doctor simply can't be trusted to do or say the right thing in crucial moments when best public health practice differs from political policy, and those are the very moments that legitimize the position's existence. The notion of seeing a Thomas Stockmann–like figure in the job, bravely sounding a health warning amid a cesspool of ignorance and selfishness, is a work of fiction.

Notes

CHAPTER I

1. Author's notes from interviews with Brenda Smith and Betty Ruth Speir, foyer of Ronald Reagan Building and International Trade Center, Washington, D.C., January 11, 2010.

2. Nurit Guttman, Daria Boccher-Lattimore, and Charles T. Salmon, "Credibility of Information from Official Sources on HIV/AIDS Transmission," *Public Health Reports,* September–October 1998, Vol. 113, No. 5, pp. 465–471; Anna Perea and Michael D. Slater, "Power Distance and Collectivist/Individualist Strategies in Alcohol Warnings: Effects by Gender and Ethnicity," *Journal of Health Communication,* October–December 1999, Vol. 4, No. 4, pp. 295–310. The author did a more recent survey of one hundred health journalists on the question, as recounted in Michael Stobbe, "The Surgeon General and the Bully Pulpit" (DrPH dissertation, University of North Carolina, 2008), pp. 177–191. Beth P. House and Kathy N. Player, *Pivotal Moments in Nursing,* Vol. 2 (Indianapolis: Sigma Theta Tau International, 2007), p. 3.

3. Daniel F. Whiteside, interview with Lynne Page Snyder, December 2, 1993, transcript p. 53. This is one of dozens of oral histories with former federal public health officials that were on file in the Office of the Public Health Service Historian, U.S. Department of Health and Human Services. The office was later closed for budgetary reasons, and its files transferred to the National Library of Medicine in Bethesda, Maryland.

4. Memoirs of Dr. Hugh Smith Cumming Sr. (unpublished), Cumming Family Papers, Albert and Shirley Small Special Collections Library, University of Virginia, accession no. 6922-a, Volume I, 8th folder, p. 307.

5. *The Daily Show,* video of January 7, 2009, broadcast, http://www.thedailyshow.com/watch/wed-january-7-2009/medicine-cabinet (accessed December 14, 2013).

6. The Harris Poll, "Positive Ratings of SEC Plunges 42 Points," February 10, 2009, press release. The online survey found that 73 percent of respondents said they understood the surgeon general's role, compared to 63 percent who understood the SEC and 58 percent the NIH. (The FDA was number one, at 94 percent.) Of those who said they knew what the position does, 68 percent said they thought the surgeon general did a good or excellent job. Only the U.S. Mint, Centers for Disease Control and Prevention, FBI, and Federal Aviation Administration got higher marks on that question.

7. To be sure, it's difficult to judge the effectiveness of a surgeon general. The job's emphasis in the last several decades has been the bully pulpit, and there is no unassailable measure of how much a single health official's speeches or education efforts influence public behavior. We could look at what happened to smoking rates while a surgeon general was hammering away at the issue, but it's impossible to distinguish the role of those harangues from the impact of other factors like tobacco taxes, local smoking bans, or crackdowns on the sale of cigarettes to minors. We could look at public opinion polls after the release of a surgeon general's report, but those can't be counted on to tell whether the message caused enduring behavior change. "With one exception . . . there is no empirical evidence on the attitudinal or behavioral impacts of the reports per se," once wrote Kenneth Warner, an esteemed University of Michigan researcher on the health dangers of tobacco, referring to the many surgeon general smoking reports. (The exception was a series of studies that showed that the famous 1964 surgeon general report on smoking caused smoking rates to go down about 5 percent.) See Kenneth E. Warner, ed., *Tobacco Control Policy* (San Francisco: Jossey-Bass, 2006), p. 21. Note also that it's not clear that the government is actually reaching out to the man in the street with some of those reports. For example, at a press conference to release a 2011 surgeon general "Call to Action" report on breast-feeding, there was an emphasis on the importance of getting more young black women to breast-feed. But the document and press conference were not really intended to persuade African American moms. Instead, the focus audience was people who work at hospitals and health departments and can institute policies to promote access to lactation consultants and other support services, said CDC official Laurence Grummer-Strawn, in an interview with the author. Speaking of surgeon general reports, he said, "I think rarely are they for the general public."

8. Michigan was the first state to create a state surgeon general, under Governor Jennifer Granholm, a Democrat. The office became vacant when the first Michigan surgeon general left office in 2010, and Granholm's Republican successor, Rick Snyder, has left the office vacant.

9. Joe Thompson, interview with the author, September 28, 2009.

10. David Sencer, interview with the author, September 25, 2007. The organization's name has changed since then to the Centers for Disease Control and Prevention. After he retired, Sencer became an unofficial historian for the CDC. He died in 2011.

11. Eric Redman, *The Dance of Legislation* (New York: Simon & Schuster, 1973; repr. Seattle: University of Washington Press, 2001), p. 141.

12. David Satcher, interview with the author, July 18, 2012.

13. The other two are C. Everett Koop and Richard Carmona. The law is 42 USC 205, "Appointment and tenure of Office of Surgeon General." The law also says a surgeon general must come from the U.S. Public Health Service Commissioned Corps, but in the last few decades presidents have gotten around that by briefly appointing an outsider to the Corps and then immediately promoting him or her to surgeon general.

14. Michael D. Tanner, "Can't We Dump This Nanny Job?" *Chicago Tribune,* June 12, 2007. Tanner was a senior fellow with the Cato Institute, a libertarian think tank in Washington, D.C.

15. Charles C. Edwards, oral history interview with Fitzhugh Mullan, October 28, 1988, transcript p. 38, National Library of Medicine (formerly on file with the now closed HHS Office of the Public Health Historian).

16. The episode, entitled "Ellie," first aired February, 21, 2001. But note that at the last moment Bartlet decided not to accept her resignation.

17. David Rutstein, interview with the author, July 22, 2012.

18. Laurence Grummer-Strawn, interview with the author, June 1, 2012. Grummer-Strawn is chief of the Nutrition Branch at the Centers for Disease Control and Prevention and was primary author of a surgeon general "Call to Action" report on breast-feeding.

19. In the wake of a nationwide recession and tightening state and federal public health budgets, local health departments shed nearly 40,000 jobs from 2008 through 2011. In twenty-six states, more than half of local health departments cut at least one program in 2011. National Association of County and City Health Officials, "Local Health Department Job Losses and Program Cuts: Findings from the January 2012 Survey" (May 2012 research brief).

20. Huong McLean, "Measles—United States, 2011," *Morbidity and Mortality Weekly Report,* April 20, 2012, Vol. 61, No. 15, pp. 253–257.

21. New York City health leaders actually had greater real power than federal health officials in the enactment of taxes and ordinances, but they also worked hard to sell their policies to the public through strong, blunt speeches and education campaigns. And they have had some success: the adult smoking rate in New York City fell from 22 percent in 2002 to 14 percent in 2010; the childhood obesity rate fell modestly from 22 percent in 2006–2007 to 21 percent in 2010–2011; the proportion of restaurants using trans fats dropped from 50 percent to 2 percent. But not every Bloomberg initiative was a success. As of this writing, there was no evidence of a dent in the adult obesity rate, for example. And some of the Bloomberg health initiatives have treaded on thin scientific ice, including a campaign against salt that has caused some experts to question whether there was sufficient scientific evidence that commonly consumed levels of sodium causes high blood pressure or other health problems. See Sarah Kliff, "Mayor Mike Bloomberg, Public Health Autocrat: A Brief History," *Washington Post's Wonkblog,* June 4, 2012; William Neuman, "Citing Hazard, New York Says Hold the Salt," *New York Times,* January 10, 2010; Ronald Mayer, David Merritt Johns, and Sandro Galea, "Salt and Public Health: Contested Science and the Challenge of Evidence-Based Decision Making," *Health Affairs,* December 2012, Vol. 31, No. 12, pp. 2738–2746.

22. As quoted in Jonathan Engel, *Poor People's Medicine* (Durham, N.C.: Duke University Press, 2006), p. 100. Note that Stewart said this in 1963, a few years before he was appointed surgeon general.

23. Anthony S. Fauci, interview with the author, March 28, 2008.

CHAPTER 2

1. John M. Woodworth, *Annual Report of the Supervising Surgeon of the Marine Hospital Service of the United States, for the fiscal year 1873* (Washington, D.C.: Government Printing Office, 1873), pp. 18, 52.

2. John M. Woodworth, *First Annual Report of the Supervising Surgeon of the Marine Hospital Service of the United States, for the year 1872* (Washington, D.C.: Government Printing Office, 1872), pp. 13, 22.

3. Margaret Humphreys, "Woodworth, John Maynard," in *American National Biography,* Vol. 23 (New York: Oxford University Press, 1999), p. 836; George Worthington Adams, *Doctors in Blue* (1952; repr., Baton Rouge: Louisiana State University Press, 1996), pp. 109–110.

4. Robert L. Pearce, "The Emerging Office of the Surgeon General," *ADF Health,* April 2002, Vol. 3, No. 1, p. 36.

5. Peter W. Bruton, "The National Board of Health" (Ph.D. dissertation, University of Maryland, 1974), pp. 15–18.

6. Unsigned article, "The United States Public Health and Marine-Hospital Service, Part I—A Historical Sketch," *Journal of the American Medical Association,* June–December 1904, Vol. 43, p. 326.

7. The term "orgy" is used by Bruton in "National Board of Health," p. 19.

8. From a report by William M. Gouge (in Senate documents from the 34th Congress), quoted in Robert Straus, *Medical Care for Seamen: The Origin of the Public Health Service in the United States* (New Haven: Yale University Press, 1950), p. 49.

9. "The United States Public Health and Marine-Hospital Service, Part I—A Historical Sketch," pp. 326–327; Bruton, "National Board of Health," p. 19; Michael D. Hammond, "Arkansas Atlantis: The Lost Town of Napoleon," *Arkansas Historical Quarterly,* Vol. 65, No. 3, Autumn 2006, pp. 213, 217–218, 220. Details about the cupola and materials used in building the hospitals come from historian Rick Bell as he gave the author a tour of the marine hospital in Louisville, Kentucky, on March 7, 2010. Bell formerly was the executive director of a project to renovate the one hundred–bed Louisville hospital. The inland marine hospitals built at the time tended to be hundred- or fifty-bed facilities, all based on a design by architect Robert Mills.

10. "The United States Public Health and Marine-Hospital Service, Part I—A Historical Sketch," pp. 326–327; Straus, *Medical Care for Seamen,* pp. 26, 38. The tax that supported the Marine Hospital Service was a monthly levy of 20 cents for every seaman who had worked on a ship since it last entered a U.S. port.

11. Charles Henry pop [*sic*] and John Arthur Loring, *Loring Genealogy* (Cambridge, Mass.: Murray & Emery Company, 1917), p. 193; Otto Juettner, *Daniel Drake and His Followers: Historical and Biographical Sketches* (Cincin-

nati: Harvey Publishing Company, 1909), p. 218; Straus, *Medical Care for Seamen*, p. 56.

12. Douglas Guthrie, *A History of Medicine* (London: Thomas Nelson and Sons Ltd., 1946), p. 400–401; Fielding H. Garrison, *John Shaw Billings: A Memoir* (New York: Knickerbocker Press, 1915), pp. 66–67, 130, 376.

13. The National Library of Medicine contains no report by Billings and Stewart, and other historians and historical collections don't have them, either. The absence of these records is also noted in Carleton B. Chapman, *Order Out of Chaos: John Shaw Billings and America's Coming of Age* (Boston: Boston Medical library, 1994), p. 87.

14. Bess Furman, *A Profile of the United States Public Health Service, 1798–1948* (Washington, D.C.: Government Printing Office, 1973), p. 119; "The United States Public Health and Marine-Hospital Service, Part I—A Historical Sketch," p. 328.

15. The theory is noted in Chapman, *Order Out of Chaos*, p. 88. The conclusion that Boutwell wanted to make Billings the first surgeon general is also noted in Furman, *Profile of the United States Public Health Service*, pp. 118–119.

16. After Woodworth and until the 1960s, all surgeons general were selected from the career ranks of the Commissioned Corps. Coincidentally, in the 1960s the surgeon general was accorded the rank of a three-star general within the Corps—a ranking equivalent to that of the U.S. Army surgeon general. Because the Commissioned Corps was founded on a navy model, however, the surgeon general came to be known unofficially as "vice admiral," to accord with navy military ranks. All that notwithstanding, for almost fifty years, nearly all the surgeons general have been civilians. Jerry Farrell, e-mail to the author, June 12, 2013.

17. Furman, *A Profile of the United States Public Health Service*, pp. 118–119. Billings's ambitious—and, to some extent, self-promoting—nature is alluded to in Wyndham D. Miles, *A History of the National Library of Medicine: The Nation's Treasury of Medical Knowledge* (Washington, D.C.: Government Printing Office, 1982), p. 105.

18. So at least one historian has concluded: Wilson G. Smillie, in *Public Health: Its Promise for the Future* (New York: Macmillan, 1955), p. 462.

19. Ralph Chester Williams, *The United States Public Health Service, 1798–1950* (Richmond, Va., Whittet & Shepperson, 1951), p. 472. Baird, who worked with John James Audubon, was one of the era's leading scientists on the study of birds and fish. Several species of birds and one species of beaked whale are named after him.

20. There are inconsistencies among sources about Woodworth's medical training. One obituary said he graduated in 1863 from the Medical College of Chicago. (Unsigned article, "A Noble Life Ended: The Death of Surgeon General Woodworth Yesterday," *Washington Post*, March 15, 1879.) But an obit in the *New York Times* gave his graduation year as 1862, as have multiple biographical summaries of Woodworth published since then.

21. Humphreys, "Woodworth, John Maynard," pp. 836–837.

22. Ibid.; "A Noble Life Ended"; Adams, *Doctors in Blue*, pp. 109, 210.

23. Furman, *A Profile of the United States Public Health Service*, p. 123; Woodworth, *Annual Report of the Supervising Surgeon, 1873*, p. 52.

24. John M. Woodworth, *Annual Report of the Supervising Surgeon, 1873*, pp. 52–59; John M. Woodworth, "Our Sick Sailors: Synopsis of the Report of the Marine Hospital Service for 1872," *New York Times*, Nov. 20, 1872; Rick Bell, interview with the author.

25. Woodworth, "Our Sick Sailors." The charge for care of foreign sailors at the time was locked at 75 cents per diem. It wasn't enough. The service was losing money on these patients.

26. Straus, *Medical Care for Seamen*, p. 65.

27. The germ theory of disease, which came to prominence in the late nineteenth century, holds that some infectious diseases are caused by microorganisms like viruses and bacteria.

28. Fitzhugh Mullan, *Plagues and Politics* (New York: Basic Books, 1989), pp. 21–22.

29. Furman, *A Profile of the United States Public Health Service*, pp. 133–134; John M. Woodworth, *Nomenclature of Diseases: Prepared for the Use of the Medical Officers of the United States Marine-Hospital Service* (Washington, D.C.: Government Printing Office, 1874), p. v.

30. The uniforms were designed by MHS surgeon Trulon V. Miller, who worked at the Chicago Marine Hospital. See Mullan, *Plagues and Politics*, p. 24.

31. "The United States Public Health and Marine-Hospital Service, Part I—A Historical Sketch," p. 401.

32. Furman, *A Profile of the United States Public Health Service*, p. 139.

33. Bruton, "National Board of Health," pp. 35–37, 40. There was, briefly, a U.S. Sanitary Commission that was staffed mainly by female volunteers. Aimed at improving health and sanitation in Union Army camps, the commission was part of a wartime operation to primarily benefit the military.

34. Smillie, *Public Health*, pp. 297, 300. The APHA was formally founded that year, 1872.

35. Woodworth, *First Annual Report of the Supervising Surgeon, 1872*, p. 22; Furman, *A Profile of the United States Public Health Service*, p. 130.

36. John M. Woodworth, *Cholera Epidemic of 1873 in the United States* (Washington, D.C.: Government Printing Office, 1875), pp. 6, 12; Furman, *A Profile of the United States Public Health Service*, pp. 130–131; "The United States Public Health and Marine-Hospital Service, Part I—A Historical Sketch," p. 401. In a short note in the 1875 report, on p. vi, McClellan acknowledged Woodworth's contributions but portrayed himself as the primary author and heartily thanked Billings for preparing an extensive bibliography on cholera "which will be found to be one of the most valuable contributions to the literature of the century."

37. The Italian scientist Filippo Pacini published a paper in 1854 identifying the cholera bacteria—thirty years before Koch arrived at the same conclusion. But Pacini's work was ignored, and it was Koch's work that was widely noted and accepted.

38. Woodworth, *Cholera Epidemic of 1873*, pp. 8, 14–15.

39. Bruton, "National Board of Health," p. 45; Margaret Humphreys, *Yellow Fever and the South* (Baltimore: Johns Hopkins University Press, 1992), p. 62; John R. Pierce and Jim Writer, *Yellow Jack: How Yellow Fever Ravaged America and Walter Reed Discovered Its Deadly Secrets* (Hoboken, N.J.: John Wiley & Sons, 2005), p. 61.

40. Smillie, *Public Health,* p. 463; "The United States Public Health and Marine-Hospital Service, Part I—A Historical Sketch," p. 401.

41. Woodworth's proposal didn't get much traction with legislators and physicians in the North. One reason: cholera was the primary epidemic threat in the North, and many thought personal hygiene and community sanitation were at least as effective as quarantines in controlling that disease. Bruton, "National Board of Health," p. 55.

Woodworth also had friends in the administration. When President Rutherford B. Hayes took office in 1877, he appointed John Sherman as his treasury secretary (and Woodworth's boss). Sherman was the younger brother of the Union Army general with whom Woodworth had marched to the sea. Woodworth also was friends with the new vice president, William Almon Wheeler. Southern legislators chose to overlook Woodworth's Civil War association with the hated General Sherman, as noted by Williams in *The United States Public Health Service,* p. 82. The relationship with Wheeler is mentioned in S.V. White, "Dr. John B. Hamilton; Career of the Late Surgeon General of the Marine Hospital Service," *Washington Post,* February 26, 1899.

42. Pierce and Writer, *Yellow Jack,* pp. 63, 69.

43. The financial toll was estimated at $100 million. Bruton, "National Board of Health," pp. 115, 120–124.

44. Ibid., pp. 143–145, 149. Bruton quotes an article in the *Medical Times* of Philadelphia, published in early 1879, entitled "National Legislation in Regard to Public Hygiene."

45. John Duffy, *The Sanitarians: A History of American Public Health* (Urbana: University of Illinois Press, 1992), p. 167; Straus, *Medical Care for Seamen,* p. 94.

46. "A Noble Life Ended"; unsigned article, "Obituary—Surgeon-General Woodworth," *New York Times,* March 15, 1879.

47. Victoria A. Harden, *Inventing the NIH: Federal Biomedical Research Policy, 1887–1937* (Baltimore: Johns Hopkins University Press, 1986), p. 12; Furman, *A Profile of the United States Public Health Service,* p. 149.

48. Unsigned article, "Consigned to Earth; Funeral of the Late Dr. Woodworth Yesterday Afternoon," *The Washington Post,* March 17, 1879; Unsigned article, "Surgeon General Woodworth; The Funeral Yesterday at Le Droit Park," *The National Republican,* March 17, 1879.

49. John Shaw Billings to H.C. Meyer, December 22, 1880, Bess Furman Armstrong Papers, 1962–1969, MS C 202, folder: Verification File for Chapter Seven 1963–64, National Library of Medicine.

50. Unsigned article, "John B. Hamilton," U.S. Department of Health and Human Services' Office of the Surgeon General website, www.surgeongeneral. gov/about/previous/biohamilton.htm (accessed January 24, 2010); S.V. White, "Dr. John B. Hamilton: Career of the Late Surgeon General of the Marine

Hospital Service," *Washington Post,* Feb. 26, 1899. The article is a first-person recollection of Hamilton's life, written by a family friend.

51. White, "Dr. John B. Hamilton"; Shari Rudavsky, "Hamilton, John Brown," in *American National Biography,* Vol. 23 (New York: Oxford University Press, 1999), p. 923.

52. Furman, *A Profile of the United States Public Health Service,* pp. 158–159.

53. White, "Dr. John B. Hamilton."

54. Bruton, "National Board of Health," pp. 162–164.

55. Cabell also had been administrator of the five hundred–bed Confederate military hospital in Charlottesville, Virginia, during the Civil War. But it's not clear whether Cabell's war history contributed to the contentious nature of the Board of Health's relationship with Woodworth and Hamilton (both Union Army veterans). Recall that Billings, too, was a Union Army vet.

56. Humphreys, *Yellow Fever and the South,* p. 6; Furman, *A Profile of the United States Public Health Service,* pp. 160–161.

57. Furman, *A Profile of the United States Public Health Service,* pp. 163, 165–166.

58. That publication was a forerunner of today's *Morbidity and Mortality Weekly Report,* published by the U.S. Centers for Disease Control and Prevention.

59. W. G. Smillie, "The National Board of Health, 1879–1883," *American Journal of Public Health,* August 1943, Vol. 33, No. 8, p. 927.

60. Article in the *New York Herald,* July 29, 1879, quoted in Bruton, "National Board of Health," pp. 238, 239, 241.

61. Hamilton was a strong believer in quarantines. "It would fill more pages in this volume than are at the writer's disposal to give brief details or perhaps even to simply enumerate all the instances where observance of strict quarantine has apparently resulted in the escape from an epidemic elsewhere prevailing," Hamilton wrote in 1885. John B. Hamilton's article "The Practice of Quarantine," quoted in Edmund Charles Wendt, *A Treatise on Asiatic Cholera* (New York: William Wood & Company, 1885), p. 346. See pages 351–353 for Hamilton's narrative of the Brownsville cordon.

62. Smillie, "National Board of Health," p. 929; Bruton, "National Board of Health," p. 337; Furman, *A Profile of the United States Public Health Service,* p. 184; Humphreys, *Yellow Fever and the South,* p. 118.

63. Bruton, "National Board of Health," pp. 385–386.

64. Furman, *A Profile of the United States Public Health Service,* pp. 194–197; Harden, *Inventing the NIH,* pp. 11–13.

65. Straus, *Medical Care for Seamen,* p. 97; John B. Hamilton, *Annual Report of the Supervising Surgeon-General of the Marine-Hospital Service of the United States, for the fiscal year 1890* (Washington, D.C.: Government Printing Office, 1890), p. 77.

66. Laurence F. Schmeckebier, *The Public Health Service: Its History, Activities and Organization* (Baltimore: Johns Hopkins Press, 1923), p. 15; Humphreys, *Yellow Fever and the South,* p. 129; Hamilton, *Annual Report of the Supervising Surgeon-General,* 1890, pp. 27, 32.

67. Unsigned article, "Dr. Hamilton Resigns; Vacancy in the Surgeon Generalship of the Marine Hospital Corps," *Washington Post,* May 30, 1891; Unsigned article, "Dr. John B. Hamilton Dead," *New York Times,* December 25, 1898.

68. Furman says she got that account from long-retired Service officers. Furman, *A Profile of the United States Public Health Service,* p. 201.

69. Unsigned article, "Dr. J.B. Hamilton Resigns; Refuses to Submit to Transfer to San Francisco," *Washington Post,* October 15, 1896; "Dr. John B. Hamilton Dead."

70. Unsigned article, "Now Rests in Arlington: Body of Dr. John B. Hamilton Brought Here for Interment," *Washington Post,* February 26, 1899; Smillie, *Public Health,* p. 304.

71. As quoted in Furman, *A Profile of the United States Public Health Service,* p. 276.

72. United States Marine Hospital Service, *Revised Regulations for the Government of the United States Marine Hospital Service: Approved November 29, 1897* (Washington, D.C., Government Printing Office, 1897), pp. 31, 66–67, 78.

73. The story of the insane man and Wyman's trip to Washington is told in Walter Wyman, *A Cruise on the U.S. Practice Ship* Salmon P. Chase (New York: Grafton Press, 1910), pp. 3–6. He delivered the roustabout to the bluntly named Government Hospital for the Insane, later renamed St. Elizabeths.

74. Furman, *A Profile of the United States Public Health Service,* pp. 202, 206; Walter Wyman, *Book of Instructions for the Medical Inspection of Immigrants* (Washington, D.C., Government Printing Office, 1903), pp. 5–9, 12.

75. Howard Markel, *Quarantine! East European Jewish Immigrants and the New York City Epidemics of 1892* (Baltimore: Johns Hopkins University Press, 1997), pp. 15–16, 87, 97, 121–122.

76. Furman, *A Profile of the United States Public Health Service,* p. 213; J.W. Kerr, "Walter Wyman (1848–1911)," in Howard A. Kelly and Walter L. Burrage, *American Medical Biographies* (Baltimore: Norman Remington Company, 1920), p. 1275.

77. Walter Wyman, "Preventive Sanitation," *American Federationist,* July 1907, Vol. 14, No. 7, p. 471. Gompers, a towering figure in American labor history, was a founder of the American Federation of Labor and leader for worker solidarity and mutual aid.

78. Furman, *A Profile of the United States Public Health Service,* pp. 248–249. The salary information comes from Straus, *Medical Care for Seamen,* p. 97.

79. Marilyn Chase, *The Barbary Plague* (New York: Random House Trade Paperbacks, 2003), pp. 12–13, 16, 28; David Morens, Victoria Harden, Joseph Kinyoun Houts Jr., and Anthony Fauci, *The Indispensable Forgotten Man* (U.S. Department of Health and Human Services monograph, August 2012), p. 28.

80. Morens et al., *The Indispensable Forgotten Man,* p. 26.

81. Charles McClain, "Of Medicine, Race, and American Law: The Bubonic Plague Outbreak of 1900," *Law & Social Inquiry,* 1988, Vol. 13, No. 3, p. 473.

82. Chase, *The Barbary Plague,* pp. 29, 47–49, 62, 71. As Chase explains, the so-called Haffkine vaccine provided only short-lived protection to people who got a dose before exposure to plague, and could actually accelerate the bacteria's attack if given to people who were already infected. "With such risks widely known, the vaccine was violently unpopular in Chinatown," Chase writes.

83. Ibid., pp. 60, 68–70, 72; The Jew Ho case—famous in the field of public health law—is summarized and excerpted in Lawrence O. Gostin, *Public Health Law and Ethics: A Reader* (Berkeley: University of California Press, 2002), pp. 217–219.

84. Furman, *A Profile of the United States Public Health Service,* pp. 247; Chase, *The Barbary Plague,* pp. 86–87, 89, 92. Kinyoun resigned from the service in anger after the transfer to Detroit.

85. Wyman has his defenders, including Richard Carmona, who was surgeon general from 2002 to 2006 and has spoken repeatedly about the political meddling surgeons general have had to endure. Carmona describes Wyman as someone who carried the banner of science against political forces in California, and in the process was labeled a heretic by those critics. Richard Carmona, "The Trauma of Politics: A Surgeon General's Perspective," *American Journal of Preventive Medicine,* December 2013, Vol. 45, No. 6, pp. 742–744.

86. Furman, *A Profile of the United States Public Health Service,* pp. 276, 279; Smillie, *Public Health,* p. 468. The Children's Bureau was created in 1912, first placed under the Department of Commerce and then made an agency within the Department of Labor. A precursor to the Social Security Administration, it was folded into the SSA in 1946.

87. Unsigned article, "Walter Wyman Dead; Surgeon General of Public Health and Marine Hospital Service," *New York Times,* November 21, 1911; Kerr, "Walter Wyman (1848–1911)," p. 1276. Marilyn Chase tells a detailed but unattributed story about Wyman's demise, saying his razor slipped while he was shaving around his mustache, and his diabetes-impaired vascular system was unable to prevent a gangrenous infection from setting in. Chase, *The Barbary Plague,* p. 200.

CHAPTER 3

1. Chase, *The Barbary Plague,* pp. 200–201.

2. Alan M. Kraut, *Goldberger's War: The Life and Work of a Public Health Crusader* (New York: Hill & Wang, 2003), p. 85.

3. That it was on MacVeagh's advice comes from Furman, *A Profile of the United States Public Health Service,* p. 283; unsigned article, "Blue to Succeed Wyman," *Washington Post,* January 6, 1912.

4. The passage and its swooning style was noted by Marilyn Chase, *The Barbary Plague,* pp. 178–179 (quoting Pauline Jacobson, "Specialist Not Blue over the Plague," *San Francisco Bulletin,* February 21, 1908).

5. John M. Barry, *The Great Influenza: The Epic Story of the Deadliest Plague in History* (New York: Viking, 2004), p. 308. The U.S. Navy's Cary Grayson, former AMA president William Henry Welch, and medical education

reformer Victor Vaughan were among the distinguished physicians who held this opinion, according to Barry. Chase, meanwhile, wrote that some doctors in San Francisco thought of Blue as little more than a public relations man. Among them was the distinguished University of California medical school professor Robert Langley Porter. He is quoted in Chase, *The Barbary Plague*, p. 179.

6. Several sources—including the U.S. Department of Health and Human Services' official biography of Blue—say he was born in 1868. But his death certificate says 1867, as does Furman, *A Profile of the United States Public Health Service*. The death certificate can be downloaded from the website Ancestry.com, South Carolina Death Records, 1821–1955 database. http://search.ancestry.com/cgi-bin/sse.dll?h=619099&db=SCDeath&indiv=1 (accessed March 21, 2010.)

7. Chase, *The Barbary Plague*, p. 37. Victor Blue went on to become a rear admiral in the navy, according to Furman, *A Profile of the United States Public Health Service*, p. 283.

8. Chase, *The Barbary Plague*, pp. 41, 102.

9. Ibid., pp. 111, 170–171, 174–177. Chase notes that not only was Rucker a better speaker but he also helped write Blue's speeches and articles. Rucker also regularly dined and drank with Blue and saw his friend through moments of depression. See also Marcos Cueto, *The Value of Health: A History of the Pan American Health Organization* (Washington, D.C.: Pan American Health Organization, 2006), p. 41.

10. Furman, *A Profile of the United States Public Health Service*, pp. 283, 286; Robert Bruere, "Uncle Sam's Plague Killer," *Hearst's Magazine*, January 1913, Vol. 23. No. 1, pp. 108–109.

11. Ibid., p. 288; Rupert Blue, *Annual Report of the Surgeon General of the Public Health Service of the United States, for the fiscal year 1913* (Washington, D.C.: Government Printing Office, 1914), pp. 261, 279.

12. Blue, *Annual Report of the Surgeon General, fiscal year 1913*, pp. 261, 269–270, 279–280.

13. Ibid., p. 252; unsigned article, "100,000 Cases of Pellagra; Surgeon General Blue's Estimate of the Possible Number," *New York Times*, October 15, 1915. The description of pellagra's symptoms comes from Kraut, *Goldberger's War*, pp. 4–5, 99–100. Some references, however, say pellagra was first reported in the United States as early as 1902.

14. Furman, *A Profile of the United States Public Health Service*, pp. 302–304; Kraut, *Goldberger's War*, pp. 170, 270; Hilary Spurling, *Pearl Buck in China* (New York: Simon & Schuster, 2010), pp. 70, 74; Sydenstricker's low-key personality is also described in an unsigned editorial marking his death entitled "Edgar Sydenstricker," *American Journal of Public Health*, May 1936, Vol. 26, No.5, pp. 526–527.

15. Jaap Kooijman, . . . *And the Pursuit of National Health* (Amsterdam: Rodopi B.V., 1999), p. 24; Daniel S. Hirshfield, *The Lost Reform: The Campaign for Compulsory Health Insurance in the United States from 1932 to 1943* (Cambridge, Mass.: Harvard University Press, 1970), p. 17.

16. Hirshfield, *The Lost Reform*, p. 35.

17. Chase, *The Barbary Plague*, p. 209.

18. Duffy, *The Sanitarians*, p. 246 (quoting from a transcript of Blue's comments that appeared in the *Journal of the American Medical Association* in 1916).

19. Alan Derickson, *Health Security for All: Dreams of Universal Health Care in America* (Baltimore: Johns Hopkins University Press, 2005), pp. 13, 29, 73; Beatrix Hoffman, "Health Care Reform and Social Movements in the United States," *American Journal of Public Health,* January 2003, Vol. 93, No. 1, pp. 75–85.

20. Furman, *A Profile of the United States Public Health Service*, p. 312.

21. Ralph Chester Williams, *The United States Public Health Service, 1798–1950* (Richmond, Va.: Whittet & Shepperson, 1951) pp. 561–562. Williams notes a 1921 attorney general opinion which concluded that Congress, not the president, holds the power to create a military force out of a civilian force. Furman, *A Profile of the United States Public Health Service*, p. 314; Rupert Blue, *Annual Report of the Surgeon General of the Public Health Service of the United States, for the fiscal year 1918* (Washington, D.C.: Government Printing Office, 1918), p. 304.

Faced with the loss of manpower, Blue cut back the Service's work on water pollution and other projects. He also pushed for creation of a Reserve Officer Corps in the Public Health Service to garner more personnel, and got his wish. The Senate passed the bill in June 1917, but the House did not sign off until late October 1918, just two weeks before the war ended. See Williams, *The United States Public Health Service*, p. 562.

22. William L. Silber, *When Washington Shut Down Wall Street: The Great Financial Crisis of 1914 and the Origins of America's Monetary Supremacy* (Princeton: Princeton University Press, 2007), pp. 11–14; Furman, *A Profile of the United States Public Health Service*, p. 319.

23. Williams, *The United States Public Health Service*, p. 579.

24. Furman, *A Profile of the United States Public Health Service*, p. 328.

25. Mullan, *Plagues and Politics*, p. 75; Furman, *A Profile of the United States Public Health Service*, p. 319.

26. That made it much faster than the so-called Russian flu pandemic of 1889–1992, which occurred in three waves that unfolded over nearly three years. See Jeffrey Taubenberger and David Morens, "1918 Influenza: The Mother of All Pandemics," *Emerging Infectious Diseases,* January 2006, Vol. 12, No. 6, pp. 15–22. Common estimates put the toll from that pandemic at 1 million worldwide, or just a small fraction of the deaths from the 1918–1919 pandemic.

27. Barry, *The Great Influenza*, pp. 94, 173–174, 310. Barry wrote that some other leading figures in medicine were much more alarmed and were intent on gathering intelligence on the new disease, such as Army Surgeon General William Gorgas and William Henry Welch, the founding dean of the Johns Hopkins School of Hygiene and Public Health. They and others faulted Blue for gathering little information about the flu as it was striking Europe, prior to its jump to the United States. In July 1918, Blue turned down a $10,000 funding request from his Hygienic Laboratory director, George McCoy, to do pneumonia research related to the flu outbreaks.

28. Susan Dominus, "In 1918 Flu Outbreak, a Cool Head Prevailed," *New York Times*, April 30, 2009. Copeland was a Tammany Hall appointee with no medical degree. He would go on to become a U.S. senator.

29. Laura Stephenson Carter, "Cold Comfort," *Dartmouth Medicine*, Winter 2006, p. 36; unsigned article, "Spanish Influenza Much Like Grippe," *New York Times*, September 22, 1918. Dover's powder, popular at the dawn of the twentieth century, contained opium and ipecac and induced sweating—as well as addiction in many patients.

30. Furman, *A Profile of the United States Public Health Service*, p. 327.

31. Duffy, *The Sanitarians*, p. 244; Alfred W. Crosby, *America's Forgotten Pandemic* (Cambridge: Cambridge University Press, 1989), p. 49; Williams, *The United States Public Health Service*, p. 598.

John Barry, in *The Great Influenza*, judges Blue more harshly. He argues that Blue—like Copeland—was passive about the pandemic until bodies were literally piling up in the street. He faults Blue for not instructing his quarantine stations to inspect ships for influenza until September 13, four days after newspapers reported a deluge of flu patients at Boston harbor hospitals. Barry also says Blue did not take concrete steps to gather national flu surveillance until September 18. Writing of Blue's September 13 circular to quarantine stations, Barry judges that it "indicated how little Blue had done—in fact he had done nothing—to prepare the Public Health Service, much less the country, for any onslaught." See Barry, *The Great Influenza*, pp. 310, 312–313. However, some other historians consider some of Barry's criticisms are unfair given the war, the evolving understanding of the epidemic, and other circumstances.

32. Quoted in Crosby, *America's Forgotten Pandemic*, p. 314.

33. Ibid., pp. 328–329; Chase, *The Barbary Plague*, p. 209; Harden, *Inventing the NIH*, p. 42.

34. Furman, *A Profile of the United States Public Health Service*, pp. 328, 330–331.

35. Chase, *The Barbary Plague*, p. 205; Blue's death certificate, downloaded from Ancestry.com, South Carolina Death Records, 1821–1955 database, http://search.ancestry.com/cgi-bin/sse.dll?h=619099&db=SCDeath&indiv=1 (accessed March 21, 2010). The document says his lungs were congested, but as to the official cause of death, the handwriting of the doctor who signed the death certificate is hard to make out.

36. Unsigned article, "Medicine: Too Much Smallpox," *Time*, Monday, December 17, 1928.

37. Bess Furman, *Washington Byline: The Personal History of a Newspaperwoman* (New York: Alfred A. Knopf, 1949), p. 76.

38. Hugh S. Cumming memoirs, Volume I, 6th folder, pp. 1, 2, 6, 8–10.

39. The U.S. eugenics movement's popularity dimmed in the 1930s when the Great Depression showed bluebloods were not immune to economic ruin. The decline accelerated in the 1940s, as some of the key leaders of the U.S. eugenics movement died off and as the horror of the German holocaust—based on the Nazi eugenics-based ideal of a "master race"—became clear.

40. Gregory Michael Dorr, *Segregation's Science: Eugenics and Society in Virginia* (Charlottesville: University of Virginia Press, 2008), pp. 36, 42; Paul A.

Lombardo and Gregory M. Dorr, "Eugenics, Medical Education, and the Public Health Service: Another Perspective on the Tuskegee Syphilis Experiment," *Bulletin of the History of Medicine,* Summer 2006, Vol. 80, No. 2, pp. 296–297, 303; Hugh S. Cumming memoirs, Volume 1, 6th folder, pp. 13–14.

41. Furman, *A Profile of the United States Public Health Service,* p. 335.

42. I viewed Lucy Booth Cumming's wedding photograph on the Ancestry.com website; Hugh S. Cumming memoirs, Volume 1, 6th folder, p. 17. Cumming met Lucy while accompanying his brother, Gordon, to the Booth home. Gordon Cumming was courting one of Lucy's relatives.

43. Cumming chose to minimize a bout of typhoid fever he'd had as a teen that sickened him for several months. Furman, *A Profile of the United States Public Health Service,* pp. 337–338; Williams, *The United States Public Health Service,* p. 482; Hugh S. Cumming memoirs, Volume 1, 6th folder, p. 10.

44. Furman, *A Profile of the United States Public Health Service,* pp. 330–331, 337–338.

45. Hugh S. Cumming memoirs, Volume I, 7th folder, pp. 210–211.

46. The growth in beds from October 1919 to December 1920 comes from an unsigned article, "Soldier Hospitals Filled," *New York Times,* December 12, 1920. Cumming's "flimsy and inflammable" description and estimate of how many beds were in unsafe structures comes from an unsigned article (apparently an editorial), "Hospital Care of War Veterans," *New York Times,* February 5, 1921. Furman, *A Profile of the United States Public Health Service,* p. 332.

47. Furman, *A Profile of the United States Public Health Service,* p. 342.

48. Unsigned article, "History of the Department of Veterans Affairs—Part 2," from the U.S. Department of Veterans Affairs website, http://www1.va.gov/opa/feature/history/history2.asp (accessed March 21, 2010); unsigned article, "Charles Forbes," Ohio Historical Society website, http://www.ohiohistorycentral.org/entry.php?rec=3034&nm=Charles-Forbes (accessed March 21, 2010); Furman, *A Profile of the United States Public Health Service,* pp. 342–346.

49. Hugh S. Cumming memoirs, Volume I, 7th folder, p. 267. The Forbes fraud was one of several scandals during Harding's short, pitiful administration. The most famous was the Teapot Dome affair, in which Secretary of the Interior Albert B. Fall was convicted of accepting bribes and illegal personal loans in exchange for leasing public oil fields to business associates.

50. Paul de Kruif, *Men Against Death* (New York: Harcourt Brace & Company, 1932).

51. Hugh S. Cumming memoirs, Volume I, 7th folder, pp. 269, 296.

52. Ibid., p. 248; unsigned article, "Dr. Cumming Urges Air Health Rules," *New York Times,* May 31, 1930.

53. As quoted in Allan M. Brandt, *The Cigarette Century: The Rise, Fall, and Deadly Persistence of the Product That Defined America* (New York: Basic Books, 2007), p. 59.

54. Cassandra Tate, *Cigarette Wars: The Triumph of "The Little White Slaver"* (New York: Oxford University Press, 1999), p. 114; John C. Burnham, "American Physicians and Tobacco Use: Two Surgeons General, 1929 and 1964," *Bulletin of the History of Medicine,* Spring 1989, Vol. 63, pp. 1–31;

Lawrence K. Altman, "Leroy Burney, 91, Early Critic of Cigarette Smoking," *New York Times,* August 4, 1998; Brandt, *The Cigarette Century,* p. 59.

55. Jamie Lincoln Kitman, "The Secret History of Lead," *The Nation,* March 20, 2000, http://www.thenation.com/doc/20000320/kitman/print (accessed March 11, 2010); Christian Warren, *Brush With Death: A Social History of Lead Poisoning* (Baltimore: Johns Hopkins University Press, 2000), pp. 116–129.

56. The Bureau of Mines agreed to an array of unusual conditions, including a press blackout and the pledge that it would submit the research results to GM for comment and criticism. See David Rosner and Gerald Markowitz, "A 'Gift of God?': The Public Health Controversy over Leaded Gasoline during the 1920s," *American Journal of Public Health,* April 1985, Vol. 75, No. 4, p. 345.

57. Unsigned article, "To End Sale Today of Leaded Gasoline," *New York Times,* May 5, 1925; Warren, *Brush With Death,* pp. 118–119; Rosner and Markowitz, "A 'Gift of God?'" p. 347.

58. Hugh S. Cumming memoirs, Volume I, 8th folder, p. 307.

59. Unsigned article, "Report No Danger in Ethyl Gasoline," *New York Times,* January 20, 1926; Warren, *Brush With Death,* p. 128.

60. Rosner and Markowitz, "A 'Gift of God?'" p. 349.

61. Environmental Protection Agency press release, "EPA Takes Final Step in Phaseout of Leaded Gasoline," January 29, 1996; Kitman, "The Secret History of Lead"; Harold M. Schmeck Jr., "Leaded Gasoline Is Termed a Peril," *New York Times,* June 9, 1966; Rogert C. Ziegenfus, "Air Quality and Health," in *Public Health and the Environment: The United States Experience,* ed. Michael R. Greenberg (New York, Guilford Press, 1987), pp. 148–149.

62. Prominent among those researchers is Richard Nevin. See John Pekkanen, "Why Is Lead Still Poisoning Our Children?" *Washingtonian Magazine,* August 2006.

63. Tom Hatfield, interview with the author, July 20, 2012.

64. The "syphilis-soaked race" notion comes from a physician named Baldwin Luche, as quoted in James H. Jones, *Bad Blood: The Tuskegee Syphilis Experiment* (New York: Free Press, 1981), p. 27.

65. John Parascandola, *Sex, Sin, and Science: A History of Syphilis in America* (Westport, Conn.: Praeger, 2008), p. 37.

66. Hugh S. Cumming memoirs, Volume I, 9th folder, p. 564.

67. Lombardo and Dorr, "Eugenics, Medical Education, and the Public Health Service," p. 310; unsigned article, "Glass Cage for Leper at His Trial Offered," *Washington Post,* December 16, 1923.

68. Susan M. Reverby, *Examining Tuskegee: The Infamous Syphilis Study and Its Legacy* (Chapel Hill: University of North Carolina Press, 2009), pp. 35, 39; Allan M. Brandt, "Racism and Research: The Case of the Tuskegee Syphilis Experiment," republished in *Tuskegee's Truths: Rethinking the Tuskegee Syphilis Study,* ed. Susan Reverby (Chapel Hill: University of North Carolina Press, 2000), p. 18.

69. H.S. Cumming, "September 20, 1932 letter to Dr. R.R. Moton, Tuskegee Institute," republished in *Tuskegee's Truths,* p. 77.

70. Jones, *Bad Blood*, p. 154; Benjamin Roy, "The Tuskegee Syphilis Experiment: Biotechnology and the Administrative State," republished in *Tuskegee's Truths*, p. 302.

71. Furman, *A Profile of the United States Public Health Service*, p. 362; unsigned article, "Mrs. Hoover Escapes Death in Auto Crash," *Washington Post*, March 18, 1928.

72. Oliver McKee Jr., "He Watches over the Nation's Health," *New York Times*, June 10, 1928.

73. Hugh S. Cumming, "The Relations of the Physician to Public Health," *Journal of the American Medical Association*, July 2, 1927, Vol. 89. No. 1, pp. 6–7; Ronald Hamowy, *Government and Public Health in America* (Northampton, Mass.: Edward Elgar, 2007), pp. 38–39.

74. Associated Press, "Hears Dr. Cumming Is Likely to Resign," *New York Times*, November 19, 1934; Furman, *A Profile of the United States Public Health Service*, pp. 370, 378–379; Warren Palmer Dearing, oral history interview with Fitzhugh Mullan, October 21, 1988, transcript p. 7, National Library of Medicine.

75. Kooijman, . . . *And the Pursuit of National Health*, p. 8; Furman, *A Profile of the United States Public Health Service*, p. 386.

76. Hugh S. Cumming memoirs, Volume I, 9th folder, pp. 554, 568–569.

77. Unsigned article, "Work of Dr. Cumming Praised by President," *New York Times*, January 29, 1936.

78. Hugh S. Cumming Sr. to Hugh Cumming Jr., May 12, 1939, Albert and Shirley Small Special Collections Library, University of Virginia, accession no. 6922, box 4, pp. 1–2.

79. Associated Press, "Dr. Hugh Cumming, Health leader, 79," *New York Times*, December 21, 1948.

CHAPTER 4

1. Parran's height and weight, as well as the description of him as a bogey-man to organized medicine, come from Alden Whitmen, "A Dynamic Fighter," *New York Times*, February 17, 1968.

2. Roy K. Flannagan, M.D., to Dr. Thomas Parran, February 26, 1938, copy from file 269, Thomas Parran Papers, University of Pittsburgh Archives.

3. Joseph V. Deporte to Dr. Thomas Parran, February 18, 1938, copy from file 269, Thomas Parran Papers, University of Pittsburgh Archives.

4. Louis Ludlow to Dr. Thomas Parran, March 2, 1939, copy from file 269, Thomas Parran Papers, University of Pittsburgh Archives.

5. Whitmen, "A Dynamic Fighter"; unsigned article, "Parran, Thomas (1860–1955)," Biographic Director of the United States Congress website, http://bioguide.congress.gov/scripts/biodisplay.pl?index=P000077 (accessed April 5, 2010); Lynne Page Snyder, "Thomas J. Parran, Jr. (1892–1968)," in *Doctors, Nurses, and Medical Practitioners: A Bio-Bibliographical Sourcebook*, ed. Lois N. Magner (Westport, Conn.: Greenwood Press, 1997), p. 209; Reminiscences of Thomas Parran (an oral history conducted by Harlan B. Phillips for the University of Pittsburgh), July 16 and 18, 1962, transcript p. 7, Columbia Center for Oral History.

6. Unsigned article, "Medicine: Great Pox," *Time*, October 26, 1936; Reminiscences of Thomas Parran, pp. 2–3.

7. Snyder, "Thomas J. Parran, Jr. (1892–1968)," p. 209; Furman, *A Profile of the United States Public Health Service*, p. 393.

8. Snyder, "Thomas J. Parran, Jr. (1892–1968)," pp. 209–210; Reminiscences of Thomas Parran, pp. 16, 45.

9. Parascandola, *Sex, Sin, and Science*, pp. 69, 71.

10. Ibid., p. 72; Allan M. Brandt, *No Magic Bullet: A Social History of Venereal Disease in the United States Since 1880* (New York: Oxford University Press, 1987), p. 125; Reminiscences of Thomas Parran, p. 76.

11. Furman, *A Profile of the United States Public Health Service*, p. 393.

12. Parascandola, *Sex, Sin, and Science*, pp. 92–93; Snyder, "Thomas J. Parran, Jr. (1892–1968)," p. 210; Reminiscences of Thomas Parran, p. 77.

13. Parascandola, *Sex, Sin, and Science*, p. 84.

14. Furman, *A Profile of the United States Public Health Service*, p. 393.

15. Ibid.; Kooijman, *. . . And the Pursuit of National Health*, p. 100.

16. Snyder, "Thomas J. Parran, Jr. (1892–1968)," pp. 210–211. The story of Parran's CBS radio address is told in several books and articles, and the details sometimes vary in the telling. My account draws mainly from Furman, *A Profile of the United States Public Health Service*, pp. 398–399.

17. Furman, *A Profile of the United States Public Health Service*, p. 399.

18. Theodore Rosebury, *Microbes and Morals: The Strange Story of Venereal Disease* (New York: Viking Press, 1971), pp. 129, 259.

19. Reminiscences of Thomas Parran, p. 90; Duffy, *The Sanitarians*, pp. 258–259; Snyder, "Thomas J. Parran, Jr. (1892–1968)," p. 211; Thomas Parran, *Shadow on the Land*, educational ed. (New York: American Social Hygiene Association, 1937), p. 260.

20. Brandt, *No Magic Bullet*, pp. 138–139, 141; Alexandra M. Lord, *Condom Nation: The U.S. Government's Sex Education from World War I to the Internet* (Baltimore: Johns Hopkins University Press, 2010), p. 53.

21. Parran speaking about Columbus, quoted in Rosebury, *Microbes and Morals*, p. 150. "He began to hear voices and to regard himself as 'ambassador of God,'" Parran said, seeing signs of syphilis-spurred madness in the famous explorer. The theory that Columbus and his crew introduced syphilis to Europe has been debated through the decades, but has been supported by several studies. See Charles Q. Choi, "Case Closed? Columbus Introduced Syphilis to Europe," *Scientific American*, December 27, 2011, http://www.scientificamerican.com/article?id=case-closed-columbus (accessed May 13, 2013).

22. Parran, *Shadow on the Land*, pp., 293–294. Among other places, human-figure illustrations can be seen on p. 146 and the page facing 248.

23. The Man of the Year and finalists were announced in the unsigned article "Generalissimo and Madame Chiang Kai-Shek," *Time*, January 3, 1938.

24. Unsigned article, "Medicine: Great Pox," *Time*, October 26, 1936; Brandt, *No Magic Bullet*, p. 141.

25. Lord, *Condom Nation*, p. 69.

26. Brandt, *No Magic Bullet*, pp. 150, 170; Theodore Rosebury, *Microbes and Morals*, pp. 217, 260.

Parran also led a successful campaign to make the prevention of pneumonia deaths a national priority. For a detailed account, see Scott H. Podolsky, *Pneumonia before Antibiotics* (Baltimore: Johns Hopkins University Press, 2006).

27. Allan M. Brandt, "Racism and Research: The Case of the Tuskegee Syphilis Study," *Hastings Center Report,* December 1978, Vol. 8, No. 6, pp. 26–27.

28. Parran's November 4, 1943, letter to the Milbank Fund's Catherine A. Doran is quoted in Reverby, *Examining Tuskegee,* p. 62.

29. Parascandola, *Sex, Sin, and Science,* pp. 120–121.

30. John Parascandola, "Quarantining Women: Venereal Disease Rapid Treatment Centers in World War II America," *Bulletin of the History of Medicine,* Fall 2009, Vol. 83, No. 3, pp. 434, 438, 442, 454.

31. Reminiscences of Thomas Parran, pp. 68, 79; Brandt, *No Magic Bullet,* pp. 155–156, 168.

32. John Douglas, comments at National STD Prevention Conference Press Briefing, March 9, 2010 (notes in the author's possession); John Douglas, clarifying comments in an e-mail from CDC press officer Scott Bryan to the author, April 14, 2010. At the time, Douglas was CDC's director of sexually transmitted disease prevention.

33. Mike Stobbe, "Shocking New Details of US STD Experiments in Guatemala," Associated Press wire, August 29, 2011; Susan M. Reverby, "'Normal Exposure' and Inoculation Syphilis: A PHS 'Tuskegee' Doctor in Guatemala, 1946–1948," *Journal of Policy History,* January 2011, Vol. 23, No. 1, p. 19; Presidential Commission for the Study of Bioethical Issues, "'Ethically Impossible' STD Research in Guatemala from 1946 to 1948" (report released September 13, 2011), p. 41, http://bioethics.gov/node/654.

34. Furman, *A Profile of the United States Public Health Service,* pp. 411–414.

The surgeon general also helped initiate a nutrition campaign in 1941 to benefit both the military and the public. That campaign included pushing millers to enrich flour with niacin and thiamine—a measure the War Food Administration mandated in 1943. Flour enrichment was one of the major steps that finally put an end to the pellagra scourge identified by Joseph Goldberger and Service officers about thirty years earlier. See Kraut, *Goldberger's War,* pp. 260–261.

35. Louis Fiset, "Public Health in World War II Assembly Centers for Japanese Americans," *Bulletin of the History of Medicine,* Winter 1999, Vol. 73, No. 4, pp. 565–566.

36. Ibid., pp. 577, 582.

37. Parascandola, *Sex, Sin, and Science,* p. 101; Reminiscences of Thomas Parran, p. 83. There was at least one early example of tension between Parran and his FSA bosses. The surgeon general was rebuked in 1941 by Miller's predecessor Paul McNutt when Parran criticized the military for not doing enough to protect soldiers from venereal disease.

38. The law was the Public Health Service Act of July 1, 1944.

39. Elizabeth W. Etheridge, *Sentinel for Health: A History of the Centers for Disease Control* (Berkeley: University of California Press, 1992), pp. 4, 12, 16.

The CDC has since changed its name but kept its initials. Today, CDC stands for Centers for Disease Control and Prevention.

40. Snyder, "Thomas J. Parran, Jr. (1892–1968)," p. 213; Furman, *A Profile of the United States Public Health Service,* pp. 398, 452–453. Furman reported that Hugh Cumming, who was director of the Pan American Sanitary Bureau after his retirement as surgeon general, fought Parran's plan and tried to keep the organization independent of the WHO.

41. Parascandola, *Sex, Sin, and Science,* pp. 109–110. A thirteen-and-a-half-minute version of the film can be seen on YouTube, at http://www.youtube.com/watch?v=bumooJ_oib8 (accessed April 12, 2010). Parascandola said one version emphasized using prophylaxis and showed male genitalia and condoms, but the YouTube version is an edited one made for mixed audiences.

42. The film can be downloaded—for a fee—from the website http:///www.ameibo.com (accessed April 14, 2010). In Mitchum's scene, he is grumbling to a character played by a young actor named Noah Beery Jr., who would enjoy a long film career before playing James Garner's father for years on the 1970s TV show *The Rockford Files.* The film also starred noted Hollywood actor Jean Hersholt. It was directed by Arthur Lubin, who directed a series of Abbott and Costello movies around that time.

43. Parascandola, *Sex, Sin, and Science,* pp. 113–115.

44. Leroy E. Burney, oral history interview with Fitzhugh Mullan, October 17, 1988, transcript p. 15, National Library of Medicine.

45. Parascandola, *Sex, Sin, and Science,* p. 114. Parran's comments at the end of the film were specifically added in response to Legion of Decency criticisms. John Parascandola, e-mail to the author, September 26, 2013.

46. Morris Fishbein, *Morris Fishbein, M.D.: An Autobiography* (Garden City, N.Y.: Doubleday, 1969), pp. 202–203.

47. Kooijman, . . . *And the Pursuit of National Health,* pp. 38, 100; Derickson, *Health Security for All,* p. 60.

48. Speech at Georgetown University, June 1, 1939, quoted in Podolsky, *Pneumonia before Antibiotics,* pp. 77, 200. Podolsky reports finding among archival materials other prepared comments from Parran that contained similar wording.

49. Kooijman, . . . *And the Pursuit of National Health,* p. 54; Derickson, *Health Security for All,* p. 66.

50. Monte M. Poen, *Harry Truman versus the Medical Lobby* (Columbia: University of Missouri Press, 1979), p. 19; Derickson, *Health Security for All,* p. 80.

51. As quoted in Derickson, *Health Security for All,* p. 82.

52. Unsigned article, "Federal Officials Back Health Bill," *New York Times,* June 3, 1939; Derickson, *Health Security for All,* pp. 81, 85.

53. Kooijman, . . . *And the Pursuit of National Health,* p. 98.

54. Ibid., pp. 100–101; Hirshfield, *The Lost Reform,* pp. 141–143.

55. Truman quoted in David Blumenthal and James A. Morone, *The Heart of Power: Health and Politics in the Oval Office* (Berkeley: University of California Press, 2009), p. 67.

56. Kooijman, . . . *And the Pursuit of National Health,* pp. 113–114.

57. Unsigned article, "Doctors Censure Surgeon General," *New York Times,* December 12, 1946.

58. Poen, *Harry Truman versus the Medical Lobby,* pp. 103–104.

59. Warren Palmer Dearing, oral history interview, transcript p. 15.

60. Derickson, *Health Security for All,* p. 108.

61. Oscar R. Ewing, oral history interview with J.R. Fuchs, May 1, 1969, pp. 201–202, electronic copy from the Harry S. Truman Library & Museum, Independence, Mo. The expanding National Institute of Health was renamed the National Institutes of Health in 1948.

62. Ibid., p. 204.

63. Unsigned article, "Parran Removal, Job Nature Linked," *New York Times,* February 14, 1948.

64. Unsigned editorial, "Dr. Parran's Retirement," *New York Times,* February 14, 1948.

65. Warren Palmer Dearing, oral history, p. 14.

66. Unsigned article, "Milestones: Feb. 23, 1868," *Time,* February 23, 1968.

67. Chang Lee, February 26, 2013, posting on ASTDA website's Thomas Parran discussion board, http://www.atsda.org/news-calendar/home-2.html (accessed May 14, 2013).

68. Bradley Stoner, president of the ASTDA, in a May 16, 2013, e-mail to the author.

69. Khalil Ghanem, February 26, 2013, posting on ASTDA website's Thomas Parran discussion board, http://www.atsda.org/news-calendar/home-2 .html (accessed May 14, 2013).

CHAPTER 5

1. Stephen P. Strickland, *Politics, Science, and Dread Disease* (Cambridge, Mass.: Harvard University Press, 1972), p. 99. Strickland's statement, made in 1972, proved premature. C. Everett Koop, surgeon general in the 1980s, enjoyed an influential eight years in office.

2. Parran is described as a friend of FDR's by several sources, including the unsigned article "Medicine: Venereal Disease Campaign," *Time,* January 11, 1937. The article says Roosevelt was "egged on" to writing an open letter to a venereal disease conference by his longtime friend and subordinate, Dr. Thomas Parran Jr. But FDR's social calendars indicate Parran was not exactly a weekly presence at the White House. From 1936 to 1943, Parran was invited to five teas, five luncheons, three dinners, and four receptions at the White House, according to the Records of the Chief of the Office of Social Entertainments, as reported by Alycia Vivona, archivist at the Franklin D. Roosevelt Presidential Library, in a February 24, 2011, e-mail to the author.

3. Jon M. Harkness, "Scheele, Leonard A.," in *American National Biography,* Volume 19 (Oxford: Oxford University Press, 1999), p. 363.

4. CDC National Center for Health Statistics, "Leading Causes of Death, 1900–1998," http://www.cdc.gov/nchs/data/dvs/lead1900_98.pdf (accessed May 20, 2013).

5. The National Cancer Institute had been created just one year earlier, in 1938, in a piece of New Deal legislation. U.S. Department of Health and Human Services, "Leonard Andrew Scheele (1948–1956)," HHS website on the history of the Office of the Surgeon General, http://www.surgeongeneral.gov/about /previous/bioscheele.htm (accessed December 29, 2005); Harkness, "Scheele, Leonard A.," p. 363.

6. Peter Schoenke, "Obituaries: Leonard A. Scheele, MD," *Journal of the American Medical Association*, December 8, 1993, Vol. 270, No. 22, p. 2749; Reminiscences of Leonard Scheele, oral history interview by Thomas F. Hogan, October 16, 1967, transcript p. 3.

7. John Gunther, *Taken at the Flood: The Story of Albert D. Lasker* (New York: Harper & Brothers, 1960), pp. 25, 169, 181, 239, 322–323. Neen Hunt, "Mary Woodard Lasker: First Lady of Medical Research," presentation at the National Library of Medicine, December 13, 2007, transcript available on Lasker Foundation website, www.laskerfoundation.org/media/firstlady.htm (accessed March 12, 2011). After Albert died in 1952, Mary Lasker became a powerful solo act.

8. The American Society for the Control of Cancer was founded in 1913 in New York City by fifteen doctors and businessmen for the purpose of raising cancer awareness. For decades it was a small organization, spending nothing on research; it had a thousand members and a $102,000 budget around the time the Laskers became involved. They raised millions and, in 1944, engineered the renaming of the organization as the American Cancer Society. See unsigned article, "The Mary Lasker Papers," in National Library of Medicine, *Profiles in Science*, http://profiles.nlm.nih.gov/ps/retrieve/Narrative/TL/p-nid/2–1 (accessed May 15, 2013).

9. Gunther, *Taken at the Flood*, p. 331; Furman, *A Profile of the United States Public Health Service*, pp. 460–461; Strickland, *Politics, Science, and Dread Disease*, pp. 52–53.

10. Reminiscences of Leonard Scheele, pp. 31, 34, Columbia Center for Oral History Collection; the author obtained a copy of this interview from the Dwight D. Eisenhower Library.

11. John A. Kastor, *The National Institutes of Health, 1991–2008* (Oxford: Oxford University Press, 2010), p. 161.

12. Reminiscences of Leonard Scheele, pp. 34–35.

13. Berton Roueché, "The Fog," *The New Yorker*, September 30, 1950, reprinted in Roueché, *Eleven Blue Men* (New York: Berkeley Medallion Books, 1966), p. 175.

14. Unsigned article, "Steel Company Pays $235,000 to Settle $4,643,000 in Donora Smog Death Suits," *New York Times*, April 18, 1951; Michael R. Greenberg, ed., *Public Health and the Environment: The United States Experience* (New York: Guilford Press, 1987), p. 140; unsigned article, "Book Notices—Air Pollution in Donora, Pa.: Epidemiology of the Unusual Smog Episode of October 1948; Preliminary Report," *Journal of the American Medical Association*, May 20, 1950, Vol. 143, No. 3, p. 323.

15. Peter C. Yeager, *The Limits of Law: The Public Regulation of Private Pollution* (Cambridge: Cambridge University Press, 1991), p. 64.

16. Roueché, *Eleven Blue Men,* p. 191.

17. Bess Furman, "Government Spurs Poisoned Air Study," *New York Times,* October 14, 1949. There have been long-standing suspicions of a government cover-up protecting U.S. Steel, which denied any responsibility and called the incident an act of God. Those suspicions were fed by investigators saying they were unable to pin down the relationship between particular contaminants and specific symptoms. That was true in the initial study as well as a follow-up study completed ten years later. See Homer Bigart, "Delayed Effects of Smog Studied," *New York Times,* November 28, 1958.

18. Michael A. Lennon, "One in a Million: The First Community Trial of Water Fluoridation," *Bulletin of the World Health Organization,* September 2006, Vol. 84, No. 9, p. 760.

19. H. Berton McCauley, "How Fluoridation Facts Were Presented to the Citizens of Baltimore, Md.," *American Journal of Public Health,* July 1954, p. 894.

20. Scheele's 1951 endorsement by no means silenced those opposed to fluoridation. In 1955, the *New York Times* reported the topic was one of the country's fiercest controversies. (See Murray Illson, "Fluoride's Value in Water Argued," *New York Times,* April 11, 1955.) Scattered battles over fluoridation would persist, and the controversy would re-emerge in 2011 when the U.S. Department of Health and Human Services announced plans to lower the recommended levels of fluoride in drinking water, after a fresh review of the science indicated many Americans were getting too much the compound.

21. Scientific study of that question would continue for many decades. In October 2013, the International Agency for Research on Cancer declared air pollution to be a cause of lung cancer. The IARC had earlier called some components of air pollution, such as diesel fumes, carcinogens. But the declaration was the first time the group had deemed the scientific evidence sufficient to give the label to collective air pollution. Maria Cheng, "WHO Agency: Air Pollution Causes Cancer," Associated Press, October 17, 2013.

22. Unsigned article, "Ernst L. Wynder, M.D.," *Morbidity and Mortality Weekly Report,* November 5, 1999, Vol. 48, No. 43, p. 987; Richard Kluger, *Ashes to Ashes* (New York, Vintage Books, 1997), p. 136.

23. Roy Norr, testimony before the U.S. House of Representatives, Committee on Government Operations, Legal and Monetary Affairs Subcommittee, July 26, 1957, http://tobaccodocuments.org (accessed March 21, 2011); Ken Warner, interview with the author, March 4, 2011.

24. Roy Norr, "Cancer by the Carton," *Reader's Digest,* December 1952, pp. 738–739, http://legacy.library.ucsf.edu (accessed March 21, 2011); Robert Proctor, *The Golden Holocaust* (Berkeley: University of California Press, 2011), p. 233; Gene Borio, "Tobacco Timeline: The Twentieth Century 1950–1999— The Battle Joined," http://www.tobacco.org (accessed March 21, 2011).

25. Advertisement, "Jan. 4, 1954: A Frank Statement to Cigarette Smokers," http://www.tobacco.org (accessed March 21, 2011).

26. Jon M. Harkness, "The U.S. Public Health Service and Smoking in the 1950s: The Tale of Two More Statements," *Journal of the History of Medicine and Allied Sciences,* April 2007, Vol. 62, No. 2, p. 179; Siddhartha Mukherjee,

The Emperor of Maladies: A Biography of Cancer (New York: Scribner, 2010), p. 244.

27. Harkness, "The U.S. Public Health Service and Smoking in the 1950s," pp. 179–181; Mark Parascandola, "Epidemiology: Second-Rate Science?" *Public Health Reports,* July–August 1998, Vol. 113, pp. 312, 316.

28. Anthony Leviero, "Eisenhower Offers Plan to Give F.S.A. Status in Cabinet," *New York Times,* March 13, 1953; unsigned article, "National Affairs: End of an Old Fight," *Time,* March 23, 1953.

29. In addition to base pay, the surgeon general got an extra $1,200 each year that was provided to all physicians and dentists in the uniformed services.

30. The first two to hold the job were Chester S. Keefer, a Boston University medical school professor, and (to the AMA's dismay) Lowell T. Coggeshall, a liberal physician and esteemed tropical disease expert from the University of Chicago.

31. Rufus E. Miles Jr., *The Department of H.E.W.* (New York: Praeger, 1974), p. 26.

32. Reminiscences of Leonard Scheele, p. 4. Scheele also had a good working relationship with White House chief of staff Sherman Adams, who tightly controlled access to Eisenhower and was considered one of the most powerful men in Washington. Adams called Scheele once every two months, on average, usually with a question for the surgeon general about public health policies or regulations. And Scheele formed a friendship with Vice President Richard Nixon. They worked together on a physical fitness initiative, and years later Scheele was an advisor to Nixon as he considered running for president.

33. Ibid., p. 29. Scheele's recollection is probably not complete. While the Commissioned Corps was untouched by the witch hunts, Public Health Service veterans have noted at least one other case involving a civilian member of the Service.

34. William H. Stewart, oral history interview by Fitzhugh Mullan, September 28, 1988, transcript p. 13, National Library of Medicine.

35. Reminiscences of Leonard Scheele, p. 28; Ted Goertzel and Ben Goertzel, *Linus Pauling: A Life in Science and Politics* (New York: Basic Books, 1995), pp. 113, 133–134.

36. Reminiscences of Leonard Scheele, pp. 25–28.

37. Unsigned article, "Medicine: Polio and Encephalitis," *Time,* August 25, 1952; James Colgrove, *State of Immunity: The Politics of Vaccination in Twentieth-Century America* (Berkeley: University of California Press, 2006), p. 115.

38. Richard Carter, *Breakthrough: The Saga of Jonas Salk* (New York: Pocket Books, 1967), pp. 8–9; David M. Oshinsky, *Polio: An American Story* (Oxford: Oxford University Press, 2005), pp. 11, 16.

39. Carter, *Breakthrough,* pp. 262; Colgrove, *State of Immunity,* p. 117; Paul A. Offit, *The Cutter Incident* (New Haven: Yale University Press, 2005), pp. 59–63.

40. Bess Furman, "6 Vaccine Makers Get Licenses," *New York Times,* April 13, 1955.

41. Carter, *Breakthrough,* pp. 295–296; Reminiscences of Leonard Scheele, p. 17.

42. These events are told in richer detail in Oshinsky, *Polio,* pp. 221–225.

43. Furman, "One Firm's Vaccine Barred; 6 Polio Cases Are Studied," *New York Times,* April 28, 1955.

44. Neal Nathanson and Alexander D. Langmuir, "The Cutter Incident: Poliomyelitis following Formaldehyde-Inactivated Poliovirus Vaccination in the Unites States during the Spring of 1955; II. Relationship of Poliomyelitis to Cutter Vaccine," *American Journal of Hygiene,* July 1963, Vol. 73, No. 1, p. 46 (table 14).

45. Ibid., p. 48; William M. Blair, "Leaders Divided on Vaccine Study," *New York Times,* June 11, 1955; Offit, *The Cutter Incident,* pp. 101–103; Reminiscences of Leonard Scheele, p. 14.

46. Leonard Scheele, "Text of Surgeon General's Statements on the Polio Inoculation Program," *New York Times,* May 9, 1955; Oshinsky, *Polio,* p. 226.

47. Reminiscences of Leonard Scheele, p. 7; William M. Blair, "President to Get New Polio Report," *New York Times,* May 20, 1955.

48. William M. Blair, "Eisenhower Hails Mrs. Hobby's Job; Says She May Quit," *New York Times,* May 19, 1955; Kay Bailey Hutchison, *American Heroines* (New York: William Morrow, 2004), p. 261.

49. Unsigned article, "Scheele Affirms Faith in Vaccine," *New York Times,* June 8, 1955; William M. Blair, "Mrs. Hobby Terms Free Vaccine Idea a Socialistic Step," *New York Times,* June 15, 1955.

50. Note that in addition to being worried about scaring people away from the vaccine, Scheele was wary of a federal statute that prohibited federal officers from detailing business practices; unsigned article, "The Nation: Polio Fog Lifts," *New York Times,* May 29, 1955.

51. Carter, *Breakthrough,* pp. 300, 323.

52. Unsigned article, "Scheele Resigns as Health Chief," *New York Times,* June 30, 1956.

53. Warren Palmer Dearing, oral history interview, transcript p. 26.

54. Schoenke, "Obituaries: Leonard A. Scheele, MD," p. 2749; Philip J. Bigger, *Negotiator: The Life and Career of James B. Donovan* (Cranbury, N.J.: Associated University Presses, 2006), p. 147.

55. Stephen J. Jay, "Leroy Burney: A Hoosier Pioneer in Public Health," *Traces of Indiana and Midwestern History,* Spring 2004, Vol. 16, No. 2, p. 23; unsigned article, "Medicine: New Surgeon General," *Time,* August 13, 1956.

56. Leroy E. Burney, oral history interview, transcript pp. 17–18; Bess Furman, "President Names Surgeon General," *New York Times,* August 4, 1956.

57. Luther Terry, oral history interview by William W. Moss, March 6, 1970, transcript p. 29, John F. Kennedy Presidential Library.

58. Leroy E. Burney, oral history interview, transcript p. 1; Jay, "Leroy Burney," pp. 17–19.

59. Leroy E. Burney, oral history interview, transcript p. 2.

60. Unsigned article, "Doctor from Indiana: Leroy E. Burney," *New York Times,* August 4, 1956.

61. Leroy E. Burney, oral history interview, transcript p. 16.

62. However, Burney wasn't formally confirmed by the U.S. Senate until January 1957.

63. Unsigned article (Associated Press), "Plans Made to Combat Asiatic Flu," *Titusville (Penn.) Herald,* August 28, 1957; unsigned article, "Medicine: Asian Flu: The Outlook," *Time,* August 12, 1957.

64. Eisenhower was reluctant because he said he didn't want to receive preferential treatment before the vaccine was widely available to the public. But Burney said the president—who had a heart attack in 1955 and was seen as at greater risk for flu complications—was among those who would be prioritized anyway. W.H. Lawrence, "Eisenhower Gets an Asian Flu Shot," *New York Times,* August 27, 1955.

65. Unsigned article, "New Type of Influenza Officially Called Asian," *New York Times,* August 24, 1957.

66. D.A. Henderson, Brooke Courtney, Thomas V. Inglesby, Eric Toner, and Jennifer B. Nuzzo, "Public Health and Medical Responses to the 1957–58 Influenza Pandemic," *Biosecurity and Bioterrorism: Biodefense Strategy, Practice, and Science,* 2009, Vol. 7, No. 3, pp. 270–272; Anne Schuchat, comments to the author, May 6, 2011.

67. Carter, *Breakthrough,* pp. 340–341; Colgrove, *State of Immunity,* p. 140.

68. O'Connor would continue to argue for the Salk vaccine, even after Burney was gone. Luther Terry, Burney's successor, signed off on the final licensing of the Sabin vaccine in 1962—and felt O'Connor's wrath. At New York's Roosevelt Hotel in 1962, Terry was interrupted during a meeting when a letter from O'Connor was hand-delivered to him. It said that if Terry licensed Sabin's vaccine, O'Connor would get the surgeon general fired. Terry read it, turned to Public Affairs Officer Stew Hunter and said "Stew, give me a cigarette." Luther Terry to David J. Sencer, December 6, 1978 (Sencer provided a copy of the letter to the author); David Sencer, interview with the author, September 25, 2007.

69. Strickland, *Politics, Science, and Dread Disease,* pp. 115, 132.

70. Arthur S. Flemming, oral history interview with Niel M. Johnson, June 19, 1989, p. 50 Harry S. Truman Library & Museum website, http://www .trumanlibrary.org/oralhist/flemming (accessed May 12, 2011); Leroy E. Burney, oral history interview, transcript pp. 24–25.

71. Unsigned article, "Bureaucracy: The Cranberry Boggle," *Time,* November 23, 1959; Bernice Flemming, *Arthur Flemming: Crusader at Large* (Washington, D.C.: Caring, 1991), pp. 197–202.

72. Miles, *The Department of H.E.W.,* pp. 38, 235–236.

73. Leroy E. Burney, oral history interview, transcript p. 19; Harkness, "The U.S. Public Health Service and Smoking in the 1950s," p. 174.

74. In his oral history interview in 1988, Burney recalled that he delivered the 1957 statement in a nationally televised press conference, and some historical articles have repeated that assertion. However, newspaper accounts make no mention of an on-air press conference.

75. Bess Furman, "U.S. Links Cancer with Cigarettes," *New York Times,* July 13, 1957; W. Kip Viscusi, *Smoke-Filled Rooms* (Chicago: University of Chicago Press, 2002), p. 140; Kluger, *Ashes to Ashes,* p. 201.

76. John Parascandola, "Cigarettes and the US Public health service in the 1950s," *American Journal of Public Health,* February 2001, Vol. 91, No. 2, pp. 201–202.

77. Alexander R. Hammer, "Sale of Tobacco Burn New Marks," *New York Times,* May 3, 1959.

78. Harkness, "The U.S. Public Health Service and Smoking in the 1950s," p. 193.

79. Leroy E. Burney, "Smoking and Lung Cancer: A Statement of the Public Health Service," *Journal of the American Medical Association,* November 28, 1959, Vol. 171, No. 13, pp. 1829–1837.

80. Jean White, "PHS Cancer Study Urges: Quit Smoking," *Washington Post,* November 27, 1959; Nate Haseltine, "Tobacco Stocks Fall as Protests Rise over PHS Warning against Smoking," *Washington Post,* November 28, 1959.

81. As noted in Harkness, "The U.S. Public Health Service and Smoking in the 1950s," p. 195.

82. As quoted by the Associated Press, "Smoking-Cancer Link is Questioned by AMA," *Washington Post,* December 12, 1959. According to the medical historian Jon Harkness, Talbott's editorial was actually based on a draft by some of Burney's subordinates. Talbott had sought input from Burney's office, but Burney was leaving for an international trip and left the matter to a subordinate. What emerged was a conservative editorial with Talbott's name attached. But the *JAMA* editorial was characteristic of Talbott, who doubted the tobacco-cancer link and also disliked government involvement in matters of public health (he wrote another editorial around that time criticizing Flemming for the cranberry warning). See Harkness, "The U.S. Public Health Service and Smoking in the 1950s," pp. 199–205; unsigned article, " 'Forthright' on Medicine: John Harold Talbott," *New York Times,* January 2, 1960.

83. Unsigned article, "Burney Disputed on Smoking Link," *New York Times,* February 28, 1960; Kluger, *Ashes to Ashes,* p. 250.

84. Leroy E. Burney, oral history interview, transcript p. 26; Wilbur J. Cohen, oral history interview with William W. Moss, May 24, 1971, p. 99, John F. Kennedy Library website, http://www.jfklibrary.org (accessed June 2, 2011).

85. Leroy E. Burney, oral history interview, pp. 9–11.

86. Lawrence K. Altman, "Leroy Burney, 91, Early Critic of Effects of Cigarette Smoking," *New York Times,* August 4, 1998; Office of the Public Health Historian, "Obituary—Leroy E. Burney, M.D. (1906–1998)," *Commissioned Corps Bulletin,* September 1998, Vol. 12, No. 9, p. 17; Jay, "Leroy Burney," p. 25.

87. David J. Bennett, *He Almost Changed The World: The Life and Times of Thomas Riley Marshall* (Bloomington, Ind.: AuthorHouse, 2007), p. 228. Marshall refused to assert power when Wilson was incapacitated by a stroke, setting the stage for a weakened White House unable to bring about ratification of the League of Nations treaty or to prevent the country from reverting to an isolationist foreign policy. The United States' isolationism is generally regarded as a contributing factor in the rapid rise of Nazi aggression in Europe and the outbreak of World War II.

CHAPTER 6

1. Unsigned article, "Celebrezze Facing Complex Job," *New York Times,* August 2, 1962; Luther Terry, oral history interview, p. 27.

2. Wilbur J. Cohen, oral history interview, p. 62; Edward Berkowitz, "Wilbur J. Cohen and the New Frontier," Social Welfare History Project, http:// www.socialwelfare history.com (accessed June 2, 1011).

3. Alvin Benn, "Terry Gave U.S. Smokers First Warning," *Montgomery Advertiser,* January 19, 2006; Kluger, *Ashes to Ashes,* p. 222.

4. Luther Terry, oral history interview, transcript pp. 14–15.

5. Ibid., pp. 17–19.

6. Ibid., p. 21.

7. Yeager, *The Limits of Law,* pp. 71, 73.

8. Wilbur J. Cohen and Jerome N. Sonosky, "Federal Water Pollution Control Amendments of 1961," *Public Health Reports,* February 1962, Vol. 77, No. 2, pp. 107, 113.

9. Wilbur J. Cohen, oral history interview, pp. 62–63.

10. The question did not come out of the blue. A spate of medical news had appeared in the preceding months about the dangers of smoking. Perhaps the most important news came from England: a March 1962 report by the Royal College of Physicians that made a strong epidemiological case against smoking and called on the British government to take steps to discourage it.

11. Kluger, *Ashes to Ashes,* p. 222; Marjorie Hunter, "U.S. Health Service to Study Cigarettes," *New York Times,* June 8, 1962.

12. Drew Pearson, "Pearson Special for Weekly Papers, 10/12/1962," printout archived at the American University Library, Special Collections, http:// dspace.wrlc.org/doc/bitsream/2041/49590/b17f21–1012xdrsplay.pdg.

13. Robert C. Toth, "Celebrezze Wary on Smoking Issue," *New York Times,* December 3, 1962.

14. Kluger, *Ashes to Ashes,* p. 243; Brandt, *The Cigarette Century,* pp. 223, 229.

15. Brandt, *The Cigarette Century,* p. 228; Ken Warner, interview with the author, March 4, 2011.

16. Eugene Guthrie, assistant surgeon general for operations, recalled forcefully urging Terry to drop the cigarette habit before the report came out. "I told him, 'You gotta quit that. I think you can get away with a pipe if you don't do it openly.' He said, 'You gotta be kidding!' I said, 'No, I'm not. It just wouldn't do. If you smoke any cigarettes, you better do it in a closet.'" Eugene Guthrie, interview with the author, December 10, 2013.

17. Ibid. Guthrie oversaw logistics for the press conference. The State Department auditorium was the same room where President Kennedy had fielded Edgar Prina's question at the press conference twenty months earlier. The temperature at noon that day was about 27 degrees with the wind chill, according to "Weather History for Washington, D.C.," wunderground.com, http://www.wunderground .com/history/airport/KDCA/1964/1/11/DailyHistory.html?req_city=NA&req_ state=NA&req_statename=NA&MR=1 (accessed December 11, 2013).

18. Marjorie Hunter, "Smoking Banned at News Parley," *New York Times,* January 12, 1964. Donald Shopland, an HEW staffer working at the press

conference, said reporters were given ninety minutes to read the report, not two hours. In spite of the elaborate setup for the press conference, Shopland recalled Terry's performance as low-key. Donald Shopland, interview with the author, December 4, 2013. Shopland provided an old, thirty-seven-page transcript of the press conference to the author that seemed to support that assessment. At one point, a reporter asked, "On the basis of this report what would you advise your patients about smoking?" His response (page 11 of the transcript) was something less than punchy: "Frankly, I would advise a person in light of the conclusiveness of this report and the clear indication of an associated health hazard that if the individual wished to smoke, one should certainly do it with the recognition that he was undertaking and subjecting himself to a definite health risk."

19. In the fourth question at the press conference, a reporter asked whether the smokers on the committee had decided to drop the habit. Three committee members answered the question, all saying no. Fieser said he still smoked Lark cigarettes, though he recommended pipes, which the report concluded were not as dangerous as cigarettes. Leonard Schuman said he had not changed his cigarette habit. Maurice Seevers said he still smoked cigars. Terry said he had quit smoking cigarettes a few weeks earlier but still smoked a pipe and an occasional cigar. Those responses are recorded on pages 5–7 of the transcript provided by Shopland.

20. Unsigned article/Associated Press, "Dr. Terry Doubts Need for Antismoking Laws," *New York Times,* January 27, 1964; John A. Osmundsen, "Follow-Up Report on Smoking Will Be Offered Today by U.S.," *New York Times,* January 11, 1965; Cabell Phillips, "Cigarette Warning Is Urged by Terry," *New York Times,* March 23, 1965.

21. Wilbur J. Cohen, oral history interview, p. 99.

22. Unsigned article, "Dr. Terry to Get Another Term as Surgeon General," *Washington Post,* February 25, 1965.

23. Alfred K. Mann, *For Better or for Worse: The Marriage of Science and Government in the United States* (New York: Columbia University Press, 2000), p. 124; Charles Miller, oral history interview with Fitzhugh Mullan, August 24, 1988, transcript pp. 6–7, National Library of Medicine.

24. Wilbur J. Cohen, oral history interview, p. 98.

25. William H. Stewart, oral history interview, transcript pp. 38, 41–42. According to Stewart, Johnson broke the news to Terry during the helicopter ride to the NIH campus that day. But Johnson announced that Terry was leaving to become vice president for medical affairs at the University of Pennsylvania, so it seems that Terry had been advised earlier to explore other opportunities and set up the transition.

26. Nan Robertson, "President Signs $280 Million Bill for Health Study," *New York Times,* August 10, 1965.

27. Joseph A Califano Jr., "Eulogy for Dr. Luther Terry, at the Funeral Services at Fort Meyer Chapel at Arlington cemetery, April 2, 1985," copy of prepared remarks faxed to the author by Califano's assistant, Sulaiman Beg, June 29, 2011.

28. Unsigned article, "Nation's Health Chief: William Huffman Stewart," *New York Times,* August 21, 1967.

29. William H. Stewart, oral history interview, transcript p. 3.

30. Etheridge, *Sentinel for Health*, p. 37.

31. William H. Stewart, oral history interview, transcript p. 8.

32. Robertson, "President Signs $280 Million Bill for Health Study"; Nate Haseltine, "Stewart Named Surgeon General," *Washington Post,* September 25, 1965.

33. William H. Stewart, oral history interview, transcript p. 36.

34. Jane E. Brody, "Smoking Is Linked to 12 Million Sick," *New York Times,* March 30, 1966; unsigned editorial, "Dr. Stewart on Cigarettes," *New York Times,* July 17, 1966.

35. *The Today Show,* August 3, 1967, episode, transcript at http://tobaccodocuments.org/ctr/HK0465009–5018.html (accessed July 25, 2011). Little's accent and sometimes-charming personality are described in Kluger, *Ashes to Ashes,* p. 141.

36. Alexander R. Hammer, "Smoking of Cigarettes Gaining Despite Attacks," *New York Times,* November 26, 1967; unsigned item, "News Summary and Index: The Major Events of the Day," *New York Times,* August 26, 1967.

37. Guthrie, the former assistant surgeon general and friend of Terry, holds that opinion. He said Stewart struck him as more "middle of the road" when it came to tobacco control, and felt Lyndon Johnson was even warier of alienating legislators from tobacco states than Kennedy had been. Kennedy's assassination cost the tobacco control movement a significant amount of White House bully pulpit support, he opined. Eugene Guthrie, interview with the author.

38. Harold M. Schmeck Jr., "U.S. Report Ranks Cigarettes by Tar," *New York Times,* November 28, 1967; Matt Schudel, "William H. Stewart: Surgeon General Condemned Smoking," *Washington Post,* April 27, 2008.

39. Alan Blum, telephone interview with the author, July 28, 2011; Kenneth Warner, e-mail to the author, December 9, 2013; Kenneth Warner, ed., *Tobacco Control Policy* (San Francisco: Jossey-Bass, 2006), p. 33. Warner writes that cigarette consumption declined by 15 percent in the months after the Terry report was released, but a *New York Times* story from the period reported the figure as 8 percent. See Associated Press, "Cigarette Industry Continues to Face a Cloudy Outlook," *New York Times,* October 1, 1964.

40. Kenneth Warner, e-mail to the author; Allan C. Erickson, Jeffrey W. McKenna, and Rose Mary Romano, "Past Lessons and New Uses of the Mass Media in Reducing Tobacco Consumption," *Public Health Reports,* May–June 1990, Vol. 105, No. 3, p. 241. The increase in smoking in the early 1970s may have stemmed at least partly from the cigarette companies cutting prices because their advertising budgets had declined.

41. See Heikki Hiilamo, Eric Crosbie, and Stanton Glantz, "The Evolution of Health Warning Labels on Cigarette Packs: The Role of Precedents, and Tobacco Industry Strategies to Block Diffusion," *Tobacco Control,* October 23, 2012, doi:10.1136/tobaccocontrol-2012–050541.

42. John F. Banzhaf III, telephone interview with the author, July 28, 2011.

43. Steven M. Spencer, "Medicare: Headache or Cure-All?" *Saturday Evening Post,* May 20, 1967, Vol. 240, No. 10, p. 23.

44. Edward D. Berkowitz, *Mr. Social Security: The Life of Wilbur J. Cohen* (Lawrence: University of Kansas Press, 1995), p. 233; P. Preston Reynolds, "The Federal Government's Use of Title VI and Medicare to Racially Integrate Hospitals in the United States, 1963 through 1967," *American Journal of Public Health,* November 1997, Vol. 87, No. 11, pp. 1852–1853.

45. John Herbers, "Medicare Funds Will Be Used to Spur Rights Act in Hospitals," *New York Times,* March 9, 1966; Reynolds, "The Federal Government's Use of Title VI and Medicare to Racially Integrate Hospitals in the United States," p. 1855.

46. Reynolds, "The Federal Government's Use of Title VI and Medicare to Racially Integrate Hospitals in the United States," p. 1853; unsigned article, "U.S. Aides Exhort Southern Hospitals on Desegregation," *New York Times,* June 10, 1966; unsigned article, "Hospital in Georgia Accused of Fooling U.S. in Bias Inquiry," *New York Times,* June 22, 1966.

47. Philip R. Lee, interview with the author, October 27, 2007.

48. Harold M. Schmeck Jr., "Medicare Is Off to Smooth Start; No Overcrowding Is Reported," *New York Times,* July 2, 1966. Of course, some places were worse than others. In Louisiana, only about 68 percent of general hospitals had desegregated. In Mississippi, only about 24 percent had.

49. Among them was Philip R. Lee, as stated in his interview with the author.

50. Jill Quadagno, *One Nation Uninsured: Why the U.S. Has No National Health Insurance* (Oxford: Oxford University Press, 2005), pp. 84–85, 88.

51. George Albert Silver, oral history interview with Fitzhugh Mullan, November 14, 1988, National Library of Medicine, transcript pp. 14, 28; Reynolds, "The Federal Government's Use of Title VI and Medicare to Racially Integrate Hospitals in the United States," p. 1855.

52. The phrase "the check-writing business" is related by John Kelso, in oral history interview with Fitzhugh Mullan, August 9, 1988, National Library of Medicine, transcript p. 63; Warren Palmer Dearing, oral history interview, transcript p. 33.

53. Paul Ehrlich, oral history interview with Fitzhugh Mullan, August 23, 1988, National Library of Medicine, transcript p. 10.

54. An assessment made by several different sources, including George Albert Silver, oral history interview, transcript pp. 25–26; Miles, *The Department of H.E.W.,* p. 193; William H. Stewart, oral history interview, transcript p. 54.

55. As quoted in Mullan, *Plagues and Politics,* p. 154. Mullan's source was *Public Health Service World,* December 1965, p. 2.

56. Technically, this change conflicted with the Public Health Service Act of 1944, which had consolidated federal public health administrative powers in the Office of the Surgeon General. But the Johnson administration had worked with key legislators to empower Gardner to snatch those powers without any formal congressional action—the reorganization plan took effect after sitting before Congress for sixty days with no objection.

57. Unsigned article, "President Asks Reorganization of PHS," *Washington Post,* April 26, 1966.

58. Richard L. Seggel, "The Organizational Roles of the Public Health Service Commissioned Corps and Surgeon General: A Monograph on Their Recent

History," November 1992, pp. 6–7, files of the Office of the Public Health Service Historian. Seggel was former HEW deputy assistant secretary for health /policy implementation. Albert W. Snoke, "The Unsolved Problem of the Career Professional in the Establishment of National Health Policy," *American Journal of Public Health,* September 1969, Vol. 59. No. 9, p. 1579.

59. John Kelso, oral history interview, transcript pp. 57–58; George Albert Silver, oral history interview, transcript p. 18.

60. By the time Lee had the job, it had been retitled assistant secretary for health and scientific affairs.

61. Stewart was a strong supporter of the smallpox eradication program that, driven by CDC staff, intensified in the late 1960s, nearly cutting the number of countries with endemic smallpox in half. During the trip in early 1968, Stewart led a U.S. delegation on a tour of Africa that included a ceremony at a soccer field in Ghana to celebrate the 25 millionth vaccination against smallpox in that region. The surgeon general danced with a local dignitary in a tribal dance that day. Horace G. Ogden, *CDC and the Smallpox Crusade* (Washington, D.C.: U.S. Department of Health and Human Services, 1987), pp. 45, 90; National Communicable Disease Center, "Smallpox Eradication Program: The SEP Report," March 1968, Vol. 2, No. 2, p. 1, http://www.globalhealthchronicle.org (an online project of the CDC and Emory University; accessed August 7, 2011).

62. David Sencer, interview with the author, September 2007.

63. John Parascandola, "History," Commissioned Officers Association of the USPHS Inc., http://www.coausphs.org/phhistory.cfm (accessed August 3, 2011); Snoke, "The Unsolved Problem of the Career Professional in the Establishment of National Health Policy," p. 1580; John Kelso, oral history interview, transcript p. 51; William Stewart, oral history interview, transcript pp. 67–68.

64. Paul Ehrlich, oral history interview, transcript p. 38.

65. Eve Edstrom, "HEW Acts to Unify Command over Its Health Activities," *Washington Post,* March 13, 1968.

66. Associated Press, "Flu Deaths Reach 3,594 in 4 Weeks," *New York Times,* January 4, 1969.

While the humiliation of Stewart's loss of power is not well recalled by the general public, he is—ironically—sometimes remembered for an embarrassment that may not have actually happened. The blunder reportedly occurred in 1967 or 1969, depending on the source. It was at a national conference of public health officials, or at a congressional hearing, or in a speech at Johns Hopkins University—again, depending on the source. Stewart reportedly proclaimed that mankind could rest easy, because scientists now knew enough that contagious illnesses were essentially conquered. "It is time to close the book on infectious diseases, and declare the war on pestilence won," Stewart has been quoted as saying. Those words were of course woefully mistaken. AIDS, SARS, swine flu, and bird flu are just a few of the many new infectious diseases that have emerged since the late 1960s, not to mention mankind's ongoing struggles with diseases that were thought to be in hand at the time of that statement but since then have developed resistance to antibiotics. The quote has become one of the hallmark examples of medical hubris, used to make a point by countless writers and lecturers, including medical historians and the editors of *Scientific American*. But later in his life, Stewart did not recall making that statement, and no witnesses to Stewart making such a statement could be found. Indeed, a growing number of scholars have come to believe he probably didn't make it. In a letter published in the medical journal *Clinical Infectious Diseases* in 2008, UCLA researcher Brad Spellberg said he tried for five years to find a primary source for Stewart's famous quotation, without success. "It appears that Dr. Stewart's now-legendary quote may be a medical 'urban legend,'" Spellberg wrote. Spellberg continued to pursue the question, in partnership with Bonnie Taylor-Blake, a researcher at the University of North Carolina. For years, they scoured scores of documents, including congressional testimony, newspaper articles, books, and speech manuscripts. Nothing like that statement appeared. On the contrary, Stewart repeatedly made statements at the time that scientists should not let down their guard against infectious diseases. "By following the trail of source documents back over the past 40 years, we can now be confident that Dr. Stewart never made any such statement," Spellberg and Taylor-Blake said. Bobby Milstein, "Hygeia's Constellation" (a booklike report, issued by the Centers for Disease Control and Prevention, based on Milstein, "Hygeia's Constellation: Navigating Health Futures in a Dynamic And Democratic World" [Ph.D. dissertation, Graduate College of Interdisciplinary Arts and Sciences, Union Institute and University, Cincinnati, 2006]), April 15, 2008, p. 34; Brad Spellberg, "Dr. William H. Stewart: Mistaken or Maligned" (Correspondence), *Clinical Infectious Diseases,* July 15, 2008, Vol. 47, No. 2, p. 294. Spellberg ended his letter with a plea to any reader who did know of a primary citation for Stewart's quote to contact Spellberg. As of August 5, 2011, no one had, Spellberg said in an e-mail to the author on that date. Spellberg also shared with the author "On the Exoneration of Dr. William H. Stewart: Debunking an Urban Legend," an unpublished manuscript that had been submitted to several medical journals but rejected because of lack of interest in the topic (August 5, 2011 e-mail to the author). It was published in 2013 in the journal *Infectious Diseases of Poverty*, under the title "On the Exoneration of Dr. William Stewart: Debunking an Urban Legend."

67. Unsigned article, "Stewart to Resign as Surgeon General," *New York Times,* May 17, 1969.

68. John Pope, "Dr. William Stewart, Past Surgeon General," *New Orleans Times-Picayune,* April 25, 2008.

CHAPTER 7

1. Roger Egeberg, oral history interview with Fitzhugh Mullan, November 2, 1988, National Library of Medicine, transcript pp. 21–22; Eric Redman, *The Dance of Legislation* (1973; repr., Seattle: University of Washington Press, 2001), p. 46.

2. Charles C. Edwards, oral history interview, transcript p. 38.

3. Jesse Steinfeld, interview with the author, November 30, 2011.

4. Jesse Steinfeld, oral history interview with Alexandra Lord, September 20, 2005, National Library of Medicine, transcript pp. 1–2.

5. Jesse Steinfeld, "Keynote Address: The Role of Government in Managing Public Health Aspects of Tobacco Dependence," Society for Research in Nicotine and Tobacco, February 1995, transcript of recording at http://legacy .library.ucsf.edu/tid/wpy06coo/pdf (accessed August 19, 2011), p. 4.

6. Jesse Steinfeld, oral history interview, transcript p. 8.

7. Jesse Steinfeld, interview with the author, March 14, 2007.

8. Roger Egeberg, oral history interview, transcript p. 20.

9. Jesse Steinfeld, oral history interview, transcript p. 25.

10. Ibid, p. 26.

11. Unsigned UPI article, "U.S. Aide Predicts Health Insurance," *New York Times,* January 9, 1970.

12. Paul Ehrlich, oral history interview, transcript p. 21. Ehrlich would fill in and carry out surgeon general duties after Steinfeld left office.

13. Unsigned article, "Sickness at HEW," *Time,* June 15, 1970; unsigned article, "Richardson Takes Over at HEW As Finch Moves to White House," *Washington Sounds,* June 18, 1970, Vol. 4, No. 5; Redman, *The Dance of Legislation,* p. 49.

14. Merlin DuVal, oral history interview, with Fitzhugh Mullan, December 15, 1988, National Library of Medicine, transcript p. 19; Roger Egeberg, oral history interview, transcript p. 20.

15. Merlin DuVal, oral history interview, transcript pp. 14–16. Apparently, that terse state of affairs did not last very long. A log of telephone messages that Steinfeld received during his years in office showed that the two spoke and even lunched together frequently after Egeberg moved to a different post. Steinfeld donated the log to the Office of the Public Health Service.

16. Darren Rovell, *First in Thirst: How Gatorade Turned the Science of Sweat into a Cultural Phenomenon* (New York: AMACOM Books, 2006), p. 60; Richard A. Merrill and Michael R. Taylor, "Saccharin: A Case Study of Government Regulation of Environmental Carcinogens," *Agriculture and Human Values,* Winter–Spring 1986, Vol. 3, Nos. 1–2, p. 45; David Sencer, interview with the author, September 25, 2007.

17. Philip D. Carter, "Marijuana Penalty Studied, *Washington Post,* January 17, 1970.

18. Harold M. Schmeck Jr., "More Federal Funds Urged for the Fight against Lead Poisoning in Children," *New York Times,* July 6, 1971; Gerald Markowitz and David Rosner, *Lead Wars: The Politics of Science and the Fate of America's Children* (Berkeley: University of California Press, 2013), p. 56.

19. UPI, "Detergents Must Drop NTA," *Wisconsin State Journal,* December 19, 1970; Detergent ingredients were a continuing controversy during Steinfeld's term. Morgens tried to stay on Steinfeld's good side, paying him courtesy calls during visits to Washington, as noted in an October 28, 1971, message from Morgens in Steinfeld's phone log.

20. Richard A. Rettig, *Cancer Crusade: The Story of the National Cancer Act of 1971* (1977; repr., New York: Authors Choice Press, 2005), p. 138.

21. In 1965, HEW leaders also moved to shutter the remaining twelve Public Health Service hospitals and transfer their patients to VA hospitals. They

dropped the plan after a comptroller general analysis found that the department lacked the statutory authority and would need congressional approval.

22. Years later, Richardson would become famous for standing up to Nixon over a personnel matter: in 1973, while serving as U.S. attorney general, Richardson would refuse Nixon's orders to fire the Watergate special prosecutor Archibald Cox (one of a series of Cox-related terminations that became known as the Saturday Night Massacre). But that was still in the future. When the Perkins report was released, Richardson was still new to the Nixon administration and less willing to fight the White House.

23. Hamowy, *Government and Public Health in America*, p. 67.

24. The smoking habits of all the surgeons general are not well recorded in history books. Certainly Steinfeld was the first surgeon general in at least fifty years who was not a smoker or regular user of tobacco. The four surgeons general before him—Stewart, Terry, Burney, and Scheele—were all smokers. Before them was Thomas Parran, who grew up on a tobacco farm. Before Parran was Hugh Cumming, also a smoker despite his famous 1929 statement before Congress that women should stop smoking because it was bad for them.

25. Jesse Steinfeld, *The Health Consequences of Smoking: A Report of the Surgeon General: 1971* (Washington, D.C., U.S. Government Printing Office, 1971), p. 281.

26. Stuart Auerbach, "Surgeon General Proposes Ban on Smoking in Most Public Places," *Washington Post,* January 12, 1971.

27. Madilyn Reynolds, "More on Public Smoking" (editorial), *Washington Post,* January 17, 1971.

28. Jesse Steinfeld, "Women and Children Last?" *New York State Journal of Medicine,* December 1983, Vol. 83, No. 13, p. 1258.

29. Unsigned article, "Smoking to Be Banned on Staten Island Ferry," *New York Times,* January 27, 1971.

30. Jesse Steinfeld to Thomas Israel, October 15, 1971, uncataloged Steinfeld personal files, Office of the Public Health Historian.

31. Jesse Steinfeld to Jack Mills, August 16, 1972. Mills, in a letter a week earlier, offered a different version. He said he had not taken a position on the future of the Corps or on whether to abolish the Office of the Surgeon General. "As I told you at Dr. Curreri's party and I repeat in this letter, we are not after your job, Jesse." Steinfeld personal files, Office of the Public Health Historian (letters not filed or catalogued at the time the author read them).

32. Christopher Lydon, "TV Chiefs Pledge Aid to Violence Study," *New York Times,* March 13, 1969; Linda Charlton, "Study Aides Voice Misgivings about Report on TV Violence," *New York Times,* February 19, 1972; Philip M. Boffey and John Walsh, "Study of TV Violence: Seven Top Researchers Blackballed from Panel," *Science,* May 22, 1970, Vol. 168, pp. 949–952. The TV networks were not explicitly promised that their objections would result in a name being dropped from the list, but that was the result. Each of the seven names that were objected to was dropped.

33. Christopher Lydon, "Hearings to Weigh TV Violence Study," *New York Times,* January 18, 1972.

34. Linda Charlton, "Surgeon General Wants TV to Curb Violence for Children," *New York Times,* March 22, 1972.

35. Jesse Steinfeld, oral history interview, transcript p. 4.

36. Ron Nessen, "Surgeon General Controversy," report on *NBC Nightly News,* February 14, 1972, Vanderbilt University Television News Archive; Bernard Gwertzman, "U.S. and the Soviet to Pool Research in 3 Health Areas," *New York Times,* February 11, 1972; unsigned article, "H.E.W. Will Study Syphilis Project," *New York Times,* August 25, 1972.

37. C. Everett Koop, interview with the author, July 7, 2006; Jesse Steinfeld, interview with the author, March 14, 2007.

38. *The Mike Douglas Show with John Lennon and Yoko Ono, Day 2* (original air date February 15, 1972), Rhino Home Video; Neil Gladstone, "The Booking of the Century," *Philadelphia City Paper,* July 9–16, 1998; 5:45 P.M. message to Jesse Steinfeld from Marvin Beers, February 16, 1972, Steinfeld phone log, now deposited with the National Library of Medicine.

39. Steinfeld quoted in Redman, *The Dance of Legislation,* p. 228.

40. Robert B. Semple Jr., "Bold Steps Hinted: President Meets Top Advisors and Then Flies to Florida," *New York Times,* November 9, 1972. The article notes that it was customary for reelected presidents to ask for resignation letters from appointees, but also that Nixon was unusually pointed in calling for the letters and said there would be a "significant" realignment of his staff and the executive departments.

41. Jesse Steinfeld, interview with the author, March 14, 2007.

42. Jesse Steinfeld, comments made to *Reader's Digest* editorial staff on January 12, 1975, during a meeting to explore development of a story on the cigarette lobby, pp. 4–5, of transcript at http://legacy.library.ucsf.edu/tid/bcx56boo/pdf.

43. Elliot Richardson to Davis S. Peoples, August 28, 1972; David S. Peoples to HEW Secretary Elliot Richardson, October 23, 1972, both on file at Office of the Public Health Service Historian (now with the National Library of Medicine).

44. Richard D. Lyons, "Ex-Surgeon General Charges 'Chaos' in Nixon Health Policy," *New York Times,* September 10, 1973.

45. Paul Ehrlich, oral history interview, transcript pp. 19, 25.

46. Victor Cohn, "Top HEW Official Quits Health Post," *Washington Post,* December 8, 1972.

47. Paul Ehrlich, oral history interview, transcript p. 33.

48. Julius Richmond, oral history interview with Fitzhugh Mullan, December 5, 1988, National Library of Medicine, transcript p. 39.

49. Victor Cohn, "New Surgeon General Chosen; Power Will Be Expanded," *Washington Post,* May 31, 1977.

50. Charles J. Bussey and Donna Bussey, "The Physician and Social Renewal: Julius B. Richmond as Role Model," *Journal of Medical Humanities,* Spring 1991, Vol. 12, No. 1, p. 27.

51. Ibid., pp. 27–28.

52. Julius Richmond, oral history interview, transcript pp. 3–4.

53. Ibid., p. 20.

54. Hale Champion, interview with the author, October 11, 2007.

55. Paul Ehrlich, oral history interview, transcript p. 54; Peter Bell, interview with the author, December 9, 2011.

56. Julius Richmond, oral history interview, transcript pp. 38–39.

57. Hale Champion, interview with the author; Peter Bell, interview with the author.

58. Julius Richmond, oral history interview, transcript pp. 39–40.

59. Charles Miller, oral history interview, transcript p. 33.

60. Julius Richmond, oral history interview, transcript p. 64.

61. Joseph Califano, interview with the author, January 16, 2008.

62. Julius Richmond, interview with the author, October 11, 2007.

63. Joseph A. Califano Jr., *Inside: A Public and Private Life* (New York: PublicAffairs, 2004), pp. 168, 354–355.

64. Ibid.; the Pat Oliphant cartoon appears among the unnumbered illustration pages in the middle of the book.

65. Don Shopland, interview with the author; Julius Richmond, interview with the author; Julius Richmond, oral history interview, transcript p. 49.

66. Kluger, *Ashes to Ashes*, p. 437; Associated Press (no byline), "HEW Cigarette War: More Smoke Than Fire?" *Santa Fe New Mexican,* January 10, 1979; Victor Cohn, "Massive New U.S. Report Blasts Cigarette Smoking," *Washington Post,* January 12, 1979.

67. Califano, *Inside,* p. 356.

68. Kluger, *Ashes to Ashes,* pp. 437–438; Joseph A. Califano Jr., *Governing America* (New York: Simon & Schuster, 1981), pp. 434–435.

69. An opinion held by several people in HEW leadership at the time, including HEW Undersecretary Hale Champion. Hale Champion, interview with the author.

70. Rosalynn Carter, comments at memorial service for Julius Richmond, October 27, 2007, Harvard Club, Boston (the author was present and took notes). Accounts differ as to the genesis of the trip. In an interview years later, Richmond said the National Security Council first proposed a surgeon general's trip to Thailand, then added Mrs. Carter as a sort of guest on the trip. See Julius Richmond, oral history interview, transcript p. 43.

71. Hale Champion, interview with the author.

72. Jacob I. Fabrikant, "Decision-Making and Radiological Protection at Three Mile Island: Response of the Department of Health, Education and Welfare," paper delivered at the Third International Symposium of Radiation Protection, Inverness, Scotland, June 1982; Barry Richmond, comments at memorial service for Julius Richmond, October 27, 2008, Harvard Club, Boston.

73. Julius Richmond, interview with the author; Julius Richmond, oral history interview, transcript p. 61.

74. Victor Cohn, "New Health Report Stresses Prevention through Diet, Habits," *Washington Post,* July 29, 1979; Rodewald quoted in Mike Stobbe, "Nation's Health Goals for Decade Unmet," Associated Press, December 31, 2009.

75. Marc Lalonde, *A New Perspective on the Health of Canadians* (Ottawa: Minister of Supply and Services Canada, 1981), pp. 67–72, http://www.hc-sc

.gc.ca/hcs-sss/alt_formats/hpb-dgps/pdf/pubs/1974-lalonde/lalonde-eng.pdf (accessed November 4, 2011); comments of Michael McGinnis, 2009 video interview aired on the Public Health Training Network, transcript available at http://adph.org/ALPHTN/assets/his_mcginnis.pdf (accessed November 3, 2011).

76. Julius Richmond, oral history interview, transcript p. 47; Joseph Califano, interview with the author, January 16, 2008; Michael McGinnis, interview with the author, December 2, 2011; William Foege, interview with the author, December 14, 2009.

77. Cohn, "New Health Report Stresses Prevention."

78. Michael McGinnis, interview with the author.

79. Julius Richmond, interview with the author.

80. David Satcher, interview with the author, September 21, 2007.

CHAPTER 8

1. Steven A. Holmes, "Jesse Helms Dies at 86; Conservative Voice in the Senate," *New York Times,* July 5, 2008.

2. In searches of newspaper and news archives, the author failed to find the phrase "the nation's doctor" in any articles about the surgeon general that predated the late 1980s. Some public health leaders said it too was their understanding that "the nation's doctor" first came into use during Koop's tenure.

3. C. Everett Koop, *Koop: The Memoirs of America's Family Doctor* (New York: Random House, 1991), p. 172.

4. Ibid., pp. 12, 23.

5. Ibid., pp. 26–27, 34–35.

6. Ibid., p. 60; C. Everett Koop, oral history interview with Fitzhugh Mullan, February 6, 1989, National Library of Medicine, transcript p. 3.

7. Edward Brandt, oral history interview with Fitzhugh Mullan, December 20, 1988, National Library of Medicine, transcript p. 32; Georges Benjamin, interview with the author, November 5, 2007.

8. Steven M. Spencer, "Surgery Saved the Day," *Saturday Evening Post,* November 7, 1953; United Press, "Surgery Separates L.I. Siamese Twins," *New York Times,* October 6, 1957; Associated Press, "Doctors Concerned on Emotional State of Separated Twins," *New York Times,* September 20, 1974; unsigned article, "The God-Fearing Surgeon Who Separated the Twins," *People,* October 4, 1974; Donald C. Drake, "The Surgery: An Agonizing Choice—Parents, Doctors, Rabbis in Dilemma," *Philadelphia Inquirer,* October 16, 1977.

9. Donald C. Drake, "The Surgery: An Agonizing Choice—Parents, Doctors, Rabbis in Dilemma"; C. Everett Koop, interview with the author, October 27, 2008. Some comedians have observed that Koop's chin beard but otherwise smooth face caused him to look the same way upside-down as right side up.

10. Koop, *Koop,* pp. 84–85.

11. Comments of Norman Koop, memorial service for C. Everett Koop, First Congregational Church of Woodstock, Vermont, March 9, 2013 (notes on the comments in author's possession); Norman Koop, interview with the author,

March 11, 2013. Years later, Koop and his wife, Elizabeth, wrote a short book about coping with David's death that extensively discussed their reliance on faith and scripture. See C. Everett Koop and Elizabeth Koop, *Sometimes Mountains Move* (1974; Grand Rapids, Mich.: Zondervan, 1995).

12. Koop, *Koop*, pp. 263–264; William Martin, *With God on Our Side: The Rise of the Religious Right in America* (New York: Broadway Books, 1996), pp. 193–194.

13. Francis Schaeffer and C. Everett Koop, *Whatever Happened to the Human Race?* (DVD; Gospel Films Distribution).

14. Unsigned editorial, "Dr. Unqualified," *New York Times,* April 9, 1981; Robert Reinhold, "The Surgeon General's Pragmatic Boss," *New York Times,* May 19, 1981.

15. Bill Peterson, "Helms' Move Is Outflanked by Speaker O'Neill," *Washington Post,* April 4, 1981; Robert Reinhold, "Health Nominee Debate Eases," *New York Times,* July 30, 1981.

16. Koop, *Koop,* p. 133. Regarding the Humphrey Building, Brutalist is the name of a fortresslike architectural style popular from the 1950s to the 1970s.

17. Edward Martin, oral history interview with Fitzhugh Mullan, March 9, 1989, National Library of Medicine, transcript pp. 27–28; C. Everett Koop, oral history interview, transcript pp. 30–31.

18. Koop repeatedly tried to promote breastfeeding. He convened the first Surgeon General's Workshop on Breastfeeding in 1984, which was followed by reports in 1985 and 1991. But it was one battle he lost: formula companies aggressively marketed their product in hospitals and elsewhere, and breastfeeding initiation rates actually fell in the late 1980s. For the trend data, see Anne L. Wright and Richard J. Schanler, "The Resurgence of Breastfeeding at the End of the Second Millennium," *Journal of Nutrition,* Vol. 131, No. 2, pp. 421S–425S.

19. Bill Peterson, "Won't Use Health Post as Pulpit, Koop Testifies," *Washington Post,* October 2, 1981; UPI, "Senate Confirms Koop, 68–24," *New York Times,* November 17, 1981.

20. C. Everett Koop, oral history interview, transcript p. 36.

21. As quoted by Frank Tursi, Susan E. White, and Steve McQuilkin, "An Ill Wind Blowing," *Winston-Salem Journal,* December 7, 1999.

22. C. Everett Koop, interview with the author, July 7, 2006.

23. Peter Schmeisser, "Pushing Cigarettes Overseas," *New York Times,* July 10, 1988; Kluger, *Ashes to Ashes,* p. 537.

24. Kluger, *Ashes to Ashes,* p. 540.

25. R. Blizzard, "U.S. Smoking Habits Have Come a Long Way, Baby," Gallup News Service, October 19, 2004, http://www.gallup.com (accessed November 28, 2013). The decline in smoking during the 1980s is also evident in an often cited chart showing adult per capita consumption in the United States from 1900 to 2006 by Kenneth Warner and David Mendez, in the article "Tobacco Control Policy in Developed Countries: Today, Yesterday and Tomorrow," *Nicotine & Tobacco Research,* September 2010, Vol. 12, No. 9, pp. 876–887; Ken Warner, interview with the author, March 4, 2011; Alan Blum, interview with the author, July 28, 2011.

26. Associated Press, "Industry Group Blasts Surgeon General's Comments on Video Games," November 10, 1982.

Koop played a pivotal and sometime underrecognized role in causing violence to be thought of as a public health issue. In the 1980s, violence still tended to be thought of as a matter for the police and courts, and only a small number of researchers were developing public health approaches to reducing injuries and slayings. In October 1985, Koop provided a breakthrough moment by holding the Surgeon General's Workshop on Violence and Public Health in Leesburg, Virginia. "It started the process of legitimizing violence as a public health issue," said Howard Spivak, a pioneer in public health violence work who would later become director of the CDC's Division of Violence Prevention. Howard Spivak, interview with the author, July 22, 2013.

27. Koop, *Koop*, pp. 240–243.

28. Glen Collins, "Physicians Criticize Rules on Newborns," *New York Times*, April 7, 1983; Edward Brandt, oral history interview with Fitzhugh Mullan, December 20, 1988,, National Library of Medicine, transcript p. 40; Cristine Russell, "Medical Groups Sue Trying to Block HHS Rule on Infant Life," *Washington Post*, March 19, 1983; Randy Shilts, *And the Band Played On: Politics, People, and the AIDS Epidemic* (New York: St. Martin's Press, 1987), p. 246; Koop, *Koop*, p. 86.

29. Russell, "Medical Groups Sue Trying to Block HHS Rule on Infant Life"; C. Everett Koop, oral history interview, transcript pp. 24–25.

30. Edward Martin, oral history interview, transcript p. 32; James Mason, interview with the author, November 12, 2007.

31. Otis Bowen and William Du Bois Jr., *Doc: Memories from a Life in Public Service* (Bloomington: Indiana University Press, 2000), pp. 193–194.

32. Not every one of the eight PHS hospitals closed. Some were turned over to community groups. John Herbers, "U.S. Seamen's Hospitals Still Open in Many Cities," *New York Times*, October 27, 1981; Robert Pear, "Budget Office Urging Sharp Cuts in Scope of Public Health Service," *New York Times*, December 1, 1982.

33. Luther Terry to C. Everett Koop, February 22, 1982, National Library of Medicine, available at http://profiles.nlm.nih.gov/ps/access/QQBCHS.pdf (accessed December 13, 2011).

34. Paul Ehrlich, oral history interview, transcript pp. 33, 35–36.

35. C. Everett Koop, oral history interview, transcript pp. 75–79; Mullan, *Plagues and Politics*, p. 207.

36. Associated Press, "Koop Plans a Shake-Up of Public Health Officers," *New York Times*, April 18, 1987; Edward Martin, oral history interview, transcript p. 46; Mary Guinan, interview with the author, December 30, 2011.

37. Edward Martin, oral history interview, transcript p. 46; Mullan, *Plagues and Politics*, p. 207.

38. Lawrence K. Altman, "New Homosexual Disorder Worries Health Officials," *New York Times*, May 11, 1982; Koop, oral history interview, transcript pp. 38–39.

39. Koop, oral history interview, transcript p. 40; Koop, *Koop*, p. 196.

40. Shilts, *And the Band Played On,* pp. 354, 398, and 456; Margaret Heckler, quoted in an interview for "The Age of AIDS," a PBS *Frontline* report that aired May 2006, www.pbs.org/wgbh/pages/frontline.aids/interviews (accessed November 7, 2011)

41. Shilts, *And the Band Played On,* p. 456.

42. Ibid., pp. 572, 586.

43. Philip M. Boffey, "Surgeon General Urges Frank Talk to Young on AIDS," *New York Times,* October 23, 1986; Cristine Russell, "AIDS Report Calls for Sex Education," *Washington Post,* October 23, 1986.

44. Shilts, *And the Band Played On,* p. 588.

45. James Mason, interview with the author, November 12, 2007.

46. C. Everett Koop, oral history interview, transcript pp. 58–59.

47. C. Everett Koop, interview with the author, July 7, 2006.

48. Anthony Fauci, interview with the author, March 28, 2008.

49. Unsigned article, "Controversial Surgeon General Never Stops," *U.S. News & World Report,* reprinted in *Albany (N.Y.) Times Union,* May 25, 1988.

50. Bernard Weinraub, "Dole Sees AIDS Issue as Key One in '88 Race," *New York Times,* March 21, 1987; Maureen Dowd, "Washington Talk: Dr. Koop Defends His Crusade on AIDS," *New York Times,* April 6, 1987.

51. Unsigned article, "Northeast Journal: Studds Mails Out U.S. AIDS Reports," *New York Times,* May 24, 1987; Dowd, "Washington Talk: Dr. Koop Defends His Crusade on AIDS."

52. U.S. Department of Health and Human Services, "C. Everett Koop (1982–1989)," SurgeonGeneral.gov, http://www.surgeongeneral.gov/about/previous/biokoop.html (accessed November 11, 2013); U.S. General Accounting Office, "AIDS Education: Activities Aimed at the General Public Implemented Slowly," December 1988 (GAO/HRD-89-2); Associated Press, "U.S. Will Mail AIDS Advisory to All Households," *New York Times,* May 5, 1988.

53. Anthony Fauci, interview with the author, March 28, 2008.

54. Bruce Lambert, "Flood of Phone Calls on AIDS Tied to Mailing," *New York Times,* July 3, 1988; N. Guttman, D. Boccher-Lattimore, and C.T. Salmon, "Credibility of Information from Official Sources on HIV/AIDS Transmission" *Public Health Reports,* 1998, Vol. 113, No. 5, pp. 465–471.

55. C. Everett Koop, interview with the author, July 7, 2006.

56. Koop, *Koop,* pp. 311–314; C. Everett Koop, interview with the author, July 7, 2006.

57. Warren Leary, "Koop Says Abortion Report Couldn't Survive Challenge," *New York Times,* March 17, 1989; Jack Anderson and Dale Van Atta, "Chilly White House Relations Kept Koop Out in the Cold," *The Oregonian,* May 24, 1989.

58. George Will, "Koop's Splendid Legacy," *Washington Post,* July 16, 1989.

59. Unsigned article, "Gunfire Shatters Peace and Lives in Washington," *New York Times,* June 11, 1992; Marian Burros, "Former Surgeon General Begins Push for Americans to Slim Down," *New York Times,* December 5, 1994.

60. The episode can be viewed on YouTube.

61. Holcomb Noble, "Hailed as a Surgeon General, Koop Is Faulted on Web Ethics," *New York Times,* September 5, 1999; C. Everett Koop, interview with the author, October 27, 2008.

62. Ken Moritsugu, interview with the author, September 1, 2006.

CHAPTER 9

1. Dan Chichester, interview with the author, February 23, 2009. The story played out in *Daredevil* issues 305 (June 1992) and 306 (July 1992). The plot was a public health nightmare: the villain's alias was Angeline Kutter, and she and her henchmen poisoned the food of a large group of office workers and then posed as an emergency response team that ambulanced them to an operating room to remove their organs—a ghastly scene that was interrupted, by Daredevil and Spider-Man.

2. David Sencer, interview with the author, September 25, 2007. Sencer opined that "she didn't talk much about anything. She did talk about child health, and that would be about it." His was perhaps an unduly harsh assessment—Novello spoke on a variety of issues while she was surgeon general.

3. Louis Sullivan, interview with the author, September 29, 2007.

4. Ivan Roman, "Humble at the Top; New Surgeon General Knows Where Her Roots Are," *Chicago Tribune,* June 3, 1990; Matt S. Meier, Conchita Franco Serri, and Richard A. Garcia, *Notable Latino Americans: A Biographical Dictionary* (Westport, Conn., Greenwood Press, 1997), pp. 270–271.

5. Unsigned article, "Interview: Antonia Novello, former Surgeon General of the United States," Academy of Achievement (a museum of living history), June 18, 1994, http://www.achievement.org/autodoc/printmember/novoint-1 (accessed December 26, 2011).

6. Ibid.; Ivan Roman, "Humble at the Top."

7. Unsigned article, "Interview: Antonia Novello"; Meier, Serri, and Garcia, *Notable Latino Americans,* p. 271.

8. Carol Krucoff, "Antonia Novello: A Dream Come True," *Saturday Evening Post,* June 1991, Vol. 263, No. 4, p. 38.

9. Ibid.; Ivan Roman, "Humble at the Top."

10. Meier, Serri, and Garcia, *Notable Latino Americans,* p. 271; Roman, "Humble at the Top."

11. Associated Press, "Antonia Novello Said in Line to Become Surgeon General," *Bowling Green (Ky.) Daily News,* October 18, 1989.

12. Charles E. Cohen, "Butt Out, Guido Sarducci! Surgeon General Antonia Novello, Your Sister-in-Law, Wants Everyone to Quit Smoking," *People,* December 17, 1990.

13. Deborah Mesce, "Lower-Profile, Less-Independent Surgeon General Sought," Associated Press wire, July 9, 1989; Mary Guinan, interview with the author, December 30, 2011.

14. Warren Leary, "Woman in the News: A Surgeon General Nominee, Antonia Coello Novello," *New York Times,* November 2, 1989; Mary Guinan, interview with the author.

15. Louis Sullivan, interview with the author, September 29, 2007.

16. Unsigned article, "Interview: Antonia Novello."

17. Ibid.

18. Roman, "Humble at the Top."

19. Louis Sullivan, interview with the author.

20. James Mason, interview with the author, November 12, 2007.

21. Gene Kramer, "Administration Squelches Health Official's Anti-Tobacco Testimony," Associated Press, May 17, 1990; Kluger, *Ashes to Ashes,* pp. 713–714.

22. Philip Hilts, "Thailand's Cigarette Ban Upset," *New York Times,* October 4, 1990.

23. Morton Mintz, "Where There's Smoke," *Washington Post Magazine,* December 3, 1995.

24. Ibid.

25. Kluger, *Ashes to Ashes,* p. 701; Stuart Elliott, "Top Health Official Demands Abolition of 'Joe Camel' Ads," *New York Times,* March 10, 1992; Stuart Elliott, "Joe Camel May Have Won a Battle, but the War Goes On," *New York Times,* June 3, 1994.

26. Joseph DiFranza et al., "RJR Nabisco's Cartoon Camel Promotes Camel Cigarettes to Children," *Journal of the American Medical Association,* December 11, 1991, Vol. 266, No. 22, p. 3151; Paul Fischer et al., "Brand Logo Recognition by Children Ages 3 to 6 Years," *Journal of the American Medical Association,* December 11, 1991, Vol. 266, No. 22, p. 3145.

27. Paul Driscoll, "Surgeon General Leads 'Dump the Hump' Parade and Rally," Associated Press wire, June 22, 1992; Elliott, "Top Health Official Demands Abolition of 'Joe Camel' Ads."

28. Desda Moss, "Surgeon General Finds Her Voice," *USA Today,* June 24, 1992; Elliott, "Top Health Official Demand Abolition of 'Joe Camel' Ads"; Kluger, *Ashes to Ashes,* pp. 702–703.

29. Emily Prager, "Joe Camel Is a Smoke Screen," *Newsday,* March 23, 1992.

30. Luz Villarreal, "'I Need Your Help,' Surgeon General Tells MADD," *Orlando Sentinel,* August 7, 1992.

31. Jeff Koplan, interview with the author, October 2, 2007.

32. Kathleen Toomey, interview with the author, February 2, 2012; Mary Guinan, interview with the author, December 30, 2011; James R. Gavin III, interview with the author, April 12, 2009. "Being a woman, I learned diplomacy," Novello once told the *Saturday Evening Post.* "We women have always learned how to listen and how to wait . . . until there comes your moment to speak. Then you take into consideration everybody's feelings and make sense of things that sound so complicated." See Krucoff, "Antonia Novello."

33. James R. Gavin III, interview with the author; Thomas Glynn, interview with the author, March 26, 2012; Walter Orenstein, interview with the author, April 8, 2010. Not everyone in public health was as appreciative of Novello's efforts against measles. In June 1991, Los Angeles County health official Dr. Shirley Fannin told a U.S. Senate panel that the measles outbreak might not have been so bad if federal officials had promptly responded to local requests for emergency funding and extra supplies of measles vaccine. Such help, Fannin

argued, would have been much more important than flying Novello and other federal health officials to various cities to speak about the importance of measles vaccinations. See Beth Hawkins, "U.S. Failed to Help in Epidemic, Doctor Says," *Los Angeles Times*, June 21, 1991.

34. Jeff Levi, interview with the author, November 6, 2007.

35. Antonia Novello, "The Modern Era Surgeon General: A Retrospective Review—A Dissertation Proposal Submitted to the Faculty of the School of Hygiene and Public Health of the Johns Hopkins University," April 2000, pp. 178–182 (photocopy in author's possession).

36. Richard Vernaci, "Surgeon General Says She Plans to Keep Her Job," Associated Press wire, December 15, 1992; Philip Lee, interview with the author, October 27, 2007.

37. State of New York, Office of the State Inspector General, "Final Report, January 27, 2009," pp. 2–4, 9, http://www.ig.state.ny.us/pdfs/Commissioner%20 Used%20Guards%20To%20Chauffeur%20Shopping%20Sprees.pdf (accessed January 5, 2012).

38. Office of the New York State Inspector General, "Press Release: Commissioner Used Guards to Chauffeur Shopping Sprees," January 27, 2009.

39. State of New York, Office of the State Inspector General, "Final Report, January 27, 2009," p. 7.

40. Glenn Blain and Kenneth Lovett, "Former State Health Commissioner Antonia Novello Pleads Guilty to Felony, Skirts Jail Time," *New York Daily News*, June 26, 2009.

41. Malcolm Gladwell, "Arkansas Health Chief May Make the Cut," *Washington Post*, December 17, 1992.

42. Nancy Kruh, "The Doctor Is In," *Dallas Morning News*, September 11, 1993; Alex Witchel, "After the Storm, Still No Calm," *New York Times*, October 24, 1996; David Nimmons, "Playboy Interview: Joycelyn Elders," *Playboy*, June 1995, Vol. 42, No. 6, p. 59; Joycelyn Elders and David Chanoff, *Joycelyn Elders, M.D.: From Sharecropper's Daughter to Surgeon General of the United States of America* (New York: William Morrow, 1996), p. 14.

43. Elders and Chanoff, *Joycelyn Elders, M.D.*, pp. 25–26, 49–50.

44. Ibid., p. 49.

45. Ibid., pp. 31, 58–59, 75, 85.

46. Ibid., p. 89; Joycelyn Elders, interview with the author, November 30, 2007.

47. Elders and Chanoff, *Joycelyn Elders, M.D.*, pp. 150, 185, 217. Clinton had already asked Elders to serve on the Arkansas Industrial Development Commission before he picked her to head the state health department.

48. Ibid., pp. 173, 223, 241–242; Steve Barnes, "The Crusades of Dr. Elders," *New York Times*, October 15, 1989; Elders quoted in Lorraine D. Jackson, "Joycelyn Elders," in *American Voices: An Encyclopedia of Contemporary Orators*, ed. Bernard K. Duffy and Richard W. Leeman (Westport, Conn.: Greenwood Press, 2005), p. 143.

49. Philip Hilts, "Surgeon General–Designate Weathers Senate Hearing," *New York Times*, July 24, 1993.

50. Joycelyn Elders, interview with the author.

51. Associated Press, "Clinton Aide Endorses Marijuana as Medicine," *New York Times*, December 20, 1992; unsigned article, "Dr. Elders Supports TV Ads for Condoms," *Chicago Sun-Times*, January 1, 1993; Beverly La Haye, "Nominee for Surgeon General Is Divisive" (letter to the editor), *New York Times*, July 22, 1993.

52. Thomas L. Friedman, "Clinton Delays Senate Hearing on Health Post," *New York Times*, July 16, 1993; Stephen LaBaton, "Abandoned by Clinton, She Finds Acceptance," *New York Times*, July 14, 1993; Patrick Riley, "Elders: Insults People of Faith," *New Orleans Times-Picayune*, July 29, 1993.

53. Hilts, "Surgeon General–Designate Weathers Senate Hearing"; Michael Wines, "Senate Confirms Elders as Surgeon General, after Months of Debate," *New York Times*, September 8, 1993.

54. Philip R. Lee, interview with the author, October 27, 2007.

55. The speech was to the Association of Reproductive Health Professionals. As quoted in Jackson, "Joycelyn Elders," p. 145.

56. Philip R. Lee, interview with the author.

57. Mary Guinan, interview with the author.

58. Kathleen Toomey, interview with the author.

59. Joycelyn Elders, interview with the author; Philip R. Lee, interview with the author; Jeffrey Koplan, interview with the author, October 2, 2007.

60. Tom Diemer, "Clinton Unwraps Health Plan: Proposes Security for Everybody," *Cleveland Plain Dealer*, September 23, 1993; Hillary Rodham Clinton, *Living History* (New York: Simon & Schuster, 2003), p. 204.

61. Nigel Hamilton, *Bill Clinton: Mastering the Presidency* (New York: PublicAffairs, 2007), pp. 225–226.

62. Merlin DuVal, oral history interview, transcript pp. 28–31.

63. Daniel Weintraub, "Wilson Calls for Clinton to Fire Surgeon General," *Los Angeles Times*, December 10, 1993; Stephen LaBaton, "Surgeon General Suggests Study on Legalizing Drugs," *New York Times*, December 8, 1993.

64. Elders and Chanoff, *Joycelyn Elders, M.D.*, p. 309; Donna Shalala, interview with the author, October 16, 2009.

65. Reuters, "Elders Still Seeks Study on Legalizing Drugs," *New York Times*, January 15, 1994; New York Times News Service, "Elders: 'White Male' Medicaid Policy Breeds Poverty," *Chicago Tribune*, February 26, 1994; unsigned article, "Surgeon General Tells Magazine Sexual Fear Causes Anti-Gay Attitudes," Associated Press wire, March 18, 1994.

66. Larry Margasak, "House Republicans Want Surgeon General to Go," Associated Press wire, June 25, 1994.

67. Ann Devroy and Charles R. Babcock, "Gingrich Foresees Corruption Probe by a GOP House," *Washington Post*, October 14, 1994.

68. James Popkin, "A Case of Too Much Candor," *U.S. News & World Report*, December 19, 1994, Vol. 117, No. 24, p. 31; Kenneth T. Walsh et al., "Charting A New Course," *U.S. News & World Report*, November 21, 1994, Vol. 117, No. 20, p. 50.

69. Popkin, "A Case of Too Much Candor"; Douglas Jehl, "Surgeon General Forced to Resign by White House," *New York Times*, December 10, 1994;

Elders and Chanoff, *Joycelyn Elders, M.D.*, p. 331; Michael Putzel, "White House Forced Elders to Resign over Remarks," *Boston Globe*, December 10, 1994.

70. Some have suggested that Shalala or someone at HHS fed Elders comments to the reporter, with the intent of forcing Elders out. That theory, without proof, is offered in Hamilton, *Bill Clinton*, p. 385.

71. Putzel, "White House Forced Elders to Resign over Remarks"; Leon Panetta, "Transcript of Remarks by White House Chief of Staff Leon Panetta, December 9, 1995," released on U.S. Newswire, available through Nexis (accessed December 15, 2007.

72. Bill Clinton, *My Life* (New York: Vintage Books, 2005), p. 348. In his autobiography, Clinton hoped that one day Elders would forgive him. Elders has said an apology wasn't necessary. "I don't think Bill Clinton, in any way, felt that I did anything wrong. I think it was just the political pressures," she said (Joycelyn Elders, interview with the author, November 30, 2007).

73. Joycelyn Elders, interview with the author.

74. Unsigned editorial, "A Surgeon General's Untimely Candor," *New York Times*, December 10, 1994. Years after she left the office, Elders faulted herself for not thinking in terms of political strategy. She suggested that if she had, she could have stayed in office longer and accomplished more. She spoke admiringly of her successor David Satcher and his release of a sexual health report that she had hoped to produce. "I didn't have enough leadership strategies to get the job done," she told an audience at Atlanta's Morehouse School of Medicine. But her regrets were limited: if she had it to do it all over again, she'd go about the job the same way, she added (to applause). Jocelyn Elders, comments at the conference "Underserved and High Risk Populations: Taking Action for Comprehensive Primary Health Care Renewal," Morehouse School of Medicine, October 3, 2013 (author's notes of the comments).

75. SNL Transcripts, "A Statement by Surgeon General Joycelyn Elders," *Saturday Night Live*, December 10, 1994, episode (hosted by Alec Baldwin), snltranscripts.jt.org (accessed January 13, 2012).

76. Roy Zimmerman (words and music), "Firing the Surgeon General," copyright 1995, Watunes (BMI), from the album *Folk Heroes* on Reprise. The chorus included the lines, "I hear you knockin' but you can't come in. / I hear you knockin' but you can't come in. / 'Cause I'm firing the Surgeon General."

77. Alison Slow Loris, "Surgeon General—Might as Well Abolish the Position," *Seattle Times*, December 18, 1994.

CHAPTER 10

1. *Congressional Record–Senate, for March 6, 1998*, p. S1523, downloaded from bulk.resource.org/gpo.gov/records/1998/1998_S01523.pdf.

2. *Congressional Record–Senate, for February 10, 1998*, p. S533, http://www.thomas.gov.

3. Damon Thompson, interview with the author, October 6, 2007.

4. David Satcher, remarks made at 2009 Case Western Reserve University graduation ceremony, News Center, Case Western Reserve University website,

http://blog.case.edu/case-news/2009/05/18/classof2009speech; David Satcher, interview with the author, October 19, 2009.

5. David Satcher, interview with the author, May 29, 2012.

6. Anne Rochell, "Dr. David Satcher, the CDC's New Chief, Is Seen as the Ideal Person in the Position," *Atlanta Journal and Constitution,* April 17, 1994; David Satcher, interview with the author, October 19, 2009.

7. Rochell, "Dr. David Satcher, the CDC's New Chief"

8. David Satcher, interview with the author, October 19, 2009; David Satcher, interview with the author, May 29, 2012.

9. David Satcher, interview with the author, October 19, 2009.

10. Ibid.; Nola Richardson, *When One Loves* (Millbrae, Calif.: Celestial Arts, 1974), p. 3. Maya Angelou wrote a blurb for the book, too. Years later—when Satcher was surgeon general—Nola was diagnosed with Alzheimer's disease, Satcher said in an interview with the author on July 18, 2012.

11. Unsigned article, "About the Council," Council on Graduate Medical Education, http://www.cogme.gov/whois.htm; David Satcher, interview with the author, September 21, 2007.

12. Amy L. Fairchild and Ronald Bayer, "Uses and Abuses of Tuskegee," in *Tuskegee's Truths,* p. 590; Jones, *Bad Blood,* pp. 215, 238.

13. The White House, Office of the Press Secretary, "President William J. Clinton's Remarks," reprinted in *Tuskegee's Truths,* p. 574. The book mistakenly says the remarks are for a ceremony held May 16, 1996. The ceremony was held May 16, 1997. David Satcher, "CDC's 60th Anniversary: Director's Perspective—David Satcher, M.D., Ph.D., 1993–1998," *Morbidity and Mortality Weekly Report,* June 15, 2007, Vol. 56, No. 23, p. 580; David Satcher, interview with the author, October 27, 2008.

14. David Satcher, interview with the author, October 19, 2009; Philip R. Lee, interview with the author, October 27, 2007.

15. Unsigned article, "The Clinton Administration's Internal Reviews of Research on Needle Exchange Programs. Part 2," Drug Policy Alliance's Lindesmith Library Web site, http://www.drugpolicy.org/library/review.cfm. (accessed October 9, 2009.)

16. David Satcher, interview with the author, September 21, 2007.

17. Donna St. George, "Nominee for Surgeon General Known as Consensus Builder," *Charlotte Observer,* February 3, 1995.

18. Donna Shalala, interview with the author, October 16, 2009; David Satcher, interview with the author, October 19, 2009.

19. Donna Shalala, interview with the author; David Satcher, interview with the author, September 21, 2007.

20. Lauran Neergaard, "CDC Chief Chosen as Surgeon General," Associated Press, September 12, 1997.

21. David Pace, "Next Surgeon General Stresses Exercise, Nutrition," Associated Press, October 8, 1997.

22. Helen Dewar, "Surgeon General Nominee Faces Opposition in Senate; Stance on 'Partial-Birth Abortion' at Issue," *Washington Post,* January 21, 1998.

23. Marcia Angell, "The Ethics of Clinical Research in the Third World," *New England Journal of Medicine,* September 18, 1997, Vol. 337, No. 12, p. 849.

24. Harold Varmus and David Satcher, "Ethical Complexities of Conducting Research in Developing Countries," *New England Journal of Medicine,* October 2, 1997, Vol, 337, No. 14, p. 1003.

25. *Congressional Record–Senate, for February 10, 1998,* pp. S532–S533.

26. Fitzhugh Mullan, "Interview: David Satcher Takes Stock," *Health Affairs,* November–December 2002, Vol. 21, No. 6, p. 158.

27. Donna Shalala, interview with the author.

28. Sheryl Gay Stolberg, "After 3-Year Void, Surgeon General Post Is Filled," *New York Times,* February 14, 1998.

29. John F. Harris and Amy Goldstein, "Puncturing an AIDS Initiative: At Last Minute, White House Political Fears Killed AIDS Funding," *Washington Post,* April 23, 1998.

30. David Satcher, interview with the author, September 21, 2007.

31. Sheryl Gay Stolberg, "Clinton Decides Not to Finance Needle Program," *New York Times,* April 21, 1998; Laura Meckler, "Surgeon General Disappointed by Needle Exchange Decision," Associated Press, April 24, 1998.

32. Donna Shalala, interview with the author.

33. Anthony Fauci, interview with the author, March 28, 2008.

34. Sheryl Gay Stolberg, "Surgeon General Warns of Rise in Ethnic Smoking," *New York Times,* April 28, 1998.

35. Through a Freedom of Information Act request to the U.S. Department of Health and Human Services, the author obtained photocopies of Satcher's schedule books during his term in office. Those records note the meetings and media interviews.

36. The textbook is David Satcher and Rubens J. Pamies, *Multicultural Medicine and Health Disparities* (New York: McGraw-Hill, 2006); David Kessler, interview with the author, October 17, 2009.

37. David Satcher, "Remarks at the Release of the Surgeon General's Call to Action to Prevent Suicide, July 28, 1999," surgeongeneral.gov, http://www.surgeongeneral.gov/library/calltoaction/remarks.htm; Patricia J. Mays, "Satcher Unveils National Suicide Prevention Strategy," Associated Press, October 21, 1998.

38. Damon Thompson, interview with the author, October 6, 2007.

39. Donna Shalala, interview with the author.

40. Robert Pear, "Mental Disorders Common, U.S. Says; Many Not Treated," *New York Times,* December 13, 1999.

41. "Evaluation of Parity in the Federal Employees Health Benefits (FEHB) Program: Final Report, December 31, 2004," U.S. Department of Health and Human Services, Office of the Assistant Secretary for Planning and Evaluation, http://aspe.hhs.gov/daltcp/reports/parity.htm; John K. Iglehart, "The Mental Health Maze and the Call for Transformation," *New England Journal of Medicine,* January 29, 2004, Vol. 350, No. 5, p. 509.

42. David Satcher, interview with the author, October 19, 2009.

43. J. Eric Oliver, *Fat Politics: The Real Story behind America's Obesity Epidemic* (Oxford: Oxford University Press, 2006), p. 40.

44. Ibid., p. 177.

45. Joe Thompson, interview with the author, September 28, 2009.

46. More than 34 percent of Americans are obese, and the percentage has been rising, according to the best available government estimates available as of this writing.

47. John Parascandola, interview with the author, October 9, 2009. A number of scholars who have written on the obesity issue have omitted any mention of Satcher or the report.

48. David Satcher, interview with the author, October, 27, 2008. The detail about Olivia Satcher came from the Satcher interview of May 29, 2012.

49. Donna Shalala, interview with the author.

50. David Satcher, interview with the author, October, 27, 2008. In the earlier, 2007 interview, Satcher made a point of not suggesting that Clinton himself had anything to do with the decision, but said that other White House officials had considered it out of the question—Satcher interview, September 21, 2007; Among the others with the same understanding of the situation was C. Everett Koop, interview with author, July 7, 2006.

51. David Satcher, interview with the author, October, 27, 2008.

52. Frank Rich, "Blame Politics, Money for Administration Gaffes," *Milwaukee Journal Sentinel,* October 30, 2001.

53. Damon Thompson, interview with the author, October 6, 2007. The author tried on three occasions to schedule an interview with Tommy Thompson for this book over the course of five years, and each time was told by his aides that he was not available at that time.

54. David Satcher, interview with the author, October 19, 2009.

55. David Satcher, interview with the author, September 21, 2007.

56. Jeffrey Koplan, interview with the author, October 2, 2007.

57. David Satcher, interview with the author, September 21, 2007.

58. Mullan, "Interview: David Satcher Takes Stock," p. 158.

59. Laura Meckler, "Controversy Is Nothing New to Surgeon General's Post," Associated Press, June 29, 2001.

60. David Satcher, interview with the author, October 19, 2009. Satcher's printed schedule confirmed his memory of his travel plans for that day. Satcher later learned that among those killed in the Pentagon crash was Paul Ambrose, thirty-two, an HHS official who was a senior editor on the nearly completed Call to Action report on obesity. Ambrose was on the plane that morning to attend an adolescent obesity conference in Los Angeles. The report was dedicated to Ambrose.

61. Damon Thompson, interview with the author.

62. "Ari Fleischer Holds White House Briefing, October 4, 2001," Federal Document Clearing House Political Transcripts, p. 2.

63. Ibid., p. 3.

64. Damon Thompson, interview with the author.

65. Jeff Nesmith, "Experts: Public Needed a Fuller Anthrax Report," *Austin American-Statesman,* November 30, 2001.

66. Jeffrey Koplan, interview with the author, October 2, 2007.

67. Georges Benjamin, interview with the author, November 5, 2007.

68. Akhter quoted in Nesmith, "Experts: Public Needed a Fuller Anthrax Report."

69. William A. Pierce, "First Words Matter: The Anthrax Attacks of 2001," in *Communicating in a Healthcare Crisis,* ed. Wayne L. Pines (Falls Church, Va.: FDAnews, 2007); William Pierce, interview with the author, November 9, 2007. Pierce was HHS deputy assistant secretary for public affairs from June 2001 through April 2005. At the time of the interview, he was senior vice president at APCO Worldwide, a communications consulting company.

70. Philip J. Hilts, "A Nation Challenged: Public Attitudes; Americans Skeptical about Bioterrorism Risk," *New York Times,* November 9, 2001; Melissa B. Robinson, "Public Health Experts Criticize Bush Administration over Early Anthrax Messages," Associated Press, November 29, 2001. The Harvard survey of more than five hundred people, conducted in late October 2001, found that 44 percent said they would view Satcher as a reliable source of information during a bioterrorism-caused outbreak of illness. That put him on higher ground than AMA president Richard Corlin (42 percent), HHS Secretary Thompson (38 percent), FBI director Robert Mueller (33 percent), Department of Homeland Security Secretary Tom Ridge (33 percent), or senior CDC scientist Stephen Ostroff (32 percent). CDC director Jeff Koplan was the only official who did better in the survey, with 48 percent deeming him a reliable source. Robert J. Blendon et al., "Public Response to the Anthrax Threats," Working Papers of the Project on the Public and Biological Security No. 1 (Harvard School of Public Health, November 8, 2001), https://www.hsph.harvard.edu /horp/files/2012/09/WP1Public_Response_Anthrax.pdf (accessed December 15, 2013).

71. Sheryl Gay Stolberg, "Surgeon General, in a Farewell, Pleads for 'a Meaningful Budget,'" *New York Times,* February 9, 2002, p. A12.

72. Jeffrey Koplan, interview with the author.

73. Elders quoted in Meckler, "Controversy Is Nothing New to Surgeon General's Post."

74. Damon Thompson, interview with the author.

75. Anthony Fauci, interview with the author, March 28, 2008.

CHAPTER 11

1. Kim Elliott, interview with the author, November 6, 2007. Elliott later left the Trust for America's Health.

2. Author's notes from a videotape of the House Committee on Oversight and Government Reform hearing, July 10, 2007, Rayburn House Office Building. U.S. Representative Henry Waxman (D-Calif.), chaired the session.

3. Jeff Levi, interview with the author, November 6, 2007.

4. Beth P. House and Kathy N. Player, *Pivotal Moments in Nursing,* Vol. 2 (Indianapolis: Sigma Theta Tau International, 2007), pp. 5–7; Carla Garnett, "New Surgeon General: 'Still a Tourist' Living the American Dream," *NIH Record,* October 29, 2002.

5. Richard Carmona, "Honoring Our Present and Leading Our Future Webcasts: Speaker, Richard H. Carmona, 9/17/2003," Library of Congress Webcasts, http://www.loc.gov/today/cyberlc/feature_wdesc.php?rec=3347 (accessed December 5, 2013).

6. Richard Carmona, interview with the author, April 9, 2012; U.S. Army, Bronze Star certificate awarded to Richard H. Carmona, copy obtained by the author from the National Personnel Records Center, National Archives and Records Administration.

7. Richard Carmona, interview with the author, April 9, 2012; Richard Carmona, e-mail to the author, April 18, 2012; Cathy Areu, *Latino Wisdom* (Fort Lee, N.J.: Barricade Books, 2006), p. 83.

8. Carmona, "Honoring Our Present and Leading Our Future Webcasts: Speaker, Richard H. Carmona, 9/17/2003"; unsigned article, "San Francisco—Traditions," University of California History Digital Archives, http://sunsite.berkeley.edu/~ucalhist/general_history/campuses/ucsf/traditions.html (accessed February 3, 2012); Ann-Eve Pedersen and Megan Garvey, "Squaring Off over Nominee: As Hearing on Bush's Pick for Surgeon General Nears, There Are Many Allies And Critics," *Los Angeles Times,* July 8, 2002.

9. Richard Carmona, e-mail to the author, April 18, 2012; Dan Nowicki, "Carmona Has a Compelling Background," *Arizona Republic,* November 12, 2011.

10. Unsigned article, "Investigators Cite Self-Defense in 2 Tucson Shootings," Associated Press wire, September 23, 1999; David Teibel, "Carmona 'Relives' Killing Daily," *Tucson Citizen,* September 28, 1999.

11. Pedersen and Garvey, "Squaring Off over Nominee."

12. Joe Salkowski, "Carmona Would Break Surgeon General Mold," *Arizona Daily Star,* June 16, 2002.

13. Ibid.; Pedersen and Garvey, "Squaring Off over Nominee"; Chris Limberis, "Medicine Man," *Tucson Weekly,* June 24, 1999.

14. Richard Carmona, e-mail to the author, April 18, 2012; Sheryl Gay Stolberg, "President Chooses 2 for Leading Posts in Health," *New York Times,* March 27, 2002. What Bush was looking for was characterized by Regina Schofield, who was involved in interviewing candidates for the surgeon general job. Regina Schofield, interview with the author, December 5, 2013.

15. Laura Meckler, "Surgeon General Nominee Defends Record before Senate Committee," Associated Press wire, July 9, 2002.

16. Jennifer Cabe, interview with the author, June 22, 2012; William Pierce, interview with the author, November 9, 2007.

17. Jeff Koplan, interview with the author, October 2, 2007.

18. Cristina Beato, comments to staff members of the House Committee on Oversight and Government Reform, November 2, 2007, transcript posted on *Politico,* May 2012, p. 40, http://www.politico.com/news/stories/0512/76543.html (accessed December 5, 2013). Beato was interviewed as part of an investigation into the politicization of the Office of the U.S. Surgeon General. In June 2013 communications through a public affairs representative at the University of New Mexico Health Sciences Center, Beato declined to speak to the author about Carmona or other HHS personnel.

19. Georges Benjamin, interview with the author, November 5, 2007.

20. Todd Ackerman, "Surgeon General Aims to Speak for Hispanics; Plans to Close Gap in Health Disparities," *Houston Chronicle,* August 17, 2002; Carla McClain, "Carmona: We Must Change Our Ways," *Arizona Daily Star,* September 28, 2002.

21. Unsigned article, "Lawmaker: Nobody Knows Surgeon General," Associated Press wire, March 27, 2003.

22. Marc Kaufman, "Surgeon General Favors Tobacco Ban," *Washington Post,* June 4, 2003. The article said Carmona's statement was the first time a surgeon general had called for an outright ban of all tobacco products, but it can be argued that Koop's campaign for a smoke-free America by 2000—made about twenty years earlier—was a far more significant declaration.

23. Georges Benjamin, interview with the author; Kim Elliott, interview with the author. Carmona himself disagreed, saying there was no single turning point but rather a series of issues and occurrences that made his term difficult.

24. Kevin Freking, "Old Feud in Bush Administration Part of Ariz. Race," Associated Press wire, May 22, 2012.

25. Carmona said an internal HHS investigation found clerical errors but no improprieties, and determined Carmona had been overpaid on travel expense. Once that was pointed out, he paid back $3,580, Carmona said. Beato, comments to staff members of the House Committee on Oversight and Government Reform, p. 13; Richard Carmona, interview with the author, June 1, 2012; John Bresnahan and Manu Raju, "Richard Carmona Draws Fire from Former Boss," *Politico,* May 21, 2012, at http://www.politico.com/news/stories/0512/76543.html (accessed June 3, 2012).

26. Arthur Lawrence to Cristina Beato and William Turenne, April 16, 2004 (e-mail); obtained from the U.S. Department of Health and Human Services through a Freedom of Information Act request. Arthur Lawrence, a Commissioned Corps veteran serving as principal deputy assistant secretary for health, was another player in the front office. The author was not able to reach Lawrence for comment. Cabe said there was no romantic relationship, and expressed unpleasant surprise when the author told her that Lawrence had referred to her as "Jennifer Babe."

27. William Turenne to Arthur Lawrence, May 30, 2004, e-mail obtained from the U.S. Department of Health and Human Services through a Freedom of Information Act request. Turenne had gotten national press attention twenty years earlier when a syndicated columnist wrote that he and another Eli Lilly official had obtained a copy of a confidential FDA report to help the company prepare its defense against allegations that the drug maker had failed to divulge thirty-two deaths related to the drug Oraflex. See Jack Anderson, "Ethics Report Is Suppressed," *Tuscaloosa News,* November 9, 1984.

Turenne had the reputation of a bully. Cabe, who ultimately filed an internal complaint against him, said he was an intimidating presence who on several occasions threw papers and walked around her desk to yell at her from as close as one foot away. He was frequently angered by Carmona's speeches, saying the surgeon general was talking about himself too much and not saying enough to promote the administration's policies, Cabe said. She also said the complaint was filed only after one of Carmona's assistants told the surgeon general about Turenne's behavior, and Carmona brought it to the attention of top HHS officials. (Cabe declined to share a copy of the complaint with the author.) Cabe had previously raised the issue with Lawrence, but he did nothing in response, she said. Jennifer Cabe, interview with the author, June 22, 2012.

28. In fact, Schofield had applied for a spokesperson job at the Tobacco Institute only a few years earlier and, in her cover letter, had described herself as a libertarian. See Regina B. Schofield to Tobacco Institute vice president Walter Woodson, June 3, 1997, and Schofield résumé, Legacy Tobacco Documents Library, University of California, San Francisco, http://www.legacy.library .ucsf.edu (accessed December 2, 2013.) The Tobacco Institute represented the U.S. tobacco industry until the institute was forced to disband in 1998 following a legal action against the industry brought by attorneys general from forty-six states. In an interview, Schofield confirmed her past with the tobacco industry but said she had no strong opinions about any of Carmona's work on smoking. Asked about the characterization that she was a political den mother, she said she disagreed because "den mothers are nice." She said her job was to make sure political appointees, including Carmona, did not embarrass the president or the HHS secretary. Regina Schofield, interview with the author.

29. In the summer of 2004, press reports detailed a series of questions about Beato's résumé. Discrepancies in her credentials included her uncorroborated claims that she had a master's degree in public health from the University of Wisconsin, that she had published a scientific paper on inert gases, and that she had been a medical attaché to the U.S. embassy in Turkey. Her Senate confirmation was delayed while senators sought answers to what increasingly appeared to be a series of fabrications that she ascribed mostly to clerical errors. (In 2005, she left the post and was replaced by John Agwunobi, a public health official from Florida.) See Ceci Connolly, "Top Health Official Awaits Hearing on Nomination," *Washington Post,* June 10, 2004; Gardiner Harris and Robert Pear, "Ex-Officials Tell of Conflict over Science and Politics," *New York Times,* July 12, 2007.

30. The source shared recollections about some of the confrontations between Carmona and Beato on the condition that the information not be attributed. For his part, Carmona said he had many confrontations with Beato, but he said he never had a screaming match, as some others have suggested. Richard Carmona, interview with the author, June 1, 2012. Cabe, his speechwriter, said she detected frostiness between Carmona and Beato but nothing more dramatic.

31. William Turenne to Regina Schofield, September 25, 2002 (e-mail), as quoted in Edward Kennedy to HHS Secretary Michael Leavitt, August 30, 2007 (letter requesting internal documents); William Turenne to Arthur Lawrence, March 2, 2004 (e-mail). Letter and e-mail obtained from the U.S. Department of Health and Human Services through a Freedom of Information Act request.

32. Sharon Eubanks, interview with the author, May 15, 2012.

33. Sharon Eubanks and Stanton Glantz, *Bad Acts: The Racketeering Case against The Tobacco Industry* (Washington, D.C.: American Public Health Association, 2012), p. 230. Meron was acting as legal counsel for HHS. Eubanks has contended that the pro-business Bush administration deliberately tried to micromanage and weaken the government's racketeering case in the late stages of the trial, and scaled back a proposed penalty against the tobacco industry from $130 billion to $10 billion.

34. Sharon Eubanks, interview with the author.

35. Richard Carmona, interview with the author, November 20, 2006.

36. The "rogue" characterization was voiced by Jennifer Cabe, in interview with the author. The author is an AP reporter who covered Gerberding while she was CDC director. However, Gerberding did not respond to a request to be interviewed for this book.

37. Robert Sullivan, "Fear Factor," *Vogue*, June 2003, Vol. 193, No. 6, pp. 252–257.

38. The summary of media mentions and the survey of journalists both come from Stobbe, "The Surgeon General and the Bully Pulpit," pp. 183–187, 205.

For his part, Carmona said he never felt he was competing with Gerberding. They had been residents together at the University of California at San Francisco—she was a year behind him—and he had commended her when Tommy Thompson was considering her for CDC director, Carmona said. Richard Carmona, interview with the author, June 1, 2012.

39. See Pew Research Center for the People & the Press, "The People and Their Government: Distrust, Discontent, Anger, and Partisan Rancor," report published online April 18, 2010. Based on a survey of about 2,500 adults conducted in March 2010, about a year after Gerberding left office, the report compared the results to a similar survey done in the late 1990s. The later survey showed a 12 percent decline in favorable ratings for the CDC, but that was in line with declines for several other agencies as well, and was interpreted as evidence of a growing overall dissatisfaction with the federal government. Despite the decline, nearly two-thirds of respondents gave the CDC good or excellent job ratings. See also Vicki S. Freimuth, Don Musa, Karen Hilyard, Sandra Crouse Quinn, and Kevin Kim, "Trust during the Early Stages of the 2009 H1N1 Pandemic," *Journal of Health Communication*, published online October 11, 2013. In that national survey of 1,500 respondents during the early days of a frightening new flu pandemic, people of all education levels ranked the CDC director as a more trusted source than the HHS secretary, the president, the media, state and local health officials, TV doctors like CNN's Sanjay Gupta, or other elected and appointed officials.

40. Union of Concerned Scientists, "Scientific Integrity in Policymaking: An Investigation into the Bush Administration's Misuse of Science," March 2004, pp. 10–12, http://www.ucsusa.org/assets/documents/scientific_integrity/rsi_final_fullreport_1.pdf (accessed February 11, 2012).

41. In May 2004, Carmona released a report on tobacco use that linked nine more illnesses to smoking, including cataracts, pneumonia, and stomach cancer. In October, out came a report giving statistics and predictions about the prevalence of osteoporosis. He also issued two abbreviated Call to Action reports, one in 2003 on oral health and another in 2005 on the health of the disabled.

42. Unsigned article, "Surgeon General Inspires Correctional Health Pros," *Correct Care*, Fall 2003, Vol. 17, No. 4, p. 5; Richard Carmona, interview with the author, June 1, 2012. The report was not Carmona's idea. Work on it began while Satcher held the office.

43. Gardiner Harris, "Ex-Surgeon General's Maverick Side Was Bound to Appear, Friends Say," *New York Times*, August 14, 2007; Christopher Lee and

Marc Kaufman, "Bush Aid Blocked Report," *Washington Post,* July 29, 2007. The *Post* also provided readers with a link to a pdf of the unreleased report, information from which is used here.

44. Lee and Kaufman, "Bush Aid Blocked Report"; unsigned article, "Steiger Picked to Be Ambassador," *Milwaukee Journal Sentinel,* January 5, 2007.

45. Judith Graham, "U.S. Sets Off Furor in Anti-obesity Fight," *Chicago Tribune,* January 20, 2004; Tom Hamburger, "White House Tries to Rein In Scientists," *Los Angeles Times,* June 26, 2004.

46. Steiger did not respond to the author's request for comment. But he has supporters who say that Steiger was unjustly painted as the primary bad guy, and that people above and below him in the organization were equally troubled by the draft Carmona first submitted. Among Steiger's supporters is William A. Pierce, a former HHS spokesman now working for a public relations firm that represents drug manufacturers and a variety of other corporations. "I don't think Bill [Steiger] had any intention of quashing reports by the surgeon general at all. I do believe he wanted there to be a vigorous debate," Pierce said, in an interview with the author, November 9, 2007. If Steiger was unimpressed with the vigor of Carmona's work, he wasn't the only one. Regina Schofield opined that while Carmona clearly sought prestige, he seemed undisciplined about setting and achieving priorities. "I don't think he had an agenda that was thwarted. I don't think he had an agenda" period, she said. Regina Schofield, interview with the author.

47. Stephen Barr, "For $117,000, Doctor Treats His Patience," *Washington Post,* June 20, 1996.

48. Jessica Gavora, "Doctor, Can I Have This Agency Removed?" *Policy Review,* January 1, 1997, p. 7.

49. Walter Orenstein, interview with the author, April 8, 2010. Thompson had HHS develop a state-of-the-art command center, placed just down the hall from his office, to track public health emergencies anywhere in the world, according to Richard Carmona, in "Surgeon General's Column," *Commissioned Corps Bulletin,* September 2003, Vol. 17, No. 9, p. 1.

The transformation of the Corps may not have been Thompson's idea originally. Kenneth Moritsugu, a Commissioned Corps leader who served as acting surgeon general between Satcher and Carmona, did much of that plotting. So said Gerard Farrell of the Commissioned Corps Officers Association of the U.S. Public Health Service, in an interview with the author, July 16, 2012.

50. The effort would involve scholarships to recruit as many as one thousand nurses and one hundred doctors to work in medically underserved areas, and change training so all Corps members were willing and ready to roll. U.S. Department of Health and Human Services news release, "Secretary Thompson to Increase Numbers and Flexibility of Public Health Services Commissioned Corps," July 3, 2003, rchive.hhs.gov/news/press/2003pres/20030703.html (accessed April 1, 2012).

51. Gerard Farrell, interview with the author, July 16, 2012.

52. Gerard Farrell, interview with the author, November 7, 2008.

53. Ibid.; Ken Moritsugu, interview with the author, September 25, 2006.

54. Three CDC sources told the author stories about such incidents.

55. Robin Toblin, interview with the author, January 10, 2009. Toblin was relating what other EIS officers had told her.

56. Thomas Glynn, interview with author, March 26, 2012; Richard Carmona, interview with the author, June 1, 2012.

57. Miriah Meyer and Jeremy Manier, "Study: No Safe Level of Secondhand Smoke," *Chicago Tribune*, June 28, 2006.

58. Charlie Gibson, comments during *ABC World News Tonight*, June 27, 2006, ABC News Transcripts; Hannah Storm, comments during *The Early Show*, June 28, 2006, CBS News Transcripts.

59. The 2006 count of states and municipalities with no-smoking laws was compiled by the group Americans for Nonsmokers' Rights. The count was cited in Jamie Kizzire and Mike Stobbe, "Small-Town USA Joins No-Smoking Trend," Associated Press, April 22, 2006; Stanton Glantz, interview with the author, April 9, 2012.

60. S. E. Schober et al., "Disparities in Secondhand Smoke Exposure—United States, 1988–1994 and 1999–2004," *Morbidity and Mortality Weekly Report*, July 11, 2008, Vol. 57, No. 27, pp. 744–747.

61. Sherry Kaiman, interview with the author, November 6, 2007.

62. Lydia Saad, "Many Americans Still Downplay Risk of Passive Smoking," Gallup News Service, July 21, 2006, http://www.gallup.com.

63. This principle of toxicology was first expressed by the Renaissance physician Paracelsus in the early 1500s. The concentrations necessary to make a chemical poisonous can vary based on a number of factors, including which chemical is being discussed, how much of it enters the body, and the size or other characteristics of a particular person that may influence his or her sensitivity or susceptibility to that chemical.

64. Michael Siegel, "In My View: Surgeon General and Anti-smoking Groups Irresponsible for Not Calling for Ban on Smoking," *The Rest of the Story: Tobacco News Analysis and Commentary*, July 10, 2006 blog posting, http://tobaccoanalysis.blogspot.com (accessed March 4, 2012).

65. Specifically, studies suggest even a brief exposure to cigarette smoke essentially can cause blood to become sticky and more prone to clotting. It also can worsen cholesterol, and degrade the body's ability to repair damaged spots in the lining of blood vessels. That all can lead to chest pain and heart attack. Repeated exposures are more dangerous, and can worsen cholesterol, increase the odds of plaque building in arteries, and raise the risk of chest pain, weakness, or heart attack. See U.S. Department of Health and Human Services, *A Report of the Surgeon General: How Tobacco Smoke Causes Disease*, 2010, p. 8, www.surgeongeneral.gov (accessed July 31, 2013).

66. Thomas Glynn, interview with author, March 26, 2012.
While there is strong consensus as to the hazards of indoor secondhand smoke, there's been a bit less unity on the dangers of outdoor secondhand smoke. Cigarette smoke dissipates more quickly in the open air, and some experts have said the evidence of serious health risk from passing smokers outdoors is flimsy. See Ronald Bayer and Kathleen E. Bachynski, "Banning Smoking in Parks and on Beaches: Science, Policy, and the Politics Of Denormalization," *Health Affairs*, July 2013, Vol. 32, No. 7, pp. 1291–1298.

67. John O'Neil, "A Warning on Hazards of Secondhand Smoke," *New York Times,* June 28, 2006; Michael Siegel, "Surgeon General's Report Publicity Focus on Risks of Minute Levels of Secondhand Smoke Exposure Belies Importance of Dose in Determining Health Risk," *The Rest of the Story: Tobacco News Analysis and Commentary,* June 29, 2006 blog posting, http:// tobaccoanalysis.blogspot.com (Accessed March 4, 2012).

68. Richard Carmona, interview with the author, June 1, 2012. Bush did not respond to a request for an interview. Carmona said he was approached about running for senator or governor. One political report said some Republicans had urged him to consider running for U.S. representative from Arizona's Eighth Congressional District. See Nathan Gonzales, "Candidates Battle for Cash in House Open Seats," *Rothenberg Political Report,* February 7, 2006, http://rothenbergpoliticalreport.com/news/article/candidates-battle-for-cash-in-house-open-seats (accessed April 15, 2012).

In Washington at the time, there were rumors about a future political career for Carmona, and some opined that the reason Carmona was not more vocal about political interference was that he worried that speaking out would jeopardize his future political aspirations. Those speculations were described by Gerard Farrell, in interview with author, November 7, 2008.

69. Karen Near, interview with the author, April 11, 2007.

70. Richard Carmona, interview with author, June 1, 2012.

71. Kevin Freking, "Surgeon General Carmona Leaves Post to Return to Civilian Life," Associated Press wire, July 31, 2006; Thomas Glynn, interview with author, March 26, 2012.

72. Richard Carmona, interview with the author, November 20, 2006; Richard Carmona, interview with the author, June 1, 2012.

73. Carla McClain, "U.S. Surgeon General to Return to Tucson after Four-Year Term," *Arizona Daily Star,* August 1, 2006.

74. Dan Christensen, "Republican Fundraiser Zachariah Testifies in Own Defense in Insider Stock Trading Trial," *Broward (County, Fla.) Bulldog,* September 8, 2010.

75. Joanne Silberner, "Challenges Await Bush Surgeon General Nominee," *All Things Considered,* National Public Radio, May 26, 2007, broadcast, http://www.npr.org/templates/story/story.php?storyId=10474698 (accessed April 9, 2012).

76. Jake Tapper, "'Homosexuality Isn't Natural or Healthy,'" *ABC News,* June 7, 2007, http://abcnews.go.com/Politics/story?id=3251663&page=1#.T4ckNiHY-8A (accessed July 8, 2007).

77. Mike Enzi, "Opening Statement, Nomination of James W. Holsinger Jr., MD, to be Surgeon General of the Public Health Service" (press release), July 12, 2007 (copy obtained by the author at the hearing).

78. James Holsinger, (brief) phone conversation with the author, January 20, 2009.

79. Carmona quoted in Harris, "Ex-Surgeon General's Maverick Side Was Bound to Appear, Friends Say."

80. Richard Carmona, interview with the author, June 1, 2012.

81. See a transcript of the hearing at http://oversight-archive.waxman.house.gov/story.asp?id=1398 (accessed December 4, 2013).

82. The former staffer spoke on condition of not being named. The source noted that the committee investigation into political meddling with the Office of the Surgeon General continued for several months but ultimately ended when Republican staffers insisted on a second interview with Carmona to discuss complaints about his travel and other issues. Carmona said, in effect, "I testified before Congress. I've had a lot of people throwing at my head and I'm not going to sit in front of those people and be a target again," the staffer recounted. But, he added, Waxman was not comfortable issuing an investigation report without a second Carmona interview.

83. C. Everett Koop, interview with the author, July 7, 2006.

84. Sharon Eubanks, interview with the author, May 15, 2012.

85. Daniel Halper, "Testimony: Carmona Took Advantage of Perks of Office When Surgeon General," *Weekly Standard,* November 1, 2012. Halper's article quoted U.S. Senator Jon Kyl, an Arizona Republican, as saying he had called Carmona in 2006 to recruit him to run. Kyl added that he was put off by Carmona's questions about what perks the office would provide him, like a house or car.

86. Brady McCombs, "Independent Voters Key to Carmona Strategy," *Arizona Daily Star,* April 11, 2012; Josh Lederman, "Democrats Strive to Swing Arizona," *The Hill,* March 6, 2012.

87. Richard Carmona, comments on *The Rachel Maddow Show,* March 22, 2012, broadcast, transcript at http://www.msnbc.msn.com/id/46836826/ns/msnbc_tv-rachel_maddow_show/t/rachel-maddow-show-thursday-march/#.T4sfVNVM7Co (accessed March 23, 2012).

88. As noted by Dan Nowicki, "Former Supervisor Speaks Out against Carmona," *Arizona Republic,* October 13, 2012.

CHAPTER 12

1. Anne Schuchat, comments to the author, April 23, 2010.

2. Frank Bruni, "Dr. Does-It-All," *New York Times Magazine,* April 18, 2010, pp. 42–45, 62.

3. Stanton Glantz, interview with the author, April 9, 2012.

4. William Schaffner, interview with the author, June 20, 2013.

5. David Satcher, comments to the author, April 20, 2012.

6. Christina Cheakalos, "Always on Call," *People,* May 13, 2002, Vol. 57, No. 18, p. 219. Biologists attribute jubilees to wedges of low-oxygen water in the bay that force marine life to the surface.

7. Regina Benjamin, interview with the author, July 30, 2012.

8. Trista Turley, "Alabama Catholic Up for Surgeon General," *National Catholic Reporter,* July 24, 2009, Vol. 45, No. 20, p. 14; Deborah Solomon, "Doctor's Orders: Questions for Regina Benjamin," *New York Times,* January 7, 2011.

9. Alice Popovici, "Nominee Puts Alabama Town on the Map," *National Catholic Reporter,* August 7, 2009, Vol. 45, No. 21, p. 9; Cheryl W. Thompson, "Surgeon General Pick's Stance on Abortion May Clash with Church's," *Washington Post,* July 18, 2009.

10. Regina Benjamin, interview with the author, January 12, 2010; Jonathan Tilove, "Obama Picks Xavier, Tulane Alumna as Next Surgeon General," *New Orleans Times-Picayune,* July 13, 2009.

11. Medical school was a five-year experience for Benjamin. To pass from the sophomore to junior year, medical students had to pass a required test. Benjamin failed it and sat out a year to study before successfully retaking the test. David Rutstein, interview with the author, July 22, 2012; Regina Benjamin, interview with the author, July 30, 2012.

12. Regina Benjamin, interview with the author, August 1, 2012.

13. Rick Bragg, "Poor Town Finds an Angel in a White Coat," *New York Times,* April 3, 1995.

14. Ibid.

15. Barack Obama, "Remarks by the President in Announcement of Surgeon General," July 13, 2009, press release, http://www.whitehouse.gov/the_press_office/Remarks-By-The-President-In-Announcement-Of-US-Surgeon-General (accessed May 3, 2012).

16. Regina Benjamin, interview with the author, January 12, 2010.

17. Doug Trapp, "Former AMA Trustee Dr. Regina Benjamin Nominated to Be Surgeon General," *AM News,* July 20, 2009, http://www.amednews.com/article/20090720/government/307209986/1/ (accessed December 6, 2013); Alicia Mundy, "Side Job for Regina Benjamin: Inspirational Speaker," *Wall Street Journal* Health Blog, posted July 15, 2009, http://blogs.wsj.com/health/2009/07/15/side-job-for-regina-benjamin-inspirational-speaker/ (accessed May 3, 2012); unsigned article, "Bayou Clinic Run by Benjamin to Go On after Pick," Associated Press wire, July 27, 2009. The Burger King position involved sitting on a nutrition advisory panel.

Benjamin was paid a salary of about $190,000 when she became surgeon general, just a bit more than she'd earned in 2007. HHS spokesperson Jennifer Koentop, comments to the author, January 12, 2010.

18. Caryn Rousseau, "MacArthur Foundation Awards 'Genius Grants,'" Associated Press wire, September 23, 2008. The author (Stobbe) visited the clinic in May 2012 and it was perhaps the fanciest building in town. The two-story building, located right next to City Hall, had marble countertops, a brass-plated water fountain, Apple computers for patient records, an elevator, a full kitchen, and a boardroom and meeting facilities, as well as a security fence.

19. Desiree Hunter and Lauran Neergaard, "From Storm-Tossed Ala. Clinic to Top Doctor Post," Associated Press wire, July 13, 2009.

20. Ceci Connolly and Howard Kurtz, "TV's Gupta Chosen for Medical Post," *Washington Post,* January 7, 2009; Joshua Drake, interview with the author, March 9, 2013. Drake was Koop's personal assistant at about the time of Gupta's visit.

21. Jeff Levi, interview with the author, January 27, 2009.

22. There was also grumbling about Gupta's hosting duties for AccentHealth, a TV network for doctor's office waiting rooms that was perceived as a credibility-eroding advertising vehicle for pharmaceutical companies. The Schwitzer quote is from Pamela Hill Nettleton, "Sick about Health Care," *Minnesota*

alumni magazine, March–April 2009, Vol. 108, No. 4, p. 20. Schwitzer's website is www.healthnewsreview.org.

23. Sarah Hampson, "Sanjay Gupta Taps into Both Sides of His Brain," *Toronto Globe and Mail*, April 16, 2012. Gupta's wife gave birth to their third daughter less than two weeks after he withdrew his name from consideration. When the author set up an interview with Gupta, a CNN spokeswoman canceled it. She said he had already given interviews on the topic and added that Gupta was not an expert on the history of the surgeon general position, "so this is probably not appropriate for [his] participation." Jennifer Dargan, e-mail to the author, June 18, 2009.

24. Jennifer Cabe, interview with the author, June 22, 2012; Political Transcript Wire, "Dr. Richard Carmona Holds a News Conference on America's Bone Health," October 14, 2004.

25. Regina Benjamin, interview with the author, August 1, 2012.

26. Claudia Kalb, "'I Understand the Challenges People Face Every Day,'" *Daily Beast*, March 15, 2010, http://www.thedailybeast.com/newsweek/2010/03/15/i-understand-the-challenges-people-face-every-day.html (accessed May 8, 2012); DupontJay, "The Checkup," *Washington Post* blog, posted 5 P.M., July 22, 2009, http://voices.washingtonpost.com/checkup/2009/07/should_the_surgeon_general_be.html (accessed July 23, 2009).

27. Michael Karolchyk, comments on Fox's *Your World with Neil Cavuto*, July 21, 2009, http://video.foxnews.com/v/3936188/she-is-obese (accessed May 3, 2012).

28. Regina Benjamin, interview with the author, January 12, 2010.

29. Jodi Kantor, *The Obamas* (New York: Little, Brown, 2012), pp. 138–140. A video of the kickoff ceremony can be seen at http://www.whitehouse.gov/photos-and-video/video/let-s-move-kick.

30. Kantor, *The Obamas,* p. 139; Jeffrey Levi, "The First Lady and the Childhood Obesity Crisis," *Huffington Post,* February 1, 2010, http://www.huffingtonpost.com/jeffrey-levi/the-first-lady-the-childh_b_445032.html (accessed May 6, 2012).

31. Michelle Obama, "Remarks by the First Lady at Grocery Manufacturers Association Conference, Grand Hyatt Hotel, Washington, D.C., March 16, 2010," transcript released by the White House, http://www.whitehouse.gov/the-press-office/remarks-first-lady-a-grocery-manufacturers-association-conference (accessed May 6, 2012).

32. Duff Wilson and Janet Roberts, "Special Report: How Washington Went Soft on Childhood Obesity," Reuters, April 27, 2012.

33. Mike Stobbe, "CDC: First National Sign of Childhood Obesity Drop," Associated Press, August 6, 2013. (Experts said it was not clear whether the same success would be seen in children not enrolled in WIC.) The findings were reported in a CDC document, "Vital Signs: Obesity among Low-Income, Preschool-Aged Children—United States, 2008–2011," *Morbidity and Mortality Weekly Report*, August 9, 2013, Vol. 62, No. 31, pp. 629–634. The CDC study found at least slight drops in childhood obesity in eighteen states.

34. Andrew Taylor, "Alabama Doctor Confirmed as US Surgeon General," Associated Press wire, October 29, 2009; Bergen Kenny, comments to the

author, October 30, 2010 (at the time, Kenny was a press secretary for U.S. Senator Tom Harkin). According to various sources, Benjamin's case was handled in that manner to get her past the blocking actions of Republican lawmakers who had bottled up the nominations of several Obama appointees.

35. Anne M. Hartman et al., "Sunburn and Protective Sun Behaviors among Adults Aged 18–29 Years—United States 2000–2010," *Morbidity and Mortality Weekly Report,* May 11, 2012, Vol. 61, No. 18, pp. 317–322.

36. Amanda Gardner (HealthDay), "Nearly Half of Americans Still Suspect Vaccine-Autism Link," *USA Today,* January 23, 2011, http://usatoday30 .usatoday.com/yourlife/health/medical/autism/2011-01-22-poll-vaccine-autism_n.htm (accessed November 17, 2013).

37. Regina Benjamin, interview with the author, January 12, 2010.

38. Gardiner Harris, "Plan to Widen Availability of Morning-After Pill Is Rejected," *New York Times,* December 7, 2011. The Obama administration ultimately stopped fighting that battle, deciding in 2013 not to appeal a federal judge's ruling in April 2012 that ordered the FDA to make it available to all women.

Health journalists came to see Obama's HHS as not much better than the message-controlling department of the Bush years. Complaints became common about slow responses to information requests and the growing intrusion of public affairs officers on any conversation between department personnel and journalists. See Curtis Brainard, "Transparency Watch: A Closed Door," *Columbia Journalism Review,* September–October 2011, http://www.cjr.org/feature/transparency_watch_a_closed_door.php?page=all (accessed December 7, 2013).

39. Regina Benjamin, interview with the author, August 1, 2012. Of course, Benjamin was not the only HHS employee to face limitations. A seven-page HHS policy statement from the time said any HHS employee approached by a reporter should coordinate their response with their immediate supervisor and with public affairs personnel. U.S. Department of Health and Human Services, Office of the Assistant Secretary for Public Affairs/News Division, "Guidelines on the Provision of Information to the News Media," March 2012.

40. David Rutstein, interview with the author, July 22, 2012. Rutstein said he retired, partly because he was frustrated with the situation. He had been in the Public Health Service for more than twenty years before Benjamin's appointment. (Coincidentally, he had known her when they were students at Morehouse together in the early 1980s.) In interviews with the author, Benjamin said little to dispel Rutstein's assessment. During one session, she said she'd been told—and believed—that a surgeon general could be appointed for one-, two-, three-, or four-year terms. Federal law clearly states that terms are four years.

41. Alan Blum, e-mail to the author, June 19, 2012. Blum also said Benjamin had offered him some advice on that day—that it was unwise to mention Philip Morris by name, because it gives the company undue attention. "Having given over 1,800 invited talks through the years on the tobacco industry and efforts to combat it, I did a double-take. What Regina was misguidedly passing along was the orders she was under not to mention any company by name—good for government bureaucrat self-preservation, but not good for advancing the effort to combat the tobacco pandemic at its source."

42. The health official, who has worked with Benjamin, spoke to the author on a not-for-attribution basis.

43. Richard Carmona, interview with the author, June 1, 2012.

44. Lori Pruett, "Surgeon General: Buying Iodide a 'Precaution,'" *NBC Bay Area*, posted March 17, 2011, http://www.nbcbayarea.com/news/local /Surgeon-General-Buying-Iodine-Appropriate-118031559.html (accessed March 20, 2011); unsigned article, "US Surgeon General Regina Benjamin Visiting Two San Mateo County Hospitals," *San Francisco Examiner*, March 15, 2011; Paul Rogers, "California's Radiation Risk Small," *San Jose Mercury News*, March 15, 2011.

45. Janet Lavelle, "Obama Says No Radiation Precautions Needed," *U-T San Diego*, March 17, 2011.

46. Anahad O'Connor, "Surgeon General Calls for Health over Hair," *New York Times*, August 25, 2011.

47. Steve Weiss, e-mail to the author, March 20, 2013. Weiss is senior director of media advocacy for the American Cancer Society Cancer Action Network. In the e-mail, Weiss said he had just been notified that Koh had referred the matter to Benjamin for a decision.

48. Ken Kelley, "Surgeon General's Warning," *Mother Jones*, January–February 1994.

49. As noted in David Hemenway, *Private Guns, Public Health* (Ann Arbor: University of Michigan Press, 2004), p. 18.

50. Benjamin worked on a report on youth violence, but it had not been released by the time she left office. Begun before Newtown, the project was envisioned as an update on a similar report by Satcher more than decade earlier, she said. Regina Benjamin, interview with the author, October 13, 2013.

51. The lawmaker was U.S. Representative Michael C. Burgess of Texas, chair of the Congressional Health Caucus. He was speaking of Sebelius's apparent disinterest in speaking to Republican legislators. Robert Pear, "Defending Law and Zeal in Push to Insure Millions," *New York Times*, July 9, 2013. The situation deteriorated when, three months later, Republican lawmakers trying to defund implementation of the Affordable Care Act forced a sixteen-day partial shutdown of the federal government.

52. Elizabeth Rigby, "How the National Prevention Council Can Overcome Key Challenges and Improve Americans' Health," *Health Affairs*, November 2011, Vol. 30, No. 11, p. 2153. The action plan can be viewed at http://www .surgeongeneral.gov/initiatives/prevention/about.actionplan.html (accessed May 19, 2013).

53. National thinking and policy on matters affecting public health "is a huge aircraft carrier that has to be turned around," he said. Georges Benjamin, interview with the author, August 28, 2013.

54. Stephanie Morain and Michelle M. Mello, "Survey Finds Public Support for Legal Interventions Directed at Health Behavior to Fight Noncommunicable Disease," *Health Affairs*, March 2013, Vol. 32. No. 3, p. 4. The survey did not ask how people thought the surgeon general was doing, because the researchers believed too few people would know what the surgeon general's role was, Mello

said in an e-mail to the author, February 28, 2013. Benjamin released two smoking reports during her time in office, one in 2010 on how smoking causes illness, and the other in 2012 on preventing youth tobacco use. But CDC staff and others did the work.

55. Nick Downes cartoon, *The New Yorker,* May 21, 2012, p. 51.

56. Mehmet Oz, "What I Learned on the Oprah Show," *Huffington Post,* posted May 10, 2009, http://www.huffingtonpost.com/dr-mehmet-oz/what-i-learned-on-the-iop_b_201390.html (accessed June 12, 2012); Paul Fucito (U.S. Patent and Trademark Office communications officer), e-mail to the author, February 29, 2012.

57. Christine Haughney, "Today's Key to Selling Magazines: A TV Doctor," *New York Times,* July 7, 2012.

58. Oz was building a constituency among the young, as well. He and his wife created an organization called HealthCorps, in which recent college graduates agree to defer medical school or graduate health studies for two years to work full-time in a public high school in an underserved community. Their task was to mentor high school kids in fitness and nutrition and in other ways to avoid obesity. In some ways it echoed the National Health Service Corps that Surgeon General Steinfeld helped create in the early 1970s, but this was a not-for-profit entity with a list of celebrity supporters that included TV news personality Diane Sawyer and actor Ben Vereen.

59. Weston Kosova and Patrice Wingert, "Live Your Best Life Ever!" *Daily Beast,* posted May 29, 2009.

60. Frank Bruni, "Dr. Does-It-All," *New York Times Magazine,* April 18, 2010, p. 45.

61. Oz also panicked viewers by attributing growing rates of thyroid cancer in women to dental X-rays and mammograms, and advocated that women who got them wear a lead neck wrap called a thyroid guard—much to the irritation of the American College of Radiology and Society of Breast Imaging. Oz barely mentioned that the death rate from thyroid cancer had not increased and that experts think the increased incidence was mainly due to better and earlier diagnosis. The American College of Radiology and Society of Breast Imaging issued a joint statement in April 2011 describing Oz's claims as "erroneous." See also Jane Brody, "Thyroid Fears Aside, That X-Ray's Worth It," *New York Times,* April 25, 2011. Oz's statements were in keeping with those of his patron, Winfrey, who told her audiences that thyroid problems should be treated with chakra balancing and soy milk.

Oz alarmed viewers again when he reported that he had commissioned private lab tests that found arsenic in several brands of apple juice. His claim quickly came under attack from experts who noted Oz's analysis failed to distinguish harmless organic arsenic from the kind of inorganic arsenic seen in pesticides. Indeed, an FDA analysis that included one of the same juice batches found much lower levels of total arsenic than Oz reported. Richard Besser, a former CDC official who had become a medical reporter for ABC, said on *Good Morning America* that Oz's broadcast was "extremely irresponsible" and the equivalent of "yelling 'Fire!' in a movie theater." Marilynn Marchione, "Dr. Oz Accused of Fear-Mongering on Apple Juice," Associated Press wire, September 15, 2011.

62. Michael Logan, "Dr. Oz Says Psychic John Edward 'Changed My Life,'" *TV Guide,* March 14, 2011. Note that Dr. Phil has had Margolis and Edward on his show as well.

63. Richard Carmona, interview with the author, June 1, 2012; Maria Poulos (publicist for *The Dr. Oz Show*), e-mail to the author, August 16, 2012. Carmona was on the April 7, 2012, show; Benjamin, the October 11, 2010, show. In her three-minute appearance, Benjamin discussed highlights of the Affordable Care Act. A contributing editor at *Bon Appétit* got nearly four minutes to talk about healthy kitchen gadgets.

64. Paul Offit, interview with the author, February 21, 2012. Through a publicist, Mehmet Oz declined an interview.

65. Note that another twitter account, @Surgeon_General, became much more active right after Benjamin left office, putting out messages on almost a daily basis. Acting surgeon general Boris Lushniak, Benjamin's interim replacement, was the person behind that account.

66. Howard Pyle, "Installing Seat Belts Isn't Enough," *Sarasota Herald-Tribune,* April 1, 1962. Pyle, who was president of the National Safety Council, wrote an editorial in which he quoted Terry's speech at a seat belt safety conference the previous June in New York City: "The wisest thing for you, and me, and everyone else who drives a car, to do is to protect ourselves with seat belts." Terry made that speech at a time when automakers resisted installing seat belts. The speech was made four years before the publication of Ralph Nader's influential book *Unsafe at Any Speed,* which detailed safety failings in autos and helped push the industry to make more safety features standard.

67. The surgeon general's "Every Body Walk!" initiative involved appearances by Benjamin in various cities in which she led one-mile walks in the middle of the day. It also involved preparation of a Call to Action to support walking and walkable communities.

The APHA's Georges Benjamin praised the effort: "She basically taught America to walk again." Georges Benjamin, interview with the author, August 28, 2013. But as of this writing, there is no CDC data yet available to show whether a significant increase in adult physical activity occurred during or after her campaign.

68. Some media reported that Benjamin was considering a run at elected office—specifically, for the seat if U.S. Representative Jo Bonner, an Alabama Republican who was not running for reelection. (See, for example, George Talbot, "Regina Benjamin to Step Down as U.S. Surgeon General," *Mobile Press-Register,* June 13, 2013, 8:01 A.M., http://blog.al.com at.) However, Benjamin said she'd decided to leave before Bonner's announcement. While admitting to being coy in answering questions about Bonner's seat, she maintained that she never said she planned to run.

69. As reported in Talbot in "Regina Benjamin to Step Down as U.S. Surgeon General" (accessed June 13, 2013). Regina Benjamin, interview with the author, October 3, 2013. Benjamin said she left because she wanted to get back to her clinic. She said she decided to step down early for two reasons. First, a number of appointees from Obama's first term were leaving, and it felt like an appropriate time for her to move on as well. Second, knowing that her

departure was a matter of when and not if, she decided to give Obama extra time to make a new appointment and help enable her successor to have as close to a full four years in office as possible.

70. Regina Benjamin statement, PHS Chat Forums for Officers of the U.S. Public Health Service," posted 4 P.M., June 12, 2013, http://www.phschat.com /forums/content.php?268-Surgeon-General-Benjamin-Stepping-Down-Effective-July-16-2013 (accessed June 13, 2013). In September 2013, she announced she had accepted the offer of endowed chair in public health sciences at her alma mater, Xavier University.

71. Reader's comment posted June 13, 2013, by Stryder73, following the article (of the same date) "Surgeon General Regina Benjamin Leaving Post," *Washington Times,* http://www.washingtontimes.com/news/2013/jun/13/surgeon-general-regina-benjamin-leaving-post/#ixzz2W6QARazB (accessed June 14, 2013).

72. The description of Murthy comes from Patricia Wen and Noah Bierman, "Surgeon General Nominee a Champion of Affordable Care," *Boston Globe,* November 16, 2013.

CHAPTER 13

1. Albert Brooks, *2030* (New York: St. Martin's Press, 2011). An influential figure, but rarely seen. The surgeon general, named Patricia Twain, is mentioned only on pages 61 and 63.

2. In recent years, according to CDC data, the U.S. adult smoking rate has hovered at around 20 percent, though it dipped to 18 percent in 2012.

3. William Schaffner, interview with the author, June 20, 2013.

4. The ranking is done by *Modern Healthcare,* which covers health care business. Benjamin ranked 31st in 2010, 26th in 2011, and 20th in 2012. Howard Koh ranked 92nd in 2011. FDA commissioner Peggy Hamburg was 73rd in 2011 and 58th in 2012. CDC director Thomas Frieden was 46th in 2012. Carmona was ranked 72nd in 2002 and 83rd in both 2003 and 2004. *Modern Healthcare* started the list in 2002. It receives thousands of nominations every year to its "Top 100" list and makes the rankings based on "50% vote and 50% expert opinion of our senior editors and reporters," said John Thomas, the magazine's chief of editorial operations. The magazine would not say how many votes Benjamin got or discuss other reasons for ranking her so high. John Thomas, e-mail to the author, August 26, 2013.

Of Regina Benjamin's very high placement on the *Modern Healthcare* list, the APHA's Georges Benjamin said, "That's a testament to people's perceptions over reality." Georges Benjamin, interview with the author, August 28, 2013.

5. Georges Benjamin, interview with the author, November 5, 2007.

6. Gerard Farrell, e-mail to the author, June 12, 2013. To be clear, I am not suggesting ending the Corps. If anything, it should be strengthened, but a surgeon general need not be person in charge.

7. David Rutstein, interview with the author, July 22, 2012.

8. Howard Markel, interview with the author, October 5, 2007.

9. Richard Carmona, interview with the author, June 1, 2012.

10. Iron pyrite, better known as fool's gold, is a gold-covered mineral sometimes mistaken for real gold.

11. Such swagger may have to come at a higher price. For decades, dynamic candidates for the surgeon general have dropped out of consideration because they determined the job simply didn't pay enough. "A lot of people are not prepared for the sacrifice" of lower income and requirements that they divest themselves of stocks or roles that might constitute a conflict of interest, said Regina Schofield, who was involved in interviewing surgeon general candidates for President George W. Bush. Regina Schofield, interview with the author.

12. C. Everett Koop, interview with the author, July 7, 2006. Carmona was still surgeon general at the time of the interview, and he had turned to Koop for advice. Koop said he was sympathetic with the challenges Carmona faced. "I never had to fight any of that," Koop said, describing the muzzling Carmona had to undergo. But Koop also said he would have handled the situation differently. "I'm a little different kind of character than Carmona. Carmona, he plays by the rules and he's afraid to get fired," Koop said.

13. Joycelyn Elders, interview with the author, November 30, 2007.

14. Nearly half are appointed by the president with Senate confirmation, and the rest are at smaller agencies and appointed by agency heads. Marcia Coyle, "Inspectors General May Get More Power," *National Law Journal,* May 5, 2008. A list of IGs is kept by the Council of the Inspectors General on Integrity and Efficiency; see http://www.ignet.gov

15. For example, a president has to notify Congress thirty days before dismissing or transferring an inspector general, and must field questions about why the step is being taken. But the 2008 law also involved measures to police IGs. IGs were prohibited from receiving cash bonuses or other awards, and the Council of Inspector Generals was charged with handling allegations of wrongdoing by IGs or their top staff members.

16. Charles C. Edwards, oral history interview, transcript p. 22.

17. Joseph Califano, interview with the author, January 16, 2008.

18. In late September 2008, the DOJ IG released a scathing report that concluded the process by which the nine attorneys had been removed was haphazard and unprofessional. One of the dismissed U.S. attorneys, David Iglesias, was fired after Republican officials argued that he was being too slow in pursuing Democrats in a corruption investigation. See Eric Lichtblau and Sharon Otterman, "Prosecutor Named on Fired U.S. Attorneys; Inspector General Issues Scathing Report," *International Herald Tribune,* September 30, 2008.

19. The former staffer spoke on condition of not being named. See note 77, chapter 11.

20. David Satcher, interview with the author, September 21, 2007.

21. Regina Benjamin, interview with the author, July 30, 2012.

22. During the shutdown of much of the federal government in autumn 2013, during a budget impasse in Congress, initially almost 70 percent of the CDC staff was placed on furlough. Yet acting surgeon general Boris Lushniak, considered essential personnel, remained on duty along with other members of the Commissioned Corps. However, he was not approved to travel for speaking

appearances. A survey conducted in 2012 found that local health departments in the United States had lost 43,900 jobs since 2008, and programs such as immunization, emergency preparedness, and maternal and child health were particularly hard hit. National Association of County and City Health Officials, "Latest NACCHO Economic Survey Reveals Local Health Departments Still Recovering from Recession," press release, July 2013.

23. The Distinguished Service Medal and the Meritorious Service Medal are both considered higher honors than the Surgeon General's Medallion. See "PHS Commissioned Corps Awards, CCPM Pamphlet No. 67—April 1998" (Department of Health and Human Services, Division of Commissioned Personnel).

24. Hale Champion, interview with the author, October 11, 2007.

25. David Sencer, interview with the author, September 25, 2007. Sencer died in 2011.

26. The wording of this line came from Arthur Miller's Americanized adaptation of Ibsen's play. Arthur Miller, *An Enemy of the People* (1950; repr., New York: Penguin Books, 1977), pgs. 84–85.

27. John Santelli, comments to the author, October 17, 2012.

28. The Pew Research Center for the People and The Press, "Scientific Achievements Less Prominent Than a Decade Ago" press release and report, released July 9, 2009, http://www.people-press.org/2009/07/09/public-praises-science-scientists-fault-public-media/ (accessed August 20, 2013). The study was based on a telephone survey of about 2,000 U.S. adults.

29. At the time of this writing, in late 2013, it's possible to argue that such a credibility-scorching event had actually befallen the Obama administration. The October 1 rollout of the HealthCare.gov website, designed to help Americans sign up for health insurance under the Affordable Care Act, had been a debacle. The website was plagued by technical glitches and other problems that for weeks made enrollment nearly impossible, and Sebelius was faulted for lack of adequate oversight. Then came another controversy. Earlier, Obama had assured Americans that no one would lose his or her current coverage as a result of the Affordable Care Act, but in the fall of 2013 millions of people with individual policies began to get cancellation notices because their policies did not meet the standards of the health care law. Sebelius had in the past sounded a caveat that current coverages could be affected if an insurer or employer made certain changes to the coverage that did not comply with standards, but those statements clearly were not absorbed by many Americans. In the midst of this uproar, Murthy was nominated to be the next surgeon general, and it's possible the Obama administration saw him as a physician spokesman who might restore some credibility with the public. Although there was reason to think Murthy might be in a position to become more visible that Benjamin or Carmona, however, there were no indications the Obama administration intended to strengthen the Office of the Surgeon General in a way to ensure ongoing independence.

Index